INFANT STRESS
UNDER
INTENSIVE CARE

INFANT STRESS UNDER INTENSIVE CARE

Environmental Neonatology

edited by
Allen W. Gottfried
California State University, Fullerton and
University of Southern California
School of Medicine

Juarlyn L. Gaiter
Children's Hospital National Medical Center and
George Washington University
School of Medicine and Health Sciences

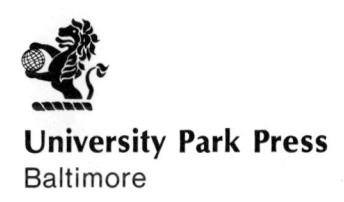

University Park Press
Baltimore

University Park Press
International Publishers in Medicine and Allied Health
300 North Charles Street
Baltimore, Maryland 21201

Copyright © 1985 by University Park Press

This book is protected by copyright. All rights, including that of translation into other languages, are reserved. No part of this book may be reproduced, stored in a retrieval system, or transmitted, in any form or by any means, electronic, mechanical, photocopying, recording, or otherwise, without the prior written permission of the publisher.

Production editor: Megan Barnard Shelton
Cover design by: Caliber Design Planning, Inc.
Text design by: S. Stoneham, Studio 1812, Baltimore

Typeset by: Ampersand Publishers Services, Inc.
Manufactured in the United States of America by: Halliday Lithograph

Library of Congress Cataloging in Publication Data
Main entry under title:

Infant stress under intensive care.

    Includes index.
    1. Neonatal intensive care—Psychological aspects. 2. Infants (Newborn)—Mental health. 3. Child development. I. Gottfried, Allen W. II. Gaiter, Juarlyn L. [DNLM: 1. Critical Care—in infancy & childhood. 2. Critical Care—psychology. 3. Intensive Care Units, Neonatal. WS 366 I43]
RJ253.5.I55   1984   618.92'01   84-7277
ISBN 0-8391-1869-4

Contents

Contributors / vii
Foreword
    Jerold F. Lucey / ix
Preface / xi

1   **Introduction** / 1
    Joan E. Hodgman

2   **Physical Structure and Functional Organization of Neonatal Intensive Care Units** / 7
    Sheldon B. Korones

3   **Environment of Newborn Infants in Special Care Units** / 23
    Allen W. Gottfried

4   **Nursery Environments**
The Behavior and Caregiving Experiences of Term and Preterm Newborns / 55
    Juarlyn L. Gaiter

5   **An Ecological Description of a Neonatal Intensive Care Unit** / 83
    Patricia L. Linn, Frances Degen Horowitz, Bonnie Johns Buddin, Janet C. Leake, and Howard A. Fox

6   **Analysis of Caregiving Events Relating to Preterm Infants in the Special Care Unit** / 113
    Susan T. Blackburn and Kathryn E. Barnard

7   **Recording Environmental Influences on Infant Development in the Intensive Care Nursery**
Womb for Improvement / 131
    Pamela C. High and Peter A. Gorski

8   **Relationships between the Distribution and Diurnal Periodicities of Infant State and Environment** / 157
    Katherine Rieke Lawson and Gerald Turkewitz

9   **Thermal Aspects of Neonatal Care** / 171
    Robert J. Moffat and Alvin Hackel

10 **Consequences of Newborn Intensive Care** / 199
  Joyce L. Peabody and Kathleen Lewis
11 **The Impact of the Environment on the NICU Caregiver**
  Perspectives of the Nurse, Pediatric House Officer, and Academic Neonatologist / 227
  Richard E. Marshall, John L. Roberts, and Joan H. Walsh
12 **Environmental Neonatology**
  Implications for Intervention / 251
  Allen W. Gottfried
13 **Ethical Considerations in the Intensive Care Nursery** / 259
  Gordon B. Avery
  Appendix Commentary 1 / 265
  Anneliese F. Korner
  Appendix Commentary 2 / 271
  John H. Kennell and Marshall H. Klaus
  Appendix Commentary 3 / 279
  T. Berry Brazelton
  Index / 285

Contributors

Gordon B. Avery, M.D., Ph.D.
Department of Neonatology
Children's Hospital National Medical
  Center
111 Michigan Avenue, N.W.
Washington, DC 20010

Kathryn E. Barnard, R.N., Ph.D.
School of Nursing
CDMRC, WJ-10
University of Washington
Seattle, WA 98195

Susan T. Blackburn, R.N., Ph.D.
Department of Parent and Child
  Nursing
School of Nursing
SC-74
University of Washington
Seattle, WA 98195

T. Berry Brazelton, Ph.D.
Department of Pediatrics
Harvard Medical School
Children's Hospital Medical Center
333 Longwood Avenue
Boston, MA 02115

Bonnie Johns Buddin, M.A.
Department of Human Development
University of Kansas
Lawrence, KS 66045

Howard A. Fox, M.D.
Department of Neonatology
University of Kansas Medical Center
39th and Rainbow Boulevard
Kansas City, KS 66103

Juarlyn L. Gaiter, Ph.D.
Department of Neonatology
Pediatric Psychology Research
  Laboratory
Children's Hospital National Medical
  Center
111 Michigan Avenue N.W.
Washington, DC 20010

Peter A. Gorski, M.D.
Department of Pediatrics
Mount Zion Hospital and Medical
  Center
Box 7921
San Francico, CA 94120

Allen W. Gottfried, Ph.D.
Department of Psychology
California State University
Fullerton, CA 92634

Alvin Hackel, M.D.
Department of Pediatrics and
  Anesthesiology
Stanford University School of
  Medicine
Stanford, CA 94305

Pamela C. High, M.D.
Department of Pediatrics, A-205
University of California
400 Parnassus Avenue
San Francisco, CA 94143

Joan E. Hodgman, M.D.
Department of Pediatrics
Los Angeles County–University of
  Southern California Medical Center
Women's Hospital
1240 Mission Road
Los Angeles, CA 90033

Frances Degen Horowitz, Ph.D.
Department of Human Development
University of Kansas
Lawrence, KS 66045

John H. Kennell, M.D.
Department of Pediatrics
Rainbow Babies' and Children's Hospital
Case Western Reserve University
2101 Adelbert Road
Cleveland, OH 44106

Marshall H. Klaus, M.D.
Department of Pediatrics and Human Development
Michigan State University
East Lansing, MI 48824

Anneliese F. Korner, Ph.D.
Department of Psychiatry and Behavioral Sciences
Stanford University School of Medicine
Stanford, CA 94305

Sheldon B. Korones, M.D.
Departments of Pediatrics and Obstetrics and Gynecology
University of Tennessee Center for the Health Sciences
853 Jefferson Avenue
Memphis, TN 38163

Katharine Rieke Lawson, Ph.D.
Department of Pediatrics
Rose Kennedy Center
Albert Einstein College of Medicine
1410 Pelham Parkway South
Bronx, NY 10461

Janet C. Leake, R.N.
Department of Neonatology
University of Kansas Medical Center
39th and Rainbow Boulevard
Kansas City, KS 66103

Kathleen Lewis, M.D.
Department of Neonatology
Children's Hospital of San Francisco
3700 California Street
Post Office Box 3805
San Francisco, CA 94119

Patricia L. Linn, Ph.D.
Cleveland Metropolitan General Hospital
Department of Obstetrics and Gynecology
3395 Scranton Road
Cleveland, OH 44109

Jerold F. Lucey, M.D.
Department of Pediatrics
University of Vermont
College of Medicine
Burlington, VT 05401

Richard E. Marshall, M.D.
Department of Pediatrics
St. Louis Children's Hospital
Washington University
500 South Kings Highway
Post Office Box 14871
St. Louis, MO 63178

Robert J. Moffat, Ph.D.
Department of Mechanical Engineering
Stanford University
Stanford, CA 94305

Joyce L. Peabody, M.D.
Department of Neonatology
Children's Hospital of San Francisco
3700 California Street
Post Office Box 3805
San Francisco, CA 94119

John L. Roberts, M.D.
Department of Pediatrics
University of Louisville School of Medicine
Louisville, KY 40202

Gerald Turkewitz, Ph.D.
Department of Psychology
Hunter College
City University of New York
695 Park Avenue
New York, NY 10021

Joan H. Walsh, R.N., B.S.N.
Department of Pediatric Nursing
St. Louis Children's Hospital
Washington University
500 South Kings Highway
Post Office Box 14871
St. Louis, MO 63178

Foreword

The human infant always begins life in a warm, peaceful, protected environment. It's a dim world of muffled sounds and gentle oscillations. The infant sleeps a great deal and perhaps even dreams. However, for some infants this idyllic life comes to an abrupt, premature halt at about 6 or 7 months. They are ejected into the world as physiologically displaced persons, facing a very unusual environment.

The prematurely born infant emerges into a hectic, cold, noisy, and bright environment filled with mysterious equipment and peopled by masked strangers who try to help. Almost everything done to or for the infant is painful and that pain can certainly be felt, although it cannot be communicated. The infant who must have an endotracheal tube cannot cry and is not fed by mouth for weeks. His or her feet are slashed periodically for blood samples. The infant's respirator roars away night and day, keeping his or her lungs inflated and sustaining life—but at what price?

This book is an attempt to describe what effects this alien environment known as the intensive care nursery may have on later development of premature infants who survive.

Jerold F. Lucey, M.D.
Professor of Pediatrics
University of Vermont
College of Medicine

Preface

This book represents the coming of age of a distinct and, we hope, applied discipline—*environmental neonatology*, the study of the environment of newborn special care facilities and its impact on the medical and developmental status of sick infants.

In recent years, there has been increased interest in the environmental characteristics associated with newborn intensive care. This interest is primarily the outgrowth of several sources: 1) neonatal environmental intervention studies; 2) iatrogenic consequences related to intensive care for newborns; 3) basic scientific investigations of the sensorimotor response systems of full-term and preterm neonates; and 4) environmental designs and characteristics of newborn special care facilities associated with staff efficiency, stress, and burnout.

We readily admit that, at this point in this new field of study, we have far more questions than answers concerning environmental influences on sick newborns. Furthermore, we recognize that the issues addressed cut across a wide range of scientific and applied disciplines. In our judgment, thorough solutions will require a multidisciplinary approach. Hence, the importance and success of this book should not be gauged by solutions put forth but by the significance of clearly defined questions and issues. If this book convinces readers that the environment of newborn special care units is worthy of investigation, then we have accomplished our initial task.

Because of the multidisciplinary nature of the subject matter, we have selected contributors to this book who represent the following professions: neonatology, pediatrics, nursing, psychology, engineering, and social work. The first chapter is a brief historical overview of the issues in the early development of newborn intensive care. The second is concerned with structure and organization of newborn intensive care facilities. Chapters 3 through 8 contain observational studies documenting the physical and social environment of newborn special care units. The ninth chapter focuses on thermal characteristics and engineering in newborn intensive care. Chapter 10 provides an extensive review of the potential adverse consequences of intensive care on the newborn. The eleventh chapter deals with the impact of newborn intensive care on the staff. In Chapter 12 some implications for intervention based on environmental data are presented. The final chapter addresses contemporary ethical issues of newborn intensive care. The appendix contains three commentaries that discuss the significance of the environmental observational studies.

We dedicate this book to the clinical staff members who work in newborn special care units. They are truly dedicated to human life.

Allen W. Gottfried
Juarlyn L. Gaiter

INFANT STRESS UNDER INTENSIVE CARE

1
Introduction
Joan E. Hodgman

Modern neonatal care originated in France with the development of the earliest infant incubator, the Tanier-Martin Couveuse, in 1880. The first special nursery for "weaklings" was established at the Paris Maternité Hospital in 1893 by Pierre Budin, a student of Tanier. Although trained as an obstetrician, he was perhaps the original neonatologist. His book, *The Nursling*, published in 1900 and translated into English in 1907, was the first text on the care of the premature infant. He emphasized support of body temperature, control of nosocomial infection, and the importance of the mother in handling and feeding (Budin, 1900). He reported a 20% neonatal mortality rate in preterm infants, a figure considered respectable in the 1950s.

In a most bizarre development, Budin's principles were spread by one of his students, Dr. Martin Couney, who exhibited living premature infants to a wondering public for a fee (Silverman, 1979). Babies were kept in incubators and carefully tended by specially trained nurses (see Figure 1.1). Strict attention was paid to infection control, but mothering was replaced by nursing. Mortality in the infants, who were not accepted until they had survived the first critical days, was very low. Because premature infants were generally not expected to live under usual circumstances, there were few objections from families. Infants for one exhibit in Berlin were supplied through the good graces of the Empress Augusta Victoria. Interestingly, Dr. Couney complained of difficulty in reuniting infants with their families at graduation time.

Dr. Couney brought his elaborate exhibition to Chicago, where it was seen by Dr. Julius Hess of Michael Reese Hospital. Dr. Hess, ably supported by the chief nursery nurse (Evelyn Lundeen), applied the principles he had observed to the hospital premature nursery (Hess and

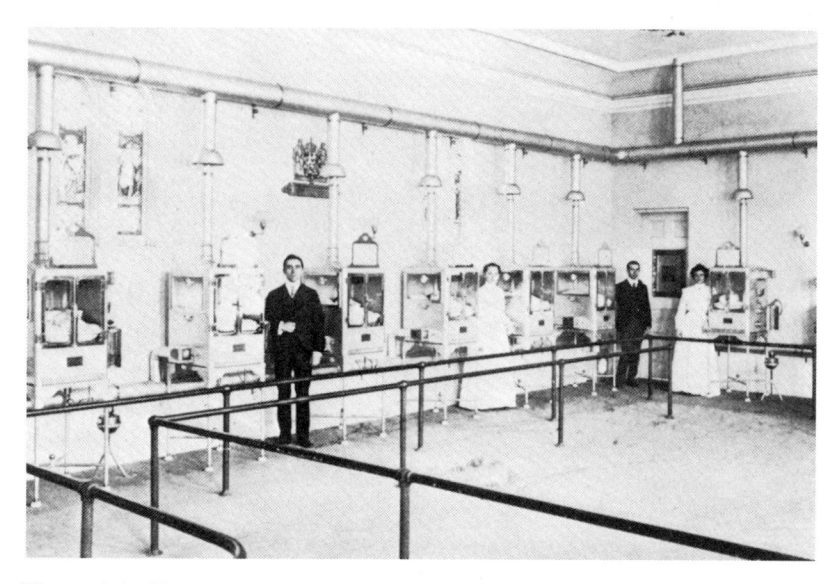

Figure 1.1. Neonatal care in the 1900s. Reprinted by permission from Silverman, 1979. Copyright American Academy of Pediatrics, 1979. (Photograph courtesy of the Buffalo & Erie County Historical Society, Buffalo, New York.)

Lundeen, 1949). Infants were dressed and nursed in incubators or heated beds in separate rooms that were devoted solely to care of the premature. Minimal handling of the infants was the goal, and infection control was rigorously enforced. Admission to the nursery was severely limited. In many nurseries, the doctor was not even allowed to enter and instead routinely examined babies in an anteroom, into which they were slid through a "pass through" constructed specifically for this purpose. Dr. Paul Wu, a graduate of the Michael Reese training program, recalled that the only duty delegated to the house officers by Miss Lundeen was signing the death certificate (Wu, 1983, personal communication). Parents, of course, were excluded. Even the viewing window, which was standard equipment in term nurseries, was not very effective because the premature infants were small, wrapped, and essentially hidden amid the equipment of the time.

Although such procedures sound antiquated, they were instrumental in reducing neonatal mortality. Figures comparable to those of Budin were achieved in Chicago, and his principles spread across the United States. The resulting mainstays of treatment were minimal handling, concentration on special nursing skills, and control of access to the infants. Nurseries were quiet, and the lights were dimmed at night as they were throughout the hospital. Although infants were housed in incubators, their ability to maintain a normal body temperature was primitive.

Stability of body temperature was the desired result, and because prematures were thought to be poikilotherms, the actual temperature was not considered important. In the 1950s, the most frequent notation for infant temperature at the large Premature Center at the University of Southern California Medical Center was "NR" (not registered) on a standard rectal thermometer on which the lowest recording temperature was 94°F. Small infants were not fed for at least 48 hours because of the fear of aspiration. Parenteral fluids were rarely administered because early weight loss was equated with the loss of excess extracellular fluid present at birth and, thus, was considered desirable.

Scientific investigation of the physical environment of the premature infant was undertaken in the late 1950s at Columbia University. In their studies of temperature and humidity Silverman et al. (1958, 1963) demonstrated that maintaining body temperature that was more nearly normal resulted in decreased early mortality, especially in smaller infants. Increased humidity, which had been added to the incubator environment for its supposed beneficial effect on breathing, actually affected outcome only through its role in enhancing temperature. Studies to support these findings followed rapidly from other centers in the United States and Europe (Day et al., 1964; Karlberg et al., 1965). Impetus for these studies came from several developments:

1. Infant mortality after 1 month of age decreased much faster than neonatal mortality; thus neonatal mortality was considered to be a more significant cause of death in the pediatric age group.
2. Follow-up studies of infants demonstrated a high incidence of handicap in survivors, which led to the questioning of established nursery routines (Drillien, 1959; Lubchenko et al., 1963).
3. A technologic explosion was beginning with microlaboratory techniques that could perform analyses on drops of blood and the availability of portable x-ray machines capable of split-second exposures. These made diagnostic studies possible in even the tiniest infants.
4. The realization that physiologic processes for control of body temperature were well developed even in small premature infants led to improvements in incubators.
5. It became evident that the preterm infant was well equipped with reflexive behavior. The main problem in controlling his or her body temperature was small physical size and limited energy reserves (Stern, 1970). Not surprisingly, provision of supportive fluids and calories improved the outcome of the premature just as similar techniques worked in older humans (Cornblath et al., 1966).

By the end of the 1960s, the nursery environment was changing rapidly. Rather than being transferred to pediatric wards, sick full-term infants were incorporated into the premature nursery for care. The number and kinds of routine observations were increased, with emphasis on temperature control, glucose utilization, and fluid balance. Fear of aspiration was replaced by a concern for caloric intake. "Early" feeding at 12 to 24 hours became routine (Wu et al., 1967). Definite improvement in neonatal mortality rates accompanied these changes. In addition, follow-up of infants born in the late 1960s revealed an improved long-term outcome for the survivors (Teberg et al., 1977). With the increased around-the-clock handling of infants necessitated by these procedures, lights were no longer dimmed in the high-risk nurseries.

The ability to manipulate the infant's environment took a quantum jump with the appearance of miniaturized monitoring equipment and the ability to provide prolonged ventilatory support (Swyer, 1969). The major goal of minimal handling was replaced by almost constant intervention by medical and nursing personnel. Nursing care was provided by a 1:1 or 1:2 nurse-to-patient ratio. Infants were repeatedly intubated for frequent gavage feedings, suctioned routinely (usually on an hourly basis), and stimulated regularly. "Early" feeding was now started between 3 and 6 hours of life. Infection control was still considered important, but seclusion of the infant had disappeared when barriers to the premature nursery were removed. Sick term infants as well as prematures were housed together, and a concept of a continuum of graduated care developed. New nurseries were needed to house the increased numbers of infants receiving high-risk care. The new intensive care techniques were difficult to provide in the existing nurseries with small rooms connected by anterooms. Construction of large nurseries for maximum efficiency in observation and manipulation of infants was recommended (Gluck, 1970).

The nursery was no longer a quiet, secluded enclave, but a busy, bustling place. Large numbers of people spent a good deal of time in the nursery. The number of nurses increased, physicians were spending full time in management of the infant, and in 1975 a new subspecialty, *neonatology*, became a reality. A variety of changes accompanied the new technology. All monitors emitted continuous noise and all had purposely abrasive alarms to warn of malfunction of the infant or machine. Infants were nursed at essentially the same intensity around the clock. Continuous cardiorespiratory monitoring and control of temperature along with other technologic advances were well-established nursery routines. Handling of infants underwent a complete transformation from minimal to almost constant. Each year during this period, neonatal mortality decreased, and long-term morbidity in survivors also decreased (Teberg et al., 1982). The concept of regionalizing expensive high-risk care developed (Committee on Perinatal Health, 1976; Subcommittee on Perinatal Mortality, 1974). Hospital nurseries were designated as capable of providing primary or routine care for the normal infant and secondary or tertiary levels were designated for the special care of the high-risk infant. Infants born in hospitals where neonatal high-risk care was not available were transferred for special care during the first hours of life. Although providing important and frequently life-saving care, the need for transfer increased the isolation of the infant from the family.

At the peak of technologic enthusiasm, the effect of separation on mother and infant began to be questioned and studied (Klaus and Kennell, 1970). With yearly decreases in mortality rate continuing, long-term outcome, especially of the very low birth weight infant, has now come under increasing scrutiny. Premature infants are known to be at higher risk for developmental delay and child abuse as well as neurologic handicap (Klein and Stern, 1971). Although neurologic sequelae are related to obstetric and neonatal medical factors, long-term developmental outcome cannot be accurately predicted from perinatal events. Some poor outcomes may have their genesis in separation of the infant from the family necessitated by high-risk nursery care. Studies of both normal and high-risk mother-infant pairs have revealed the inter-reactions necessary in order for normal development to proceed. Increased understanding of the needs of parents and how this influences the progress of the infants had led to the reintroduction of the mother into the nursery (Kennell et al., 1974). The sensitivity of the normal infant to his or her environment and the ability of the very young infant to learn have been well established (Fantz, 1963). It is evident that the small preterm infant is also capable of responding to his or her environment (Hack et al., 1976). Thus, reactions between the infant and the nursery environment must influence the infant's performance while in the nursery. The long-term behavioral effects of nursery routines are mostly unknown. However, it seems reasonable to suppose that nursery stays of several weeks, which are common for the very low birth weight infant, may have a significant effect on their later behavioral performance.

The 1980s may well be the decade of correlation between physical and psychological needs of the high-risk infant. Already, the immediate and dramatic effect of the handling of infants on their blood oxygen levels has been reported (Long et al., 1980). The importance of minimal handling for fragile infants has resurfaced. The appropriate interface between stimulation and medical and nursing intervention has not as yet been defined for this population. Descriptive data of the nursery environment must be established. One of the future directions for neonatal care is further exploration of this *terra incognita*.

References

Budin P. 1900. Le Nourisson. Octave Dion, Paris. (English translation by Maloney, W. J. 1907. *The Nursling*. Caxton Publishing Co., London.)
Committee on Perinatal Health. 1976. Toward Improving the Outcome of Pregnancy. March of Dimes Birth Defects Foundation, White Plains, NY.
Cornblath, M., Forbes, A., Pildes, R., et al. 1966. A controlled study of early fluid

administration on survival of low birthweight infants. Pediatrics 38:547–556.

Day, R. L., Caliguiri, L., Kamenski, C., and Ehrlich, F. 1964. Body temperature and survival of premature infants. Pediatrics 34:171–181.

Drillien, C. M. 1959. Physical and mental handicap in the prematurely born. J. Obstet. Gynaecol. Br. Commonw. 66:721–735.

Fantz, R. 1963. Pattern vision in newborn infants. Science 140:296–297.

Gluck, L. 1970. Design of a perinatal center. Pediatr. Clin. North Am. 17:777–791.

Hack, M., Mostow, A., and Miranda, S. 1976. Development of attention in preterm infants. Pediatrics 58:669–674.

Hess, J., and Lundeen, E. 1949. The Premature Infant, 2nd ed. Lippincott, Philadelphia.

Karlberg, P., Moore, R. E., and Oliver, T. K. 1965. Thermogenic and cardiovascular responses of the newborn baby to Noradrenaline. Acta Paediatr. Scand. 54:225–238.

Kennell, J. H., Jerauld, R., Wolfe, H., Chester, D., et al. 1974. Maternal behavior one year after early and extended post-partum contact. Dev. Med. Child Neurol. 16:172–179.

Klaus, M. H., and Kennell, J. H. 1970. Mothers separated from their newborn infants. Pediatr. Clin. North Am. 17:1015–1037.

Klein, M., and Stern, L. 1971. Low birth weight and the battered child syndrome. Am. J. Dis. Child. 122:15–18.

Long, J. G., Philip, A. G. S., and Lucey, J. F. 1980. Excessive handling as a cause of hypoxemia. Pediatrics 65:203–207.

Lubchenko, L. O., Horner, F. A., Reed, L. H., Hix, I. E., Metcalf, D., Cohig, R., Elliott, H. C., and Bourg, M. 1963. Sequelae of premature birth. Evaluation of premature infants of low birth weights at 10 years of age. Am. J. Dis. Child. 106:101–110.

Silverman, W. A. 1979. Incubator-baby side shows. Pediatrics 64:127–141.

Silverman, W. A., Agage, F. J., Jr., and Fertig, J. W. 1963. Sequential trial of the nonthermal effect of atmospheric humidity on survival of newborn infants of low birth weight. Pediatrics 31:719–724.

Silverman, W. A., Fertig, J. W., and Berger, A. P. 1958. Influence of the thermal environment upon survival of newly born premature infants. Pediatrics 22:876–886.

Stern, L. 1970. The newborn infant and his thermal environment. Curr. Prob. Pediatr. 1:1.

Subcommittee on Perinatal Mortality. 1974. Goals for Regionalized Perinatal Care. California Medical Association, San Francisco.

Swyer, P. 1969. An assessment of artificial respiration in the newborn. Report of the 59th Ross Conference on Pediatric Research, p. 25. Ross Laboratories, Columbus, OH.

Teberg, A., Hodgman, J. E., Wu, P. Y. K., and Spears, R. L. 1977. Recent improvement in outcome for the small premature infant: Follow-up of infants with a birthweight of less than 1,500 grams. Clin. Pediatr. 16:307–313.

Teberg, A., Wu, P. Y. K., Hodgman, J. E., Mich, C., et al. 1982. Infants with birth weight under 1500 g: Physical, neurological, and developmental outcome. Crit. Care Med. 10:10–14.

Wu, P., Teilmann, P., Cabler, M., et al. 1967. "Early" versus "late" feeding of low birth weight neonates. Pediatrics 39:733–739.

2
Physical Structure and Functional Organization of Neonatal Intensive Care Units

Sheldon B. Korones

Perspective

Newborn intensive care units (NICUs) were designed to sustain life and enhance the possibility of intact survival. All other considerations have been afterthoughts, their importance notwithstanding. Beginning in the mid-1960s, phenomenal changes in bedside care gave rise to new nursery design and to an array of equipment, both of which were conceived as means to lifesaving ends (Gluck, 1976). The allocation of one nursery for prematures and another for term infants gave way to a facility in which personnel and equipment were concentrated for the treatment of all sick neonates, regardless of their maturity. Several small rooms for six to eight infants each were replaced by fewer and larger rooms or by a straightforward unicameral arrangement. Environmental considerations were primarily geared to optimal performance of personnel. Deployment of beds, cabinets, and counters were planned to accommodate lifesaving equipment and to facilitate nursing activity. The intensity and spectrum of light were aimed at undistorted visual evaluation by personnel; a neutral color for walls was recommended to avoid distortion of infants' skin tones, particularly for evaluation of cyanosis, jaundice, and pallor. Avoidance of excessive noise was considered essential because of its disturbing impact on the nursery staff.

These early considerations, still valid in the 1980s (Basler and Hager, 1977), were extended to include the direct effects of environmental factors upon the infant. In addition to an interest in the tone and intensity of light for visual monitoring, there arose an added interest in the lack of circadian variation and its effect on infant behavior. To anxiety about the disturbing impact of noise on personnel was added concern for its potential to impair infant hearing (American Academy of Pediatrics, 1974). Moreover, recent observations have suggested that excessive noise is an unrecognized cause of hypoxemia (Long et al., 1980a). Thus the approach to physical factors in the nursery environment has evolved from a primary concern for personnel function to concern about direct effects on the infant. A single exception to this evolutionary pattern was the early interest in thermal environment and its influence on the infant's capacity to maintain body temperature.

The importance of physical factors in the environment has been further expanded to include ecologic considerations—the interplay among personnel, between personnel and babies, and between both of them and the physical environment. Thus, an enlarging literature describes, analyzes, and speculates on the emotional stress experienced by caretakers in the newborn intensive care unit, particularly among nurses and, less frequently, among social workers and physician trainees. There are also reports on fatigue associated with the long working hours of physician trainees—its effect upon the quality of care and on the trainees themselves (Tyson et al., 1979).

The effects of tactile stimulation on infants have been explored during recent years. We first focused attention on the frequency with which babies were disturbed within a 24-hour period. A mean of 132 hands-on events among 11 infants was recorded (Korones, 1976). The results showed that sick infants were thoughtlessly disturbed more often than was necessary and certainly more often that had been the case with sick adults. A later study (Long et al., 1980b) demonstrated the significance of frequent disturbance more concretely than we did. The disturbances in the Long et al. study were associated with hypoxemic episodes. Hypoxemia was considerably more frequent as handling of the infant increased; 75% of the total time in hypoxemia was associated with handling of infants by personnel.

The paucity of stimulation from the environment of intensive care units was deplored in publications that appeared during the early 1970s (Rice, 1977). However, later, more accurate assessments concluded that there was indeed an abundance of stimulation from light, noise, and touch, but that these "stimuli" were purposeless, unplanned, and disorganized (Gottfried et al., 1981). They did not stimulate; they merely disturbed.

Thus, there has been a mounting interest in the influence of environmental and ecologic factors on the status of infants who survive the life-threatening aftermaths of their unfortunate births. Such interest is provocative because its global approach seeks to characterize the effects of human behavior (personnel) and physical phenomena (light, noise, temperature, and touch) on immediate and long-term outcomes of surviving infants. The effects are difficult to measure, and the causes are hard to define. If the NICU environment is to be altered in response to valid conclusions that indicate that the existing environment is a suboptimal state-of-the-art, then there must first be an understanding of the factors that contribute to the success of these units.

Regionalization of Perinatal Care

The advances in neonatal intensive care were like a show of fireworks— spectacular to behold, despite numerous fizzles. As the effectiveness of therapeutic modalities gained credibility, diminished neonatal mortality at the major centers began to contrast sharply with the unchanging experience of smaller hospitals. The concept of regionalization arose in response to a demonstrated need for the delivery of advanced levels of care to smaller communities and to smaller hospitals in large communities. The improved care provided by research had not yet been delivered to the bedside, except in the major centers where most of the research had transpired.

In simplest terms, regionalization is a formalized contemporary version of the pattern of medical practice that has long pervaded this country. Physicians in small communities have referred patients with complex problems to the "big city specialists" for years; they have attended conferences at medical centers habitually. Obviously, regionalization of perinatal care is a considerably more complex arrangement, but the fundamental idea is to deliver advanced levels of health care to all patients, regardless of geographic factors, and to impart new information to perinatal caretakers everywhere. The professional advice and supervision that constitute perinatal care in the 1980s should be available to every pregnant woman and newborn child. Although the vast majority of newborn babies are healthy, intact survival is jeopardized in a substantial number, who require complex care for their severe illnesses. In many instances, neonatal complications can be anticipated, ameliorated, or eliminated by special management of their high-risk mothers. This brand of care entails recruitment of a variety of professional personnel who are generally concentrated in densely populated communities. It is in these large communities that the full spectrum of medical consultants, nurse specialists, laboratory capabilities, and facilities with equipment are found. That perinatal mortality and morbidity are significantly reduced by the best contemporary technology has been plainly demonstrated for at least two decades. Thus, there is an urgency to make the technology available to all mothers and infants, to eliminate any existing inaccessibility to complex care, and to ensure optimal quality of medical attention in every hospital, regardless of its geographic location or the complexity of care it can provide.

Optimal care can be planned for a region as a whole. The region is defined geographically according to preexisting patterns of medical referrals, commercial ties, and sociocultural bonds. Personnel and money can be allocated to avoid duplication of facilities and to ensure proper utilization of services. Theoretically, the needs of individual patients should be met within a perinatal region, with all levels of care available. The sole determinants of the care given to mother and infant should be the severity and complexity of their illnesses. Services are best offered in facilities that are close to home, but the transfer of patients from one hospital to another is inevitable if an appropriate level of care is to be delivered.

A coordinated regional system requires designation of hospitals by the level of care that they provide. Beyond the designation of care levels, activation of effective communication for consultation and for transport of patients provides functional continuity between the diverse hospitals in a region. Fundamental to all these activities is a plan for continuing education of personnel; without it, any system will falter. Although guidelines are usually addressed to hospitals because they are institutional providers of care, the real pitch is to physicians, nurses, and other personnel as the personal providers of care.

Types of Facilities

The regionalized system provides three types of facilities: Levels I, II, and III. Hospitals are designated by these three levels of care according to the *extent* of their respective capacities. These designations do not grade the *quality* of care; they indicate only the *extent* of care.

Level I The Level I facility has three principal functions: 1) management of normal pregnancy, labor, and delivery; 2) earliest feasible identification of high-risk pregnancies and high-risk neonates; and 3) provision of competent emergency care in the event of unanticipated obstetric and neonatal emergencies. These hospitals are usually located in small communities, where they are vital to the health care of the area. They are defined as primary (Level I) care centers by virtue of their limited capacity to manage perinatal complications. There is little justification for Level I facilities in densely populated (urban) areas. Approximately 500 to 750 annual live births occur at these hospitals. By virtue of a small number of births, complications are infrequent. Staff and equipment needs are therefore less demanding than for Level II and III units.

Level II Level II facilities are larger perinatal facilities in hospitals that generally serve urban and suburban communities. The ideal Level II facility is capable of managing 75% to 90% of maternal and neonatal complications. However, this capacity must necessarily vary from one hospital to another. A Level II facility should care for most perinatal complications and for uncomplicated patients as well. As in the Level I unit, activities of the Level II facility are of the highest possible quality for that level of care.

Level III Level III facilities have the capacity to manage the most complex perinatal disorders in addition to offering care for uncomplicated maternity and newborn patients. For neonatal disorders, the Level III facility should have at its disposal a complete roster of pediatric subspecialists, pediatric surgeons, pediatric radiologists, geneticists, and hospital epidemiologists. This facility should deliver all modalities of care that comprise contemporary practice. In a densely populated region where there is more than one Level III unit, only one may be designated as a *regional center*. The regional center is responsible for the coordination of perinatal activities in its region. It is also responsible for maintaining consultation services for obstetricians, pediatricians, and the respective nursing services. At all Level III units and at regional centers in particular, a staff of *perinatal social workers* should be available to manage the psychosocial problems that arise in families whose infants receive intensive care. The regional center must conduct ongoing education programs intramurally, and additionally to other hospitals of the region (outreach). The Level III unit, whether or not it is a designated regional center, has at least one full-time obstetrician who is a subspecialist in maternal/fetal medicine and a full-time pediatrician who is a subspecialist in neonatal/perinatal medicine. Nurse specialists in obstetric and newborn care should deliver their respective nursing services in consonance with physicians and social workers.

Referral for Transport

Level III units usually maintain a system of transport for mothers and infants. Alternatively, such a system may be maintained in a region by cooperative responsibility of its constituent hospitals. In either case, transport (by ground or air) requires nurses and physicians who are specifically educated for this purpose. In numerous localities, clinical nurse specialists manage the entire process of infant transfer; in most areas, physicians (often advanced trainees) are charged with this responsibility. Transport vehicles for infants vary from ambulances of standard size that carry incubators with monitors and ventilators to larger vehicles that are as fully equipped as the nursery itself. At the University of Tennessee Newborn Center we use the latter type, which is 30 feet in length with two radiant warmer beds, ventilators, monitors, blood gas apparatus, a sink with running water, and a complete supply of consumable items. Air transport (usually fixed-wing aircraft) is used in regions that are spread over a large area and in some large cities where heavy vehicular traffic creates problems that are surmountable only by helicopters. Maternal transport is the referral modality of choice. Adept screening at any hospital should predict 60% to 70% of the infants who will be in jeopardy at birth. Referral of these high-risk mothers for delivery of their babies at a tertiary care unit constitutes the best contemporary care available.

Educational Programs

The regional center is responsible for the dissemination of information to the staffs of all hospitals within its region. These educational activities have been largely directed to practicing physicians and nursing staffs. Structured series of lectures and demonstrations or single sessions devoted to a specific topic are the usual formats of presentation. Instruction is usually given at the outlying hospitals but often at the regional centers as well. In Tennessee, extensive compilations of educational objectives have been circulated throughout the state for nurses, physicians, and social workers. Nurses' objectives are organized by specific care levels ("Educational Objectives for Nurses—Levels I, II, III, Neonatal Transport Nurses," 1982). The guide for physicians is directed to pediatricians and family practitioners ("Outlines of Courses for Physicians," 1982). The social workers' material is intended for Level II and Level III facilities ("Educational Objectives in Medicine for Perinatal Social Workers," 1982). Courses and sessions offered by each of the four regional centers in the state are based upon these educational objectives. Regionalized professional education programs are emphasized throughout the country because the quality of perinatal care is ultimately dependent upon the effectiveness of its educational efforts.

Maximal Care Units (Level III)

An accurate national inventory of intensive care units has yet to be produced, because mailed surveys have yielded a paucity of responses and realistic definitions of Level II and III care are not universally understood. Some useful estimates are available, however—they show approximately 300 Level III units among the 4800 birthing hospitals in the United States. Approximately 100,000 infants are admitted to these units annually, one-third of whom are transported from other hospitals. Mean length of stay is estimated at approximately 15 days; total annual baby days are thus calculcated at 1.5 million per year (Sheridan, 1983). In a 1980 survey, 32 of 253 units (12.7%) indicated no full-time neonatologists on their staffs, yet they claimed Level III status. Approximately one-half of the 253 respondents reported three to more than six neonatologists on their staffs; 52% allowed practicing physicians who are not certified neonatologists to care for infants (Sheridan, 1983).

Of particular pertinence to ecologic considerations and to the behavioral inclinations of personnel in Level III units is the constant ratio of nurses to patients that is maintained around the clock. They work with little respite; the time of day is not a high priority. Maximal care is given by three nurses for every two infants during each shift of the day; intermediate care is administered by one nurse to every three babies, and convalescent care by one nurse to four infants. In the aggregate, intensive care units employ 11 different types of health professionals and support personnel besides physicians and registered nurses.

The nurse-patient ratios reported in this survey seem to belie the widespread complaints regarding nurse shortages and the frustrations of attempts to maintain adequate staffing ratios. Our unit is one of the largest; in 1983 1500 infants for three levels of care were admitted to 80 beds. A total of 27,000 baby days were recorded for the year. Approximately 35% of these days were given to maximal care. As a consequence, there is ongoing difficulty in the maintenance of a nurse-patient ratio that approaches 1.5, as reported in the 1980 survey, and these frustrations are suspected to be common in other localities. These staffing shortfalls should be borne in mind when considering ecologic phenomena. In all probability, the interplay among personnel and between personnel, babies, and their families is influenced profoundly by slim staffing patterns. In these circumstances, for sheer lack of time, preoccupation with infant survival may unfortunately displace important ecologic considerations.

Structural Elements

Those of us who have designed Level III nurseries have had the needs of personnel uppermost in mind, particularly the needs of nurses. Beds are thus deployed to accommodate the management of their patient assignments. Placement of major equipment (monitors, respirators, incubators, and radiant warmers) is planned for effective use by the nursing staff. Consumable items are virtually always in reach. Although reserve supplies are located more remotely, they must be readily accessible and in quantities that are adequate for several days' use. Preparation of medications and intravenous fluids is best performed within the nursery (or close to it) by a pharmacist whose principal obligation is to the intensive care unit. Medications and fluids thus prepared are delivered to the nurse or are placed in convenient proximity to the nurse's assigned patient area. If, as in most facilities, the nurse must prepare medications, counter space for that purpose is planned as close as possible to assigned patients.

The earliest consideration in planning a neonatal unit is a determination of its location within the hospital. It should be juxtaposed to the delivery room or at least close to it. The next decision concerns the number and configuration of infant rooms. The two most prevalent floor plans utilize a single large room or smaller multiple rooms, usually two or three in number. Configuration is most often dictated by the design of the building if new construction is involved or by a preexisting arrangement if renovation is utilized. A square room is best. A number of centers have opted for a single large room. We designed one for maximal and intermediate care (60 beds in 6600 square feet) and a second, smaller room was added for convalescent care (20 beds in 1000 square feet). The large room was chosen because of its flexibility for patient assignments to nurses, the cross-coverage it facilitates when several hands are required for emergencies, and the ease of surveillance that is possible at all times.

Spacing is the single most important element of structural design; its fundamental determinant is patient census. Most publications recommend

80 to 100 square feet per infant, but it is more effective to begin by planning for bed arrangements with respect *to the space that separates them* (Korones, 1983). In terms of operational effectiveness, bed intervals and aisles are the least amenable to compromise. Bed intervals that are less than 5 feet wide and aisles that are less than 6 feet wide will result in situations that range from inconvenience to impossibility. Intervals greater than 6 feet and aisles of more than 8 feet are impractical, particularly for nurses who must care for more than one patient. Planning for deployment of beds should begin by considering interval and aisle space requirements rather than primary assignment of square feet per bed, because a number of space-occupying variables ultimately impinge upon bed spread. These variables include: 1) the width and number of island cabinets for infant care; 2) the number and size of counters and cabinets for supplies; 3) preparation of medication; 4) clerical functions; and 5) the space that must remain unoccupied at entry ways. Furthermore, generous yet practical allocation of space between beds is essential for placing equipment and using x-ray and ultrasound apparatus. Because today's state-of-the-art is tomorrow's anachronism, effective planning must also provide adequately for the use of equipment that has yet to be devised.

Using this approach, we distributed 60 beds for both intensive and intermediate care in a single large room of 6600 square feet. We had vacated a previous facility in which 41 babies were placed in a single room of 2000 square feet. In that unit, the presence of permanent and visiting personnel of all sorts eventually took its toll. On some occasions during morning teaching rounds, one could count 55 individuals in this infant care room. These individuals included attending physicians, trainees, technicians from our own laboratory and from the hospital's as well, x-ray technicians, and the nursing staff. Crowding was stressful, even though it waxed and waned. Bedside procedures and the taking of x-rays entailed substantial inconvenience. "Rubbing elbows" was inescapable, and a significant noise factor was unavoidable. The crowding and noise incurred an identifiable psychological burden on personnel. In contrast, spread of beds in the facility now occupied provides each nurse with adequate turf that is rarely encroached upon. Furthermore, wide spacing in a very large room has serendipitously resulted in an unusually low noise level, presumably because of its dilution within a large air space.

Outside windows are important; a windowless room is depressing to personnel. Windows must be effectively insulated, especially if infants are housed close by. During periods of extremely cold weather, those who are placed nearly poorly insulated windows will be seriously cold-stressed. Curtains are inadvisable because they gather dust that is ultimately wafted into room air. Room temperature should be maintained at approximately

75°F. In a large room, a steady temperature can be maintained only by zonal control, with thermostats in several locations.

Lighting must be bright at all times. Although standard recommendation is 100 foot-candles, we have found 150 foot-candles to be preferable. Circadian variation of light intensity is inconsistent with any level of cautious care, and this applies to well-baby nurseries as well. Adequate surveillance is impossible in dim light. Pallor, cyanosis, abnormal respiration, seizure activity, and vomiting require immediate attention. They are less likely to be discerned in semidarkness (they are occasionally missed even when a nursery is brightly illuminated).

Unobstructed visibility is indispensable. Infants on monitors must be visible from a distance. Monitoring devices should have both visual and auditory alarms. The usual audible alarms fill a room with nondirectional sound, making it difficult to identify the source. To combat this problem red lights can be installed in the ceiling above each infant. They flash when tripped by the monitor and identification of the affected infant is instantaneous.

Cabinets in a variety of designs can be placed along the wall and elsewhere throughout an infant care room, where they are free-standing islands. They serve several pivotal functions: outlets for electricity, suction, oxygen, and air are built into their vertical panels. Incubators and radiant warmers are docked to them for connection to gas and power lines. The cabinets are primarily a center of activity for infant care. Counter tops serve as repositories for equipment, as work surfaces to prepare for procedures, and as surfaces for recording notes. A second surface is provided by a shelf that is mounted above the counter top for placement of monitors at eye level, about 5 feet above the floor. Shelving and drawers beneath the counter tops are for immediate accessibility of consumable supplies. These cabinets are designed to concentrate intensive care activity within each infant's circumscribed, yet spacious, area. The area must be circumscribed and relatively self-contained because speed is often the essence of effectiveness. The nurse should not find it necessary to leave frequently for the multiplicity of small items that are constantly used and discarded. The area should be sufficiently spacious for several caretakers to operate simultaneously around three sides of an infant's incubator or radiant warmer, and it should accommodate large pieces of equipment such as x-ray, ultrasound, portable radioactive scanners, and apparatus for electroencephalography and electrocardiography. For contrasting yet appealing needs, a comfortable upholstered stool and a rocking chair should be close by for the quieter moments that inevitably follow intense activity. Rocking chairs are indispensable in the intermediate and convalescent care areas of the nursery, where a larger proportion of time is appropriately devoted to social interaction with infants.

Sinks must be installed at strategic intervals throughout the nursery. There should be one sink conveniently accessible for every four to six patients in a given room. The spread of infection in an intensive care unit is often life-threatening. The most effective procedure for prevention of infection and its spread is hand-washing between patient contacts. An adequate number of sinks throughout the nursery is thus mandatory.

Support Services

Laboratory services must be structured to respond to recurrent urgencies. Turn-around time for laboratory data must be as short as possible. Larger units usually include some type of laboratory facility that is situated within them. Alternatively, a central laboratory that serves the entire hospital provides services for the NICU. It should be staffed around the clock by medical technologists who are an integral part of the staff. The staff of the laboratory should be impressed with the priorities and exigencies of intensive care, having been instructed in the clinical significance of their efforts.

Radiology Services

A portable apparatus is used for virtually all x-rays. In most units, the radiology department processes, interprets, and stores films in its own central area. In some nurseries, x-rays are kept on the premises in a designated viewing area. Our patient volume justifies incorporation of an imaging service within the unit. X-ray and ultrasound equipment is stored in a room that opens into the infant care area, where films are also processed and interpreted by the radiologist. Each infant's x-ray films are kept at the bedside for the duration of the nursery stay. Multiformat copies of intracranial ultrasound images are also stored at the bedside. X-ray view boxes are installed throughout the infant care area so that films may be viewed during rounds as a baby is discussed. The daily presence of a radiologist promotes ongoing contact with clinicians, and the result of all these factors is a well-integrated program of diagnostic imagery. Ours is but an example of a scheme that has proved appropriate for a large unit.

Personnel

The series of events that is triggered by the admission of a sick neonate involves a sizable cohort of people who are well versed in the functions they must perform. When the birth of a distressed infant is anticipated, a *physician* and a *nurse* from the intensive care unit await the baby in the delivery room. The *obstetrician* is prepared to provide resuscitation at birth, and the nursery is notified of the impending admission of a severely depressed infant. The *respiratory therapist* sets up a ventilator; a *nurse* and an *aide* prepare the radiant warmer bed. Upon arrival of the baby, *three nurses* perform admission procedures, ranging from determination of blood pressure, body temperature, blood sugar, and weight to adjustment of the warmer, starting intravenous fluids, and unpacking a tray for umbilical artery insertion. The *physician* provides assisted ventilation with a bag until the baby is placed on the respirator. The *ward clerk* notifies radiology and the laboratory that they are needed immediately. A *blood collector* takes samples for the laboratory, and a *medical technologist* performs the tests requested. An *x-ray technologist* takes the film that was ordered, develops it, and submits it to the *radiologist*. A *social worker* visits the baby's family as soon after birth as feasible. This typical admission, which occupies a period of approximately 1 hour, already involves 12 individuals. The ongoing care of this baby will involve more personnel with similar or varying expertise. This is not solely a matter of numbers of personnel. In no instance can any individual, from physicians and nurses to ward clerks, be drafted abruptly from another area of the hospital to fill a gap in the NICU.

A staff of physicians in the Level III unit has at its core an appropriate number of board-certified neonatologists. If the unit is an integral part of a university program, fellows in neonatal/perinatal medicine are also part of the staff. The university program provides residents who spend 5 to 6 months in the NICU during the course of their 3-year training in pediatrics, and in some units, as in ours, residents in obstetrics, anesthesiology, and family medicine are also regularly present. In a large university unit, therefore, 6 to 10 physicians may be present during regular hours; most of them are trainees under the supervision of senior physicians. At most nonuniversity centers, there are fewer physicians but all are likely to be senior. Trainees are subjected to an overbearing work schedule. They are on duty every third or fourth night and, in a large unit, this translates into 1 or 2 hours of sleep, if any at all. A considerably reduced level of effectiveness can be expected from them as the night wears on and during the day that follows.

More so than any other type of personnel, the quality of nurses is the most critical determinant of the overall quality of an intensive care unit.

The role of the registered nurse has changed dramatically during the past 15 years. In the late 1960s and even into the very early 1970s, there was a real need to decry the "handmaiden" concept of nursing that was then pervasive. Burgeoning activity and new knowledge precipitated an urgent need for increased nursing responsibility and enhanced expertise to activate it. "Handmaiden" changed to "colleague" as postgraduate courses arose for the specific education of neonatal intensive care nurses. There soon followed a movement to develop clinical nurse practitioners and specialists whose responsibilities were more like those of a physician than those of the traditional nurse. The cohort of nurses in the average Level III unit of the 1980s is remarkably heterogeneous. There are instructors who deal primarily with in-service and outreach education of nurses, practitioners who manage selected babies as physicians do, transport nurses who manage infants from outlying hospitals during their transfer, research nurses who knowledgeably assist physicians in clinical research and conduct their own as well, and staff nurses whose expertise in caring for sick infants hour by hour cannot be duplicated by others who are neither educated nor dedicated to the purpose.

The urgent need to alleviate the emotional crises of parents caused by the severe illness of their newborn infants became apparent early in the history of neonatal intensive care. Social and emotional support for parents is an essential component of total neonatal care. Temperamentally and professionally, no one is better equipped for this task than the neonatal social worker. In essence, social workers are compassionate activists. Their list of functions is lengthy, and the scope of nonmedical support is broad. The social worker is a parent advocate to the nursery staff, an interpreter of medical jargon and concepts to parents, a procurer of tangible necessities for parents, a coordinator of the staff's efforts at emotional support, a counselor in all forms of grief, a source of information on available community facilities, a facilitator of conferences, an arranger of postdischarge follow-up, an advisor on financial problems, and a vocal conscience on the ethical dilemmas.

Overlap of the roles of physicans, nurses, and social workers is quite easily identified. We consider this to be an advantage. The separate disciplines, utilizing their primary responsibilities as a focal point of parental contact, reinforce each other in the total effort. Ultimately, the social worker is responsible for the coordination of psychosocial care. There is neither time nor reason for interdisciplinary friction because of overlapping functions. For instance, the nurse, who is often the first to encounter parents, briefs them about the medical situation, assesses their reactions, attempts to comprehend their attitudes, and supports them during stressful moments. The nurse functions similarly during subsequent parental visits and vigils. During these encounters, the nurse has roles that ordinarily accrue to physicians or social workers. Nevertheless, these encounters are effective with few exceptions. The physician, who also plays multiple roles, draws upon explanations of biologic disorders and upon predictions of outcome, but effectiveness would be incomplete if these contacts with parents were devoid of psychosocial elements.

If the psychosocial concerns of physicians and nurses tend to reinforce the social worker's primary commitment, the latter's concern with medical matters is also reciprocally constructive. Neonatal social work requires sufficient knowledge of medical events to relate these to psychosocial difficulties. Without such knowledge, there is little basis for most of the social worker's counseling activities in an intensive care unit. Explanations of medical difficulties by physicians and nurses are too often replete with scientific terms that impair parental understanding. The social worker minimizes or eliminates confusion by offering explanations that are more easily understood. Also, parents are less restrained and self-conscious in the presence of the social worker; they more readily acknowledge confusion and ask more questions. The social worker is also an intermediary, relaying to the physician the parental anxieties that arise from an overtechnical explanation of an infant's biologic disorder. We have had a historic commitment to social work in our unit, having 9 full-time perinatal social workers on our staff. Social work, like medicine and nursing, is indispensable to such totality.

Other disciplines are significantly active, each with a unique indispensability. The respiratory therapist has been educated to the singular characteristics of neonatal ventilatory support. The therapist whose principal responsibilities are to adults, or even to older pediatric patients, is not as expert as one who is specifically trained and experienced in tending to neonates. The same can be said for the physical therapist, who must be knowledgeable in the characteristics of infant development, the peculiarities of neonatal neuromuscular disorders, the effects of an environment that necessarily neglects psychosocial contacts during acute life-threatening illness, and the multiple aspects of infant management that indirectly influence the areas of concern to the physical therapist.

In recent years, the philosopher has been summoned to the scene—not by any particular individual but rather by the well-known sequence of events that has increased the capacity to sustain the lives of smaller and more severely ill infants. This medical ethicist has brought knowledge to the bedside that is farther removed from endotracheal tubes, respirators, and catheters than any other discipline thus far recruited to the purposes of total neonatal intensive care. Added to intense anxieties for the infant's intact survival are the ethics of decisions, demeanor, and motivation. At one end of the spectrum is the question of who dies and who decides. On the other extreme is the contention that no one dies by decision and therefore no one need decide. Medical ethicists are consulted regularly in a number of centers; for some protocols have been written requiring such consultations, and in others the ethicist is periodically present during rounds in the nursery. Many institutions are planning the establishment of an Infant Bioethics Committee that will be comprised of representatives of nonmedical disciplines as well as physicians to assist in the resolution of ethical problems.

Summary

The milieu of the neonatal intensive care unit is best described as "ordered chaos." Recurrent emergencies preclude a smooth routine. Situations vary from severely stressed infants (a primary concern) and emotionally stressed parents to shortages of critical equipment and personnel to iatrogenic misadventures that are inevitable in such a setting. Structural components thus far have proved to be appropriate means to fundamental ends. A multidisciplinary cohort of personnel, predominantly oriented toward intact survival, has now become aware of the environmental contributions to "intactness." The time is right for a systematic acquisition of ecologic data and observations in the nursery environment.

The patient is sensitive and fragile. Physical elements in the environment, such as excessive noise, are hazardous and should be minimized or eliminated. Psychosocial factors are significant and their neglect is an impediment to optimal outcome, so rectification is mandatory. Random disturbance can be minimized, and coordinated stimulation can be enhanced. Neonates are unique, but not so unique that we can be mindless of their status as patients whose environmental needs must be met and whose human needs require thoughtful social interaction.

Acknowledgments

I would like to thank Marion Haynes and Rosalind Griffin for their expert preparation of the manuscript and for their editorial contributions. Thanks, too, to Susan Poo.

References

American Academy of Pediatrics, Committee on Environmental Hazards. 1974. Noise pollution: Neonatal aspects. Pediatrics 54:476–478.

Basler, D. S., and Hager, D. E. 1977. Planning and Design for Perinatal and Pediatric Facilities. Ross Laboratories, Columbus, OH.

Educational Objectives in Medicine for Perinatal Social Workers. 1982. Task Force on Educational Objectives for Perinatal Social Workers, Tennessee Perinatal Care System, Tennessee Department of Public Health, Division of Maternal and Child Health, Nashville, TN.

Educational Objectives for Nurses—Levels I, II, III, Neonatal Transport Nurses. 1982. Task Force on Nurse Education, Tennessee Perinatal Care System, Tennessee Department of Public Health, Division of Maternal and Child Health, Nashville, TN.

Gluck, L. 1976. Preventing obsolescence in the design of a perinatal unit. Clin. Perinatol. 3:349–351.

Gottfried, A. W., Wallace-Land, P., Sherman-Brown, S., King, J., Coen, C., and Hodgman, J. E. 1981. Physical and social environment of newborn infants in special care units. Science 214:673–675.

Korones, S. B. 1976. Disturbance and infants' rest. In: T. D. Moore (ed.), Iatrogenic Problems in Neonatal Intensive Care: Report of the Sixty-Ninth Ross Conference on Pediatric Research, pp. 94–97. Ross Laboratories, Columbus, OH.

Korones, S. B. 1983. Evolution of nursery design and function: The Memphis story. Clin. Perinatol. 10:127–40.

Long, J. G., Lucey, J. F., and Philip, A. G. S. 1980a. Noise and hypoxemia in the intensive care nursery. Pediatrics 65:143–145.

Long, J. G., Philip, A. G. S., and Lucey, J. F. 1980b. Excessive handling as a cause of hypoxemia. Pediatrics 65:203–207.

Outlines of Courses for Physicians. 1982. Task Force on Courses for Physicians, Tennessee Perinatal Care System, Tennessee Department of Public Health, Division of Maternal and Child Health, Nashville, TN.

Rice, R. D. 1977. Neurophysiological development in premature infants following stimulation. Dev. Psychol. 13:69–76.

Sheridan, J. F. 1983. The typical perinatal center: An overview of perinatal health services in the United States. Clin. Perinatol. 10:31–47.

Tyson, J., Schultz, K., Sinclair, J. C., and Gill, G. 1979. Diurnal variation in the quality and outcome of newborn intensive care. J. Pediatr. 95:277–280.

3

Environment of Newborn Infants in Special Care Units

Allen W. Gottfried

Each year an estimated 2% to 9% of all live births in the United States require intensive care. This is a total annual rate of approximately 200,000 to 250,000 newborns. The average length of stay in special care units is from 15 to 20 days, with infants weighing from 1000 to 1500 grams averaging 40 to 50 days (Budetti et al., 1981; Donahue, 1981).

The majority of these infants fare well. However, prospective investigations continue to show cognitive and sensory deficits in very small prematures (Broman et al., 1975; Field, 1979; Friedman and Sigman, 1980). These impairments in prematures have been attributed to brain damage. Recently, it has been suggested that environmental stimulation in newborn intensive care units (NICUs) may contribute to the deficits associated with prematurity. Researchers and clinicians working in these units began raising issues regarding potential medical and developmental consequences of environmental stimulation in NICUs. It has been proposed that contemporary management of newborns in NICUs may be responsible for iatrogenic complications and may not be conducive to optimal development.

Various conceptualizations about the nature of the NICU environment have been advanced. Several investigators put forth the view that intensive care provides an environment that is sensorily depriving for

---

The preparation of this chapter and the research presented herein were made possible in part by a grant from the Thrasher Research Fund and a California State University, Fullerton, President's grant.

newborns (Barnard, 1973; Freedman et al., 1966; Katz, 1971; Leib et al., 1980; Powell, 1974; Rice, 1977; Scarr-Salapatek and Williams, 1973; Segall, 1972; Solkoff et al., 1969; White and LaBarbara, 1976). Specifically, these investigators assumed that newborns in these units are deprived in amount and/or pattern of stimulation of various types (i.e., visual, auditory, tactile, vestibular-kinesthetic, and socioemotional). This assumption provided a major underlying basis and impetus for the proliferation of environmental intervention studies during the 1970s. Contrary to the view that infants in NICUs are sensorily deprived, Cornell and Gottfried (1976) contended that:

> As a consequence of the personnel, equipment, and activity present in most modern high-risk nurseries, one can as readily assert that the premature infant is exposed to a variety and large amount of sensory experiences. (p. 33)

In line with this conceptualization were the arguments of Korones (1976) and Lucey (1977) that intensive care may have become too intense and may be accountable for newly recognized clinical problems. Lawson et al. (1977) supported the hypothesis that prematures in NICUs do not suffer from an inadequate amount of stimulation. They suggested that newborns receiving intensive care are exposed to a pattern of stimulation that is disjunctive (also see Newman, 1981). In summary, the various conceptualizations about the nature of the NICU environment described newborns as: 1) being sensorily deprived or isolated; 2) being exposed to various sorts and large amounts of stimulation; or 3) receiving disintegrated or inappropriate patterns of stimulation.

Knowledge about the environment of NICUs has important psychological, medical, and occupational implications. First, basic environmental information is necessary in order to design the most appropriate and effective type of sensory intervention for premature infants. All of the newborn environmental intervention programs have operated under the assumption that either premature infants are sensorily deprived or that increases in stimulation ameliorate developmental status. Based on the various preceding conceptualizations of the NICU environment, it is conceivable that environmental intervention programs may involve reduction and reorganization of environmental stimulation as well. Furthermore, evidence indicates an interaction between the efficacy of sensory intervention programs and concurrently existing environmental factors in NICUs (Katz, 1971; Neal, 1968).

Second, the Committee on Environmental Hazards of the American Academy of Pediatrics (1974) expressed a strong concern about the consequences of noise pollution for newborns. Of particular concern was the possible hearing loss attributable to high-intensity sounds and the potentiation between these sounds and ototoxic medication. In the only controlled clinical trial or experimental study, Kitchen et al. (1979) in Australia randomly assigned prematures between 1000 and 1500 grams to routine or intensive care units. At an 8-year follow up, it was found that compared to the children who received routine care, those receiving intensive care had fewer severe handicaps but more ocular abnormalities and sensorineural deafness. Sound levels, among other environmental characteristics in the NICU, may have adverse consequences on the medical status of the newborn premature (see Chapter 10 of this volume).

Third, in view of the undue stress and demands placed upon the professional staff in the NICU and the burnout and turnover of nursing personnel in these units (Gribbins and Marshall, 1982; Marshall et al., 1982), environmental characteristics for staff as well as infants must be given serious consideration.

Aim and Research Setting

This chapter presents a series of studies by the author and his colleagues, who investigated the environmental stimulation available to infants in special care units of a Level III facility. The aim of these studies was to assess the nature of physical and social stimulation in both the NICU and the newborn convalescent care unit (NCCU). The research was conducted at the Los Angeles County–University of Southern California Medical Center Women's Hospital. At Women's Hospital there are currently some 17,000 births per year, and approximately 2000 of the infants are admitted to the NICU or NCCU. The area of each unit where observations were conducted measures approximately 14.6 by 8.5 meters and houses an average of 20 to 25 infants. The ratio of staff to infants is 1:1–2 and 1:5 in the NICU and NCCU, respectively.

Study I—Physical and Social Environment: A Time-Sampling Analysis (Investigators: Allen W. Gottfried, Patricia Wallace-Lande, Susan Sherman-Brown, Jeanne King, Carolyn Coen, and Joan E. Hodgman)

This initial study sought to determine the amount of physical stimulation (illumination and sound) and the frequency, type, and organization of social contacts received by infants, and the diurnal rhythmicity of both physical and social stimulation (Gottfried et al., 1981). The following questions were addressed:

1. What are the magnitudes of illumination and sound levels in the NICU and NCCU?

2. What is the occurrence of speech, nonspeech, and radio sounds in these units?
3. What is the frequency of medical-nursing care, feeding, social touching, rocking, and talking in these units?
4. Are there differences between the units in amount and frequency of physical and social stimulation?
5. Are social sensory experiences organized or coordinated (e.g., co-occurrence of talking and handling of infants or infant in position to see caregiver when handled)?
6. Is there diurnal regularity across days in the level of physical and social stimulation?

Method Observations were conducted in designated locations in the NICU and NCCU. Three locations were selected in each unit that were comparable across units. In each unit, 3-minute observations were conducted (1 minute at each location) at the same time every hour for a duration of 24 hours over 3 nonconsecutive days (Tuesday, Thursday, and Saturday of the same week). Each observation required two researchers—one recorded physical data while the other recorded social data.

The physical data included illumination levels (Gossen Luna Pro light meter), characteristic and peak sound levels (Bruel and Kjaer sound meter 2203), a frequency analysis of the sound spectra (Bruel and Kjaer octave filter set 1613), and the occurrence of speech, nonspeech (i.e., inanimate), and radio sounds. Additionally, these data were collected by means of the light and sound meters and by a tape recorder placed in an operating incubator located in the center of each unit. The social data included the frequency of medical-nursing care, bottle feeding, social touching, rocking, talking when in contact with an infant (not necessarily to the infant), and whether the infant was in a position to see the caregiver (vision). It was also noted whether the caregiver was a professional or a family member. For all physical and social variables, interobserver reliabilities exceeded 97% and 92% agreement, respectively.

Results

Physical The physical data (see Table 3.1) included 405 measurements for each variable taken in the units (204 and 201 in the NICU and NCCU, respectively). Analysis of the sound spectra was based on 18 recordings in the units and in the incubators. Illumination and sound levels in incubators were also based on 18 recordings. A total of 9 hours of tape-recordings from incubators were collected at various time intervals. Observations of infants totaled 1551 (NICU = 846, NCCU = 705), of which 292 (18.8%) involved contacts with infants. There were no significant differences among the 3 days in the magnitude or frequency of

Table 3.1. Physical data of Study I.

Variable	NICU		NCCU
In Units[a]			
Illumination levels (lumen/m^2)			
Mean	530		508
Range	344–1400		243–1400
Sound characteristics (dB)			
Mean	77.4	*	74.5
Range	66.0–109.0		62.0–109.0
Sound peak (dB)			
Mean	85.8	*	82.0
Range	69.0–118.0		65.0–118.0
Speech (%)	92.2	*	69.2
Nonspeech (%)	100.0		100.0
Radio on (%)	79.4	*	54.2
In Incubators			
Illumination levels (lumen/m^2)			
Mean	486		448
Range	344–699		344–699
Sound characteristics (dB)			
Mean	81.1	*	78.8
Range	72.0–106.0		71.0–90.0
Sound peak (dB)			
Mean	88.7	*	83.6
Range	74.0–116.0		77.0–98.0

*$p < .01$.
[a] This portion of the table is reproduced by permission from Gottfried, A. W., et al. 1981. Physical and social environment of newborn infants in special care units. Science 214:674. Copyright 1981 by the AAAS.

physical and social recordings (all data are combined across the 3 days).

Ambient cool-white fluorescent lighting was continuously present with little variation. The highest levels recorded occurred during mid-afternoon hours, probably because of the addition of sunlight. Sound levels averaged in the 70 to 80 dB range (linear) with high upper levels. A sample of recordings using A-weighting were collected. The mean characteristic and peak levels in the NICU were 63.2 dB and 70.3 dB; in the NCCU, they were 53.0 dB and 60.4 dB, respectively. The overall noise environment was comparable to light auto traffic and at times reached a level of large machinery and engines (Peterson and Gross, 1974). Sound levels fluctuated continuously. The high sound levels were not brief but were elevated for durations of 4 to 6 hours. Nonspeech sounds were heard during all observations, and speech and radio sounds

28 Gottfried

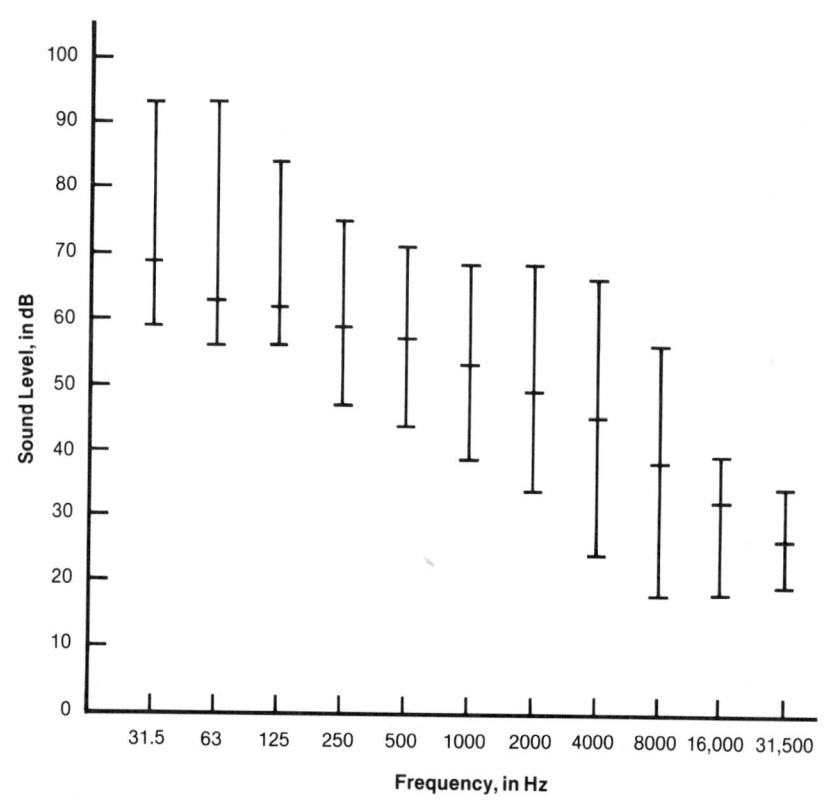

Figure 3.1. Frequency analysis of the sound spectra.

were heard during the large majority of observations with no discernible patterns of occurrence.

The frequency analysis of the sound spectra taken at each octave band from 31.5 to 32,000 Hz (see Figure 3.1) revealed that the acoustic energy was distributed in the lower frequencies. The acoustic environments of the NICU and NCCU are characterized as high intensities at low frequencies.

The light and sound data in the incubators presented a virtually identical picture to that of the units proper. Illumination levels were slightly lower and sound levels slightly higher, with comparable upper peak sound levels. The slightly higher sound levels were probably attributable to the motor inside the incubator. Nonspeech sounds, including the continuous white noise emanating from the incubator itself, were picked up on all tape recordings. Human speech sounds were identifiable on the tape recordings but were somewhat muffled and indistinct. The frequency analysis of the sound spectra inside the

Table 3.2. Social data of Study I.[a]

Variable	NICU		NCCU
Medical-nursing care	15.5	*	3.8
Bottle feeding	0.02	**	8.5
Social touching	0.02	**	5.8
Rocking	0.001	**	2.6
Talking	13.0	*	7.9
Handling	17.8		15.3

All data are presented as percentages.
*$p < .01$.
**$p < .001$.
[a] Reproduced by permission from Gottfried, A. W., et al. 1981. Physical and social environment of newborn infants in special care units. Science 214:674. Copyright 1981 by the AAAS.

incubators showed the same distribution of acoustic energy as measured in the units. These data indicate that the visual and auditory stimulation in the units penetrated the incubator Plexiglas and were continuously available to the infants.

Statistical analyses were conducted to determine whether the intensity of the physical environment differed between the two units. With the exception of illumination levels and percentage of nonspeech sounds, values in the NICU were significantly higher than those in the NCCU (for parametric data: $t_{403} \geq 3.33$, $p < .01$; for frequency data: $\chi_1^2 \geq 7.37$, $p < .01$).[1] These data indicated an overall greater noise level in the NICU than in the NCCU. Kendall's coefficient of concordance was conducted on each physical variable to test whether there was diurnal rhythmicity across the 3 days in each of the units. The results showed no temporal stability on any of the variables (W $< .51$, $k = 3, j = 24$, NS).[2]

Social The social data are shown in Table 3.2. As previously noted, 18.8% of the observations involved nursery personnel contacts with infants. In the NICU and NCCU, 21% (178) and 16.2% (114) of the observations included contacts, respectively, with the proportion of

---

[1] The same significant findings were obtained when analyses were conducted by tests of differences between proportions (Hoel, 1976).

[2] The differences between the present findings and those of Lawson et al. (1977) concerning rhythmicity of illumination across days may be due to two factors. First, windows in the units at Women's Hospital faced south, whereas those at Jacobi Hospital faced west. The latter, in contrast to the former, is subject to greater intensity and regularity of illumination resulting from the sun. Second, recordings of illumination in the Lawson et al. study were conducted with light meters directed toward the windows. In the present study, recordings of illumination were conducted at each location with light meters directed toward the center of each aisle of incubators, all of which were parallel to the windows. However, in both studies the highest levels of illumination were recorded during midafternoon hours.

contacts significantly greater in the NICU ($p < .05$). Eighty-five percent of the contacts involved staff only. Family members alone accounted for 14% of the contacts, and 1% of the contacts involved both staff and family members. The most frequent type of contact was (not unexpectedly) medical-nursing care, and the least frequent contact was rocking. Medical-nursing care and talking occurred at a significantly greater frequency in the NICU than in the NCCU ($\chi_1^2 \geq 8.56$, $p < .01$), whereas bottle-feeding, social touching, and rocking occurred significantly more in the NCCU ($\chi_1^2 \geq 19.00$, $p < .001$).[3] Handling was a variable generated to provide an index of the occurrence of tactile stimulation. Handling was defined as the occurrence of one or more nontalking contacts during a single observation of an infant. Some form of handling occurred in 16.7% of the observations (across units). Although handling occurred at a slightly higher rate in the NICU than in the NCCU, there was no statistical difference in frequencies between the units. Of contacts in the NICU and NCCU, 84.8% and 94.4%, respectively, involved handling. The difference between these two percentages was significant ($p < .05$). Infants in the NCCU received a relatively greater proportion of handling compared to infants in the NICU. For each social variable, Kendall's coefficient of concordance was used to test for diurnal rhythmicity across the 3 days in each of the two units. The results showed no temporal consistency for any of the variables ($W < .47$, $k = 3$, $j = 24$, NS).

The co-occurrence of social events with talking and vision was also studied (see Table 3.3). This analysis determined the frequency of sensory coordinated, or integrated, experiences available to infants. Compared with the magnitude of visual, auditory, and tactile stimulation, sensory coordinated experiences occurred infrequently. To help explain these low co-occurrences, the occurrence of talking and vision was analyzed according to each social event (see Table 3.4). This analysis sought to determine not the occurrence of sensory coordinated experiences in the total number of observations (as in the preceding analyses) but rather the occurrence of talking and vision, given the occurrence of a social event (i.e., conditional probabilities or percentages). For example, in 51.1% of the occurrences when NICU infants were given medical-nursing care, caregivers were talking. A trend that emerges is that the percentages of sensory coordinated experiences were relatively lower when infants were given medical-nursing care and being bottle fed than when they received social touching and rocking. Assuming that the latter two events are relatively more social than the former two events because they are not necessary for survival and are voluntarily initiated, it seems reasonable to

---

[3] The same significant findings were obtained when analyses were conducted by tests of differences between proportions (Hoel, 1976).

Table 3.3. Co-occurrence of social events.

Variable	Talking NICU	Talking NCCU	Vision NICU	Vision NCCU	Talking and vision NICU	Talking and vision NCCU
Medical-nursing care	7.9	1.8	8.0	2.3	3.8	1.3
Bottle feeding	1.1	2.8	1.2	7.0	0.6	2.6
Social touch	1.7	3.7	0.9	4.3	0.9	3.1
Rocking	0.1	1.1	0.1	2.1	0.1	0.9
Handling	9.6	7.2	9.6	11.7	4.8	5.5
Talking			7.1	5.4		

Statistical analyses were not conducted on these data because the percentages were very small. All data are presented as percentages of total observations.
[a]Reproduced by permission from Gottfried, A. W., et al. 1981. Physical and social environment of newborn infants in special care units. Science 214:674. Copyright 1981 by the AAAS.

Table 3.4. Conditional probabilities of social events.

Variable	Talking NICU	Talking NCCU	Vision NICU	Vision NCCU	Talking and vision NICU	Talking and vision NCCU
Medical-nursing care	51.1	48.1	51.9	59.3	24.4	33.3
Bottle-feeding	56.3	33.3	62.5	81.7	31.3	30.0
Social touching	93.3	63.4	53.3	73.2	53.3	53.7
Rocking	100.0	44.4	100.0	83.3	100.0	33.3
Handling	53.6	47.2	53.6	76.9	27.2	36.1
Talking			54.5	67.9		

Statistical analyses were not conducted on these data because they are based on the small co-occurrence percentages. All data are presented in percentages.

assert that the more social the contact the greater the sensory coordinated experience.

Summary The results of this study indicated that infants in NICUs and NCCUs are exposed to a variety of stimuli. The data pertaining to physical types of stimulation showed that infants in these units were not sensorily deprived but received a considerable amount of ongoing stimulation. With respect to social contact, the data suggested that infants received a negligible amount of social experiences throughout the course of their hospitalization. Furthermore, there were a minimum of coordinated social sensory experiences and a lack of rhythmicity in physical and social stimulation.

Because the present study involved a time-sampling analysis, the actual amount and frequency of social stimulation received by individual infants in a given day is not known. Time-sampling analysis permits only a global description of the occurrences of social contacts; it does not provide information as to what absolutely and continuously occurs for the infants. Hence, definitive conclusions concerning the social stimulation available to infants in NICUs and NCCUs cannot be advanced. A second study was conducted to provide a thorough diurnal analysis of the quantity and quality of social events received in a typical day by infants in NICUs and NCCUs.

Study II—Contacts between Caregivers and Infants: A Diurnal Microanalysis (Investigators: Allen W. Gottfried, Kathleen W. Brown, April M. Kazarian, Richard S. Hagene, and Joan E. Hodgman)

This investigation focused on the nature of social stimulation available in a typical day to individual infants in NICUs and NCCUs by determining frequencies, duration, regularities, sequences, contingencies, and organization of caregiver-infant contacts during 24-hour continuous recordings. The following questions were addressed in this research:

1. What are the average frequencies of contact, hours of contact, duration of individual contacts, and intervals between contact for infants in the NICU and NCCU?
2. Are there differences in the amount and type of contacts received by infants in these units?
3. Are there gender differences in the contacts that infants receive, and do male and female staff differ in the social contacts they provide?
4. Is there systematic variability across work shifts in the amount and type of contacts?
5. Is there diurnal regularity across days in the hourly frequency and amount of contact with infants?

6. In a sequential analysis, does talking to infants at the onset of contacts predict talking to infants subsequently during contacts?
7. What are the contingency responses of caregivers when infants cry during contact? Does talking at onset of contacts also predict whether caregivers respond to infants' cries during contacts and, if so, what is the type of response?
8. To what extent are social sensory experiences organized or coordinated during contacts?
9. Is there a relationship between acute medical status and the frequency of medical-nursing and social contacts?
10. Based on the answers to the above questions, what statements seem reasonable to put forth about the social environment of infants in NICUs and NCCUs?

Method Two nonconsecutive (Thursday and Saturday within the same week), 24-hour continuous recordings (beginning 7 AM) were conducted in the NICU and NCCU. Infants observed were randomly selected from a group considered by the Director of Newborn Services (Joan E. Hodgman) to be typical of premature infants in these units. A total of nine infants were observed (five males, four females; three blacks, four Hispanics, two whites). However, an equal number (eight) were observed on each day and in each unit (four per unit). One infant was discharged from the NICU; one was transferred from the NICU to the NCCU; and one was added to the NICU to equalize the observational schedule across days and units. Six of the nine infants were in the same unit across the 2 days of observation. All infants were of low birth weight (mean = 1427 grams; range = 810–2190) and preterm (mean = 30 weeks gestational age; range = 25–34). Their 1- and 5-minute Apgar scores were: 1, 6; 9, 10; 6, 8; 8, 10; 3, 7; 1, 6; 3, 6; 5, 9; and 9, 9. Their medical status typically included conditions such as respiratory distress syndrome, hyperbilirubinemia, intracranial hemorrhage, and patent ductus arteriosus. The infants' average chronological and conceptional ages were 22 days (range = 1–74) and 33 weeks (range = 30–37), respectively. Staff-infant ratios for the infants in the NICU and NCCU were 1:2 and 1:5, respectively.

To obtain detailed recordings of contacts, each of eight trained observers attended to only two infants. Each contact was recorded on a checklist containing predefined situational and person variables. The situational variables included the time contact occurred, the duration of the contact (in seconds), the unit in which the contact occurred, and whether the contact occurred with the infant in or out of the incubator. The person set of variables included whether: 1) the infant was handled and, if so, the type of handling (i.e., medical-nursing, bottle or gavage feeding, social touching, or rocking); 2) medical-nursing contact occurred that did not require handling the infant (e.g., adjusting equipment or tubes); 3) the infant was talked to at onset of (within five 5 seconds) and/or subsequently during contact; 4) the caregiver responded (by talking and/or social touching) if the infant cried during contact; 5) the infant was in a position to see the caregiver (and whether his or her eyes were open or closed); and 6) the caregiver was staff (male or female) or family (male or female).[4] Interobserver reliability exceeded 93% on all variables.

Results The data base was comprised of 384 hours of infant observations, which resulted in 47.9 hours of contact (combined across units and days). There was a total of 891 contacts (NICU = 556, NCCU = 335), of which 97% were accounted for by staff exclusively. Of contacts involving staff, there was a greater percentage with female (89.2%) than male staff (10.8%). One percent of the contacts included both staff and family, and 2% of the contacts involved family members only. Six of the nine infants had contact with family. Of a total of 19 family contacts, one mother accounted for 11 contacts. Because of the small numbers involving family, analyses of contacts with family members were not conducted. There was a significant reduction of 15% (in each unit) in the number of contacts on Saturday compared to Thursday. As reported above, there was no difference across the weekend day and weekdays in the initial study. The reason for the reduction in this second study is not known. There was no change in the number of staff except for supervisory staff. Although there was a reduction in the number of contacts, the distribution of the different types of contacts remained unchanged across days. Hence, the data presented are combined across days.

Frequency Analyses of Daily Contacts The data were reduced to provide information on the contacts an infant received daily in the NICU and NCCU. These data are presented for the major variables in Table 3.5. On the average, the frequency of contacts for infants in the NICU was approximately two-thirds greater than the frequency of contacts for infants in the NCCU. However, the average duration of contacts for infants in the NCCU was slightly more than twice as long as the duration of contacts for infants in the NICU. A three-way ANOVA (2 units × 2 days × 3 shifts) was conducted separately for frequency and duration of contacts. There were significant main effects for units (for frequency, $F_{(1,84)} = 35.42$, $p < .001$; for duration, $F_{(1,885)} = 32.98$, $p < .001$) and days (for frequency, $F_{(1,84)} = 6.01, p < .05$; for duration, NS). There were

---

[4] In contrast to the initial study, in this study we delineated medical-nursing contacts by those requiring and not requiring handling, recorded talking only to infants, and included gavage feeding in our observations of feeding.

Table 3.5. Average frequency of daily contacts.

	NICU Mean	NICU Range		NCCU Mean	NCCU Range
Total contacts	69.5	29–106	**	41.9	29–55
Average duration of contact (minutes)	2.2	0.02–42.1	**	4.8	0.02–103.5
Average interval between contacts (minutes)	18.3	0.03–238.1	**	29.7	0.02–272.0
Hours of contact[a]	2.5	1.9–3.4		3.3	1.5–3.8
Medical-nursing contacts	68.1	5–78	**	36.8	0–44
Handling	53.0	22–78	**	33.9	24–44
No handling	15.1	5–30	**	2.9	0–5
Social contacts					
Talking at onset of contact	10.3	2–21		8.8	5–10
Talking during contact	17.1	8–29		16.3	11–32
Social touching	5.9	1–10	*	11.5	1–30
Rocking	0.4	0–1	**	4.4	0–12
Handling	57.1	22–82	**	39.7	27–51

Data on the occurrence of feeding are not included because babies were fed on an individually prescribed schedule; feeding schedules ranged from 2 to 3 hours.

*$p < .01$.
**$p < .001$.

[a] A statistical analysis was not conducted on hours because of the very small degrees of freedom.

no significant main effects for shift nor any significant interactions. Infants in the NICU received significantly more contacts compared to infants in the NCCU, but their contacts were significantly shorter. The nonsignificant effects involving shift indicated that the average frequency and duration of contacts with infants did not differ from shift to shift. Hence, there was a lack of systematic variability across days on these variables for the three work time-blocks (i.e., 7 AM until 3 PM, 3 PM until 11 PM, and 11 PM until 7 AM).

Additional evidence showed a lack of diurnal regularity across the two days for frequency and duration of contacts based on an hourly analysis. Frequency and duration of contacts for each hour by day were aggregated across infants in the same unit. Pearson product moment correlations were conducted on corresponding hours across days for each unit. For frequency of contact, the correlations were .08 and .24 for the NICU and NCCU, respectively. For duration of contact, the correlations were .01 and .06 for the NICU and NCCU, respectively. All correlations were nonsignificant.

An analysis of the average interval between contacts showed that the interval was significantly shorter for infants in the NICU than for infants in the NCCU ($t_{875} = 4.53, p < .001$). As a consequence of the differing temporal structure of contacts in the NICU and the NCCU, infants in the NCCU (in contrast to infants in the NICU) received a greater duration of time per day in contact with caregivers. However, for infants in both units, there was no rhythmicity or pattern to the contacts.

Contacts were divided into two major rubrics: medical-nursing and social. Within each category, there were further delineations. Medical-nursing contacts included the mutually exclusive subdivisions of medical-nursing care that required handling of infants and medical-nursing care that did not necessitate handling of infants. The results of the three-way ANOVAs on these data yielded significant main effects for unit (medical-nursing, $F_{(1,84)} = 49.35, p < .001$; medical-nursing—handling, $F_{(1,84)} = 23.72, p < .001$; medical-nursing—no handling, $F_{(1,84)} = 30.75, p < .001$) and for day (medical-nursing, $F_{(1,84)} = 4.17, p < .05$; medical-nursing—handling, $F_{(1,84)} = 12.48, p < .001$; medical-nursing—no handling, $F_{(1,84)} = 4.62, p < .05$). There were no significant main effects for shift nor any significant interactions. As inferred in the definition of intensive care and as found in Study I, infants in the NICU received a greater frequency of medical-nursing contacts than did infants in the NCCU.

Social contacts comprised the non-mutually exclusive categories of talking at onset of contact, talking subsequently during contact, social touching, and rocking. Three-way ANOVAs on these data revealed no significant differences between the units for the talking variables (only a significant day main effect for talking during contact; $F_{(1,84)} = 11.04$, $p < .001$). However, there were significant unit main effects for social touching ($F_{(1,84)} = 7.52, p < .01$) and rocking ($F_{(1,84)} = 35.84, p < .001$). There was a significant day main effect only for social touching ($F_{(1,84)} = 9.66, p < .01$). There were no significant main effects for shift or interactions. Infants in the NCCU received significantly more social touching and rocking compared to infants in the NICU.

As previously noted, handling was a variable generated to provide an index of the occurrence of tactile contact or stimulation. Handling comprised one or more of the following variables: medical-nursing care requiring handling, feeding, social touching, and rocking. Infants in the NICU received significantly more handling than infants in the NCCU ($\chi_1^2 = 24.66, p < .001$).

Table 3.5 also shows the ranges for each contact variable. The range gives the daily limits (i.e., lowest to highest) of the occurrence or duration of contacts for the infants in each unit. Examination of these data revealed that the ranges of contacts in the NICU tended to be greater than the ranges in the NCCU and that the ranges of contacts across the two units overlapped (e.g., some infants in the NICU received more social touching than infants in the NCCU). The greater variability in contacts for infants in the NICU compared to infants in the NCCU was probably attributable to the greater variability in medical status for infants in the NICU. The medical condition of infants in the NCCU was probably more stable and, consequently, there was less variation in their care. The finding that the range or distribution of contacts overlapped between the units suggested that there were factors other than stability of medical status accounting for the various contacts (particularly social contacts). These factors may include family contact, attraction, attachment, detachment, and so on.

Proportion Analyses of Daily Contact Another important way of viewing and analyzing the data involves the use of percentages (i.e., proportions) of contacts. Converting the data to percentages provides direct information on the distribution of contacts and also corrects or takes into account differences in total number of contacts when comparing data across units or reference groups (e.g., gender). For example, infants in the NICU received significantly more handling per day than did infants in the NCCU. However, this is a function of infants in the NICU receiving a greater total number of contacts per se. When the percentages of handling were compared between units (total contacts in each unit served as denominators in computing percentages), infants in the NCCU received proportionately a significantly greater amount of handling compared to infants in the NICU. Hence, despite the fact that NICU infants received a greater absolute frequency of handling than did NCCU infants, the latter compared to the former group received a relatively greater amount of handling (see Table 3.5). This was due to infants in the NCCU receiving relatively less medical-nursing care not requiring handling and receiving relatively more social contacts than infants in the NICU.

Once the actual or absolute amount of daily contacts infants received in each of the units was known, percentages and statistical comparisons between percentages (Hoel, 1976) could be presented. The percentages for the major variables are shown in Table 3.6. Contacts in both units predominately involved medical-nursing care. In fact, virtually all of the contacts were for this purpose. There was a significantly greater percentage of medical-nursing contacts in the NICU than in the NCCU. This was accounted for not by the percentage of medical-nursing care requiring handling but by the significantly greater percentage of medical-nursing care not requiring handling in the NICU. As anticipated, all medical-nursing contacts occurred with infants in incubators.

The environment of infants in the NCCU was more social compared to infants in the NICU. There was significantly more social touching and rocking of infants (both in absolute and relative frequencies) and a relatively higher frequency of talking during contacts in the NCCU than in

Table 3.6. Percentages of daily contacts.

	NICU		NCCU
Total medical-nursing contacts	98.0	*	87.8
Medical-nursing (handling)	76.3		80.9
Medical-nursing (no handling)	21.7	**	6.9
Social contacts			
Talking at onset of contact	14.7		20.8
Talking during contact	24.6	**	38.8
Social touching	8.5	**	27.5
Rocking	0.5	**	10.4
Handling	80.8	**	93.1

All data are presented in percentages.
*$p < .01$.
**$p < .001$.

the NICU. Although the social climate for infants was greater in the NCCU than in the NICU, social contacts (regardless of type) occurred infrequently in either unit. Social activities were exhibited in no more than approximately one-fourth of the total contacts in the NICU and around one-third of the total contacts in the NCCU. The large majority of contacts with infants in both units were devoid of social events. The location of social contacts differed significantly between the units (all comparisons, $p < .05$). In the NICU, 94.6% of the social contacts occurred in the incubator, 2.7% occurred out of the incubator, and 2.7% involved a change from one location to the other. The comparable percentages for the NCCU were: 74.4% of contacts occurred in the incubator, 8.3% occurred out of the incubator, and 17.3% involved a change in location. In both units, the preponderance of social contacts was restricted to infants situated in the incubator.

Further analyses of social activities involved caregivers' talking to infants and responses to infants' cries during contacts. Analyses were conducted on sequential and contingency probabilities of these data (units combined). The occurrence or base rate of caregivers' talking subsequently during contacts with infants (as noted previously, subsequent to 5-second onset) was 30.9%. If caregivers did not talk to infants at the onset, the probability that talking occurred subsequently during contact was 15.0%. However, if at the onset caregivers did talk to infants, the probability was significantly ($p < .001$) and substantially increased to

Table 3.7. Caregiver responses to infants' cries during contact.

	Percentages of responses		
No response to cries	58.1		
Respond by talking	29.2		
Respond by social touching	5.5		
Respond by talking and social touching	7.2		
	Talk at onset		No talk at onset
No response to cries	9.8	***	76.7
Respond by talking	62.7	***	16.8
Respond by social touch	11.8	*	2.9
Respond by talking and social touching	15.7	**	3.6

All data are presented as percentages.
$*p < .05.$
$**p < .01.$
$***p < .001.$

88.7% that talking occurred subsequently. Hence, whether caregivers emitted a verbal greeting to infants at the initial phase of a contact served as a powerful predictor of whether infants were directly exposed to language stimulation by caregivers subsequently during contact.

The average daily frequency of contacts in which infants cried was 11.8 (range = 2–27; in NICU, mean = 15.3, range = 2–27; in NCCU, mean = 8.3, range = 2–12). This represented 21.2% of the contacts across units. The caregivers' responses to infants' cries during contact are presented in Table 3.7. The data showed that more than one-half of the time when infants cried caregivers did not attempt to soothe them. When caregivers did attempt to soothe infants, it was done primarily by talking to the infant and seldom by social touching or by both modalities. Further analyses revealed that talking or not talking at the onset of contacts was related to caregivers' responses to infants' cries. If caregivers talked at the onset, and if infants cried, the probability of no response to the infants' cries was significantly lower and the probability of soothing responses by all modalities was significantly greater. These data imply that the sociability of caregivers toward infants at the onset of contacts seemed to be an important moderator variable in providing language stimulation to infants and in responding to infants' distress.

On all variables, there were no gender differences between infants in the amount or type of contacts. However, male and female staff differed significantly in the occurrence of social contacts displayed toward infants (Table 3.8). As shown, females exhibited a higher percentage of social responses across these variables. It is not apparent why male professionals were consistently less socially responsive toward the infants.

Table 3.8. Gender differences between staff in social contacts with infants.

	Male staff		Female staff
Talking at onset of contact	7.6	*	16.9
Talking during contact	12.0	***	29.8
Social touching	4.3	*	13.8
Rocking	0.0		3.9
Social response to cries (talking, social touching, or both)	12.5	**	43.9

All data are presented as percentages.
*$p < .05$.
**$p < .01$.
***$p < .001$.

Whether it was attributable to socialized characteristics of "maleness" or whether most males in the units were physicians and therefore did not consider it their responsibility to interact socially with infants cannot be determined in this study. A study assessing and analyzing differences in staff status (and having a larger number of male and female family members to compare) could resolve this provocative finding.

To determine the extent to which sensory experiences received by infants were organized or coordinated during contacts, the co-occurrence of each type of contact with talking and vision (i.e., whether the infant was in a position to see the caregiver) was calculated separately for each unit. These data are displayed in Table 3.9. The data are presented in percentages, which were computed by dividing the frequency of the co-occurring events by the total number of contacts in that unit. The overall results showed that the percentages of sensory coordinated experiences were not impressively high. The best way of viewing these data is by examining the co-occurrence of handling (a generated index variable) with talking, vision, and these last two variables combined. Except for one isolated situation (handling and vision in the NCCU), the percentages of these sensory coordinated experiences tended not to exceed around one-third of the contacts. Although virtually all of the percentages in the NCCU were significantly greater than in the NICU, most of the contacts in both units did not include sensory coordinated experiences.

As noted, whether infants' eyes were open or closed when infants were in a bodily position to view the caretaker was recorded. Thus, the co-occurrence of each event with the infants' eyes being open could be ascertained. These percentages are also presented in Table 3.9. Again, the percentages in the NCCU were in almost all situations significantly greater than in the NICU. Infants in the NCCU had their eyes open significantly more often during contacts than did infants in the NICU.

Table 3.9. Co-occurrence of events.

	Talking			Vision			Talking and vision			Eyes open		
	NICU		NCCU	NICU		NCCU	NICU		NCCU	NICU		NCCU
Medical-nursing (handling)	20.7		31.3	35.2	***	73.7	11.2	**	29.8	19.0	**	43.2
Medical-nursing (no handling)	1.4		1.4	8.0		5.7	1.1		1.4	3.4		2.4
Feeding (gavage and bottle)	4.3	*	15.0	5.6	**	24.1	3.9	*	15.0	3.6	*	17.9
Social touching	7.2	**	20.3	5.8	**	25.3	5.2	**	19.6	3.4	**	19.6
Rocking	0.3	*	9.8	0.3	**	10.5	0.3	*	9.8	0.1	*	8.6
Talking				14.1	**	38.2				9.5	*	26.7
Handling	23.7		38.2	38.0	***	85.4	13.5	**	36.8	20.3	***	51.2

All data are presented as percentages.
*$p < .05$.
**$p < .01$.
***$p < .001$.

However, in no more than approximately one-half of the situations in which infants were in a position to see the caregivers during contact did they have their eyes open. Hence, the low occurrence of sensory coordinated experiences received by infants is a function of not only the unit the infant is in and the type of contact (including the sociability of caregiver) but also the state (sleep/awake) of infants when contacts occur.

The conditional probabilities (i.e., percentages) of talking, vision, and eyes open by each contact are presented in Table 3.10. The percentages were computed by dividing the frequency of the co-occurring events by the frequency of the particular contact event. It is important to note that a different denominator was used in each computation, in contrast to the constant denominator (total number of contacts) used in determining the percentages of co-occurring events in Table 3.9. There are three major findings in these data:

1. The probabilities in the NCCU tended to be higher (usually significantly) than those in the NICU. The probability is greater that talking, vision, and eyes open will occur given a contact in the NCCU than is the case given the same contact in the NICU. Hence, the course of hospitalization for infants in special care units seems to correspond with greater increases and probabilities of receiving organized or integrated sensory experiences. However, as noted previously, the occurrence of sensory coordinated experiences was not high.
2. There was considerable variation in the magnitude of the probabilities. The variability depended on the type of contact.
3. As found in Study 1, there was a trend for the probabilities of social touching and rocking to be higher than medical-nursing contacts and feeding.

Another conditional probability analysis of interest was the occurrence of social touching, talking, and rocking during a contact when the infant was bottle or gavage fed. This analysis was limited to data from the NCCU because the infants in the NICU were primarily gavage fed. These data are in shown in Table 3.11. The data show that bottle feeding, compared to gavage feeding, did elicit a higher frequency of social activities (not necessarily simultaneously) toward infants during the contact. The lower percentage of rocking during contact when the infants were gavage fed was probably because these infants were less well than bottle-fed infants. However, it is unlikely that this factor accounted for the lower percentages of social touching and talking. Hence, bottle feeding facilitates the origins of social eating compared to gavage feeding.

Table 3.10. Conditional probability of events.

	Talking			Vision			Talking and vision			Eyes opened		
	NICU		NCCU	NICU		NCCU	NICU		NCCU	NICU		NCCU
Medical-nursing (handling)	27.1	**	38.7	46.2	***	91.1	14.6	***	36.9	25.0	***	53.5
Medical-nursing (no handling)	6.6	*	21.7	37.2	***	82.6	4.9		21.7	15.7	*	34.8
Feeding (gavage and bottle)	58.8		60.4	76.5	**	100.0	52.9		62.4	49.0		74.2
Social touching	85.1		73.9	67.8	***	92.1	61.0		71.3	25.2	***	54.8
Rocking	66.7		94.3	66.7	***	100.0	66.7		94.3	33.3	*	82.8
Talking				56.9	***	96.2				38.7	**	69.2
Handling	29.4	***	41.0	47.0	***	91.7	16.7	***	39.4	25.2	***	54.8

All data are presented as percentages.
*$p < .05$.
**$p < .01$.
***$p < .001$.

Table 3.11. Caregiver responses during feeding.

	NCCU		
	Bottle		Gavage
Social touching	43.2		29.7
Talking	79.5	***	40.5
Rocking	54.5	***	10.8

All data are presented as percentages.
***$p < .001$.

The last analysis concerned the relationship between acute medical status and the frequency of medical-nursing and social contacts. The medical status of the infants was evaluated and ranked by the chief physicians on service. Inter-ranking agreement was 90%. This ranking was correlated with the total frequency of medical-nursing and social contacts in each unit separately (the sample size on which these correlations are based is very small). A correlation of .9 emerged with frequency of medical-nursing contacts in the NICU. As expected, infants who were more ill received more medical-nursing contacts. In the NCCU, the correlation between these variables was .0, indicating that the frequency of medical-nursing contacts was unrelated to the medical status of infants. This was probably because infants were more stable in the NCCU and received more routine types of medical-nursing care. Also, there was less variability in contacts (mentioned previously) in the NCCU compared to the NICU. The correlations between acute medical status and social contacts revealed no reliable pattern, suggesting again that social factors, such as family contact, attachment, and/or attractiveness of infants, may play a significant role in the occurrence of social contacts.

Summary This study showed that infants in NICUs and NCCUs receive a considerable amount of contact with persons, both in daily frequency and duration. Contacts predominantly involved medical-nursing care, with social events occurring infrequently. The occurrence of the various types of contacts and their temporal structure differed between the units. In the NICU, there was a greater frequency of medical-nursing care, and in the NCCU, there was a relatively higher occurrence of social events. There were no differences among the work shifts in the amount or frequency of contacts and no hourly or work shift regularities across days in the contacts infants received in either unit. How caregivers verbally greeted infants predicted the occurrence of language stimulation and caregivers' responses to infants' cries during contacts. In most instances, caregivers did not respond to infants' cries. Although social sensory integrated experiences occurred more often in the NCCU than in the NICU, the rate of occurrence was not impressively high in either unit. The co-occurrence of sensory experiences varied according to the type of contact, with the probability of integrated experiences tending to be greater for social touching and rocking than for medical-nursing care and feeding. Bottle feeding elicited more social experiences for the infant than did gavage feeding. Ratings of acute medical status correlated with frequency of medical-nursing care in the NICU but not in the NCCU. The relationships between these ratings and frequency of social contacts bore no systematic pattern in either unit. The overall findings suggested that the occurrence, regularity, quality, and organization of social contacts in special care units are not impressively high.

Discussion

The data from these studies indicate that conceptualizations about the environment of special care units need refinement. Global descriptions or hypotheses that suggest that infants in special care units are sensorily deprived are not accurate. Infants were exposed to many kinds of stimulation (including light, sound, tactile, vestibular-kinesthetic, and social) that varied considerably from one unit to the next. The evidence strongly suggests that conceptualizations of newborn special care unit environments must be variable specific (also see Gottfried, 1984; Wachs and Gruen, 1982). Furthermore, there were significant differences in environmental stimulation betwen NICUs and NCCUs. Differences between units were found in: 1) noise level; 2) the frequency and type of contacts; 3) the way in which various contacts were proportioned; and 4) the temporal characteristics of contacts. Infants in both units were exposed to constant light, high sound levels, numerous brief handling contacts. There were relatively low frequencies of social stimulation and integrated social sensory experiences, minimal direct verbal stimulation, and a lack of diurnal rhythmicity across days in physical and social stimulation. The data also revealed vast individual differences in medical-nursing and social contact experiences received by infants. These findings can be integrated in a comprehensive model of special care unit environments.

To obtain a precise understanding of the environment of special care units and the impact of environmental stimulation on premature infants, each type of stimulation must be considered and evaluated individually. With respect to visual stimulation, infants were exposed continuously to cool-white fluorescent lighting. Illumination varied minimally and was monotonous throughout the day. The rationale for constant lighting is that it allows immediate and ongoing visibility of infants. Although it is not known whether continuous cool-white fluorescent lighting has negative consequences on premature infants, there is a considerable body of evidence with infrahumans (as well as with children and adults) indicating that such lighting conditions have adverse biochemical and physiologic effects. There are experimental studies showing that prolonged exposure to cool-white fluorescent lighting may lead to alternations in endocrine functions, increased incidence of hypocalcemia, cell transformations, immature gonad development, and chromosome breakage (Gantt, 1979; Hakanson and Bergstrom, 1981; Kennedy et al., 1980; Mayron and Kaplan, 1976; Wurtman, 1975; Wurtman and Weisel, 1969). Furthermore, there is evidence suggesting a synergistic effect of the vibratory phenomena of light and sound on newborn animals (e.g., Wallace-Lande et al., 1981). Because there is no convincing rationale for premature infants to be continuously exposed to cool-white fluorescent light and because there is evidence indicating possible harmful effects, modification of such lighting conditions in NICUs and NCCUs units is warranted.

A decade has passed since the American Academy of Pediatrics expressed a formal concern about noise pollution in newborn special care units. However, noise levels continue to be intense and aversive (at least to personnel). High noise levels have been documented in units worldwide (Bess et al., 1979; Blennow et al., 1974; Gaiter et al., 1981; Lawson et al., 1977; Newman, 1981; Perlstein, 1983). In this study there were several hours per day when noise levels were unduly high and potentially hazardous. Infants were exposed incessantly to nonspeech or mechanical sounds and much of the day to speech sounds. Infants in incubators were not protected from the noise. On the contrary, infants in incubators were exposed to slightly higher noise levels and unclear speech sounds. Infants received no periods of relief from this noisy atmosphere. Epidemiologic data and continuing reports associate prematurity with hearing impairment; studies indicate a relationship between intensive noise levels and extraauditory effects in young infants and children (Cohen and Weinstein, 1981; Douek et al., 1976; Drillien, 1961; Falk and Farmer, 1973; Falk and Woods, 1973; Long et al., 1980a; Mills, 1975). Environmental interventions aimed at abating noise in special care units need to be conducted for the sake of infants and personnel.

In Studies I and II, the absolute frequency of handling infants was greater in the NICU than in the NCCU (statistically greater in Study II). However, the proportion of contacts involving handling to total number of contacts was significantly higher for infants in the NCCU than for infants in the NICU in both studies. Across both investigations, contacts including handling ranged from 81% to 85% in the NICU and 93% to 94% in the NCCU. The data reliably showed that in both units almost all contacts included handling of infants. Handling was task oriented, that is, for the purpose of medical-nursing care. The typical infant in the NICU and NCCU was handled on an average of 57 and 40 times per day, respectively. Some infants received as many as 82 and 51 handling contacts daily in the NICU and NCCU, respectively.

Normative data do not exist that specify how much tactile stimulation is appropriate for newborns to receive. These data show that premature infants in special care units are not deprived of this type of stimulation. In fact, infants in the NICU may be overstimulated. Research has shown that routine handling of sick newborns by nursery personnel may cause hypoxemia in these infants (Long et al., 1980b; Speidel, 1978). The mechanism accounting for this adverse consequence of handling has not been determined. Speidel (1978) hypothesized that crying, whether induced or spontaneous, causes arterial pO_2 to fall. Because crying is a common reaction of sick newborns to handling, it may be the mediating mechanism between handling and the reduction in arterial pO_2. Evidence also suggests that numerous tactile contacts of infants throughout the day may disturb their rest and normal sleep patterns (Korones, 1976). Although REM or nonREM sleep was not recorded in the present research, Study II showed that when infants were handled their eyes were closed in approximately 75% and 50% of the contacts in the NICU and NCCU, respectively. The implication of these findings is that any handling may be deleterious, and unnecessary handling should be avoided when infants are in the NICU. Furthermore, these findings emphasize the necessity of transcutaneous oxygen monitoring (Long et al., 1980b) and the use of soothing techniques (such as talking and social touching), which were seldom observed in this research, when infants cry during handling.

Although handling of infants in the NICU may have harmful effects, handling or rocking of NCCU infants whose condition is healthy may have positive outcomes. In view of the clinical findings, not rocking infants in the NICU is understandable and recommended. However, the lack of rocking of infants in the NCCU is surprising. A number of experiments show that vestibular-kinesthetic types of stimulation enhance development in young premature infants (see Gottfried, 1981). Thus, when the condition of infants is stable, handling and rocking may prove to be advantageous.

In contrast to the high magnitudes of visual, auditory, and tactile stimulation that infants were exposed to in special care units, infants received infrequent social experiences. Infants did not lack, either in frequency or duration, contact with persons. On the average, infants in the NICU received 70 contacts per day, with one infant receiving as much as 106 contacts, and infants in the NCCU received 42 contacts per day, with an upper range of 55. Contacts were equally distributed across the work shifts (Korones, 1976). Contacts typically occurred two to three times per hour, were brief (each usually lasting 2 to 5 minutes), and totaled a duration of 2 to 3 hours daily.

Although persons were constantly in contact with infants throughout the 24 hours, the preponderance of contacts between caregivers and infants may be appropriately described as nonsocial. Many infants in NICUs and NCCUs may indeed be sensorily deprived with respect to social stimulation. Several aspects of the data support this contention. First, most contacts involved medical-nursing care and seldom included social activities. Approaching an infant for the sole purpose of providing social stimulation was a rare event. If social stimulation was provided, it was included in routine care. The occurrence of talking to infants at the onset or subsequently during contacts, socially touching infants, or rocking infants was minimal. Social behaviors have been found to have developmental significance. The impact and importance of speech in eliciting newborns' vocal exchanges and social behaviors have been demonstrated (see Rheingold and Adams, 1980; Rosenthal, 1982). Social touching of infants (by parents) can be a particularly important behavior in the formation of attachment (Klaus and Kennell, 1983). Rocking or vestibular-kinesthetic stimulation not only can accelerate certain types of development (e.g., motor skills and muscle tone) but is very effective in soothing or consoling crying infants (see, e.g., Byrne and Horowitz, 1981). These social activities occurred infrequently, and with no diurnal regularity to their occurrence.

Second, in addition to the low frequency of the preceding social activities, caregivers often neglected to attempt to soothe crying infants during contact. This finding is interesting in view of the hypothesis of Speidel (1978) that crying may be the mediating factor in hypoxemia. The lack of responsiveness to infants' cries may also serve to delay the development of contingencies between infants' behavior and social environmental reactions.

Third, the co-occurrence or integration of social sensory experiences for infants was infrequent. It was common for infants to be handled and not talked to, or positioned in a way so as not to have the opportunity to see the caregiver. The infrequency of coordinated sensory experiences received by premature infants was not entirely a function of the caregiving environment. Quite often when infants were in a position to see the caregiver, their eyes were closed. These experiences occurred independent of the infants' state. The effect of these dissociated sensory experiences is unknown; however, this finding is significant in view of evidence showing a deficit in the ability of premature infants up to 1 year of age to integrate tactile-visual sensory information (Gottfried et al., 1977; Rose et al., 1978). Whether there is a delay or deficit in audiovisual integration in premature infants remains to be determined.

Fourth, although family were welcomed and encouraged to visit their infants in the special care units, family members accounted for a negligible portion of the contacts in both studies. The reason for their lack of contact is not clear (see Jones, 1982). Mothers have been found to provide an important source of stimulation to their infants compared to nursery personnel (Marton et al., 1981; Minde et al., 1975, 1978) and usually serve as the primary caregiver when infants are discharged from the hospital. Studies have shown that: 1) normal patterns of interaction are difficult to establish in premature infants (Goldberg, 1979); 2) nurses are accurate predictors of subsequent parent-infant interactions (Allen et al., 1982); and 3) the social home environment of prematurely born children is the most powerful determinant of their developmental outcome (Beckwith and Cohen, 1984). In view of these findings, the extent to which the social activities of staff with infants in special care units inadvertently encourage or discourage family members from visiting their infants and the extent to which staff serve as models for interacting with premature infants are important issues that should be given serious attention.

As knowledge about the physical and social environments of infants in special care units grows rapidly, the impact of specific types of stimulation on neurophysiologic and behavioral organization, medical and developmental status, and social interactions of premature infants needs to be established. On the one hand, there is the view that the progression of neurophysiologic and behavioral organization is genetically regulated and that the immaturity of the central nervous system of the premature infant protects it from aberrant environmental conditions (Parmelee, 1975, 1981; also see Schulte et al., 1977). However, there is emerging evidence that infants' behavior and organization of behavioral states may be related to environmental factors in special care units (see Chapters 6 and 8, this volume; also see Holmes et al., 1982). Furthermore, the environment of and certain types of medical treatment in special care units may have adverse consequences on the medical status of premature infants (see Chapter 10, this volume). However, definitive conclusions concerning the relationship between the environment of special care units and the development of premature infants cannot as yet be put forth.

Solutions will require carefully designed intervention studies in which environmental information serves as the foundation for the experimental manipulations.

Acknowledgments

The author thanks Dr. A. Parmelee, Jr., for reviewing the manuscript.

References

Allen, D. A., McGrade, B. J., Affleck, G., and McQueeney, M. 1982. The predictive validity of neonatal intensive care nurses' judgments of parent-child relationships: A nine-month follow-up. J. Pediatr. Psychol. 7:125–133.
American Academy of Pediatrics, Committee on Environmental Hazards. 1974. Noise pollution: Neonatal aspects. Pediatrics 54:476–479.
Barnard, K. 1973. A program of stimulation for infants born prematurely. Paper presented at the meeting of the Society for Research in Child Development, March, Philadelphia.
Beckwith, L., and Cohen, S. E. 1984. Home environment and cognitive competence in preterm children in the first five years. In: A. W. Gottfried (ed.), Home Environment and Early Cognitive Development: Longitudinal Research, pp. 235–271. Academic Press, New York.
Bess, F. H., Peek, B. F., and Chapman, J. J. 1979. Further observations on noise levels in infant incubators. Pediatrics 63:100–106.
Blennow, G., Svenningsen, N. W., and Almquist, B. 1974. Noise levels in infant incubators (Adverse effects?). Pediatrics 53:29–32.
Broman, S. H., Nichols, P. L., and Kennedy, W. A. 1975. Preschool IQ: Prenatal and early developmental correlates. Erlbaum, Hillsdale, NJ.
Budetti, P., Barrand, N., McManus, P., and Heinen, L. A. 1981. The Implications of Cost-Effectiveness Analysis of Medical Technology: The Costs and Effectiveness of Neonatal Intensive Care. Office of Technological Assessment, Washington, DC.
Byrne, J. M., and Horowitz, F. D. 1981. Rocking as a soothing intervention: The influence of direction and type of movement. Infant Behav. Dev. 4:207–218.
Cohen, S., and Weinstein, N. 1981. Nonauditory effects of noise on behavior and health. J. Soc. Issues 37:36–70.
Cornell, E. H., and Gottfried, A. W. 1976. Intervention with premature human infants. Child Dev. 47:32–39.
Donahue, C. L. 1981. A review of planning methods and criteria for neonatal intensive care units. Report HRA 231-77-0108. Department of Health and Human Services, Hyattsville, MD.
Douek, E., Bannister, L. H., Dodson, H. C., Ashcroft, P., and Humphries, K. N. 1976. Effects of incubator noise on the cochlea of the newborn. Lancet 2:1110–1113.
Drillien, C. M. 1961. The incidence of mental and physical handicaps in school-age children of very low birth weight. Pediatrics 27:452–464.
Falk, S. A., and Farmer, J. C. 1973. Incubator noise and possible deafness. Arch. Otolaryngol. 97:385–387.

Falk, S. A., and Woods, N. F. 1973. Hospital noise-levels and potential health hazards. N. Engl. J. Med. 289:774–780.

Field, T. (ed.). 1979. Infants Born at Risk. Spectrum, New York.

Freedman, D. G., Boverman, H., and Freedman, N. 1966. Effects of kinesthetic stimulation on weight gain and smiling in premature infants. Paper presented at the Annual Meeting of the American Orthopsychiatric Association, April, San Francisco.

Friedman, S., and Sigman, M. (eds.). 1980. Preterm Birth and Psychological Development. Academic Press, New York.

Gaiter, J. L., Avery, G. B., Temple, C. J., Johnson, A. A. S., and White, N. B. 1981. Stimulation characteristics of nursery environments for critically ill preterm infants and infant behavior. In: L. Stern (ed.), Intensive Care in the Newborn. Masson Publishing, New York.

Gantt, R. 1979. Fluorescent light-induced DNA cross linkage and chromatid breaks in mouse cells in culture. Proc. Natl. Acad. Sci. 75:3809–3812.

Goldberg, S. 1979. Premature birth: Consequences for parent-infant relationship. Am. Sci. 67:214–220.

Gottfried, A. W. 1981. Environmental manipulations in the neonatal period and assessment of their effects. In: V. L. Smeriglio (ed.), Newborns and Parents, pp. 55–61. Erlbaum, Hillsdale, NJ.

Gottfried, A. W. (ed.). 1984. Home Environment and Early Cognitive Development: Longitudinal Research. Academic Press, New York.

Gottfried, A. W., Rose, S. A., and Bridger, W. H. 1977. Cross-modal transfer in human infants. Child Dev. 48:118–123.

Gottfried, A. W., Wallace-Lande, P., Sherman-Brown, S., King, J., Coen, C., and Hodgman, J. E. 1981. Physical and social environment of newborn infants in special care units. Science 214:673–675.

Gribbins, R. E., and Marshall, R. E. 1982. Stress and coping in the NICU staff nurse: Practical implications for change. Crit. Care Med. 10:865–867.

Hakanson, D. O., and Bergstrom, W. H. 1981. Phototherapy-induced hypocalcemia in newborn rats: Prevention by melatonin. Science 214:807–809.

Hoel, P. G., 1976. Elementary Statistics. John Wiley, New York.

Holmes, D. L., Magy, J. N., Slaymaker, F., Sosnowski, R. J., Prinz, S. M., and Pasternak, J. F. 1982. Early influences of prematurity, illness, and prolonged hospitalization on infant behavior. Dev. Psychol. 18:744–750.

Jones, C. L. 1982. Environmental analysis of neonatal intensive care. J. Nerv. Ment. Dis. 170:130–142.

Katz, V. 1971. Auditory stimulation and developmental behavior of the premature infant. Nurs. Res. 20:196–201.

Kennedy, A. R., Ritter, M. A., and Little, J. B. 1980. Fluorescent light induces malignant transformation in mouse embryo cell cultures. Science 207:1209–1211.

Kitchen, W. H., Rickards, A., Ryan, M. M., McDougall, A. B., Billson, F. A., Keir, E. H., and Naylor, F. D. 1979. A longitudinal study of very low-birthweight infants: II. Results of controlled trial of intensive care and incidence of handicaps. Dev. Med. Child Neurol. 21:582–589.

Klaus, M. H., and Kennell, J. H. 1983. Bonding: The Beginning of Parent-Infant Attachment. Mosby, St. Louis.

Korones, S. B. 1976. Disturbance and infants' rest. In: T. D. Moore (ed.), 69th Ross Conference on Pediatric Research: Iatrogenic Problems in Neonatal Intensive Care. Ross Laboratories, Columbus, OH.

Lawson, K., Daum, C., and Turkewitz, G. 1977. Environmental characteristics of

a neonatal intensive care unit. Child Dev. 48:1633–1639.
Leib, S. A., Benfield, G., and Guidubaldi, J. 1980. Effects of early intervention and stimulation on the preterm infant. Pediatrics 66:83–90.
Long, J. G., Lucey, J. F., and Philip, A. G. S. 1980a. Noise and hypoxemia in the intensive care nursery. Pediatrics 65:143–145.
Long, J. G., Philip, A. G. S., and Lucey, J. F. 1980b. Excessive handling as a cause of hypoxemia. Pediatrics 65:203–207.
Lucey, J. L. 1977. Is intensive care becoming too intensive? Pediatrics: Neonatol. Suppl. 59:1064–1065.
Marshall, R. E., Kasman, C., and Cape, L. S. 1982. Coping with Caring for Sick Newborns. Saunders, Philadelphia.
Marton, P., Minde, K., and Ogilvie, P. 1981. Mother-infant interactions in the premature nursery: A sequential analysis. In: S. L. Friedman and M. Sigman (eds.), Preterm Birth and Psychological Development. Academic Press, New York.
Mayron, L., and Kaplan, E. 1976. Bioeffects of fluorescent light. Acad. Ther. 12:75–90.
Mills, J. H. 1975. Noise and children: A review of literature. J. Acoust. Soc. Am. 58:767–779.
Minde, K., Ford, L., Celhoffer, L., and Boukydis, C. 1975. Interactions of mothers and nurses with premature infants. Can. Med. Assoc. J. 113:741–745.
Minde, K., Trehub, S., Corter, C., Boukydis, C., Celhoffer, L., and Marton, P. 1978. Mother-child relationships in the premature nursery: Observational study. Pediatrics 61:373–379.
Neal, M. V. 1968. Vestibular stimulation and developmental behavior of the small premature infant. Nurs. Res. Rep. 3:2–5.
Newman, L. F. 1981. Social and sensory environment of low birth weight infants in a special care nursery. J. Nerv. Ment. Dis. 169:448–455.
Parmelee, A. H., Jr., 1975. Neurophysiological and behavioral organization of premature infants in the first months of life. Biol. Psychiatry 10:501–512.
Parmelee, A. H., Jr., 1981. Auditory function and neurological maturation in preterm infants. In: S. L. Friedman and M. Sigman (eds.), Preterm Birth and Psychological Development. Academic Press, New York.
Perlstein, P. H. 1983. Physical environment. In: A. Fanaroff and R. Martin (eds.), Behrman's Neonatal-Perinatal Medicine, pp. 259–277. Mosby, St. Louis.
Peterson, A., and Gross, Jr., S. 1974. Handbook of Noise Measurement. General Radio, Concord, MA.
Powell, L. F. 1974. The effect of extra stimulation and maternal involvement on the development of low birth-weight infants and on maternal behavior. Child Dev. 45:106–113.
Rheingold, H. L., and Adams, J. L. 1980. The significance of speech to newborns. Dev. Psychol. 16:397–403.
Rice, R. D. 1977. Neurophysiological development in premature infants following stimulation. Dev. Psychol. 13:69–76.
Rose, S. A., Gottfried, A. W., and Bridger, W. H. 1978. Cross-modal transfer in infants: Relationship to prematurity and socioeconomic background. Dev. Psychol. 14:643–652.
Rosenthal, M. K. 1982. Vocal dialogues in the neonatal period. Dev. Psychol. 18:17–21.
Scarr-Salapatek, S., and Williams, M. L. 1973. The effects of early stimulation on low-birth-weight infants. Child Dev. 44:94–101.

Schulte, F. J., Stennert, E., Wulbrand, H., Eichhorn, W., and Lenard, H. G. 1977. The ontogeny of sensory perception in preterm infants. Eur. J. Pediatr. 126:211–224.

Segall, M. E. 1972. Cardiac responsivity to auditory stimulation in premature infants. Nurs. Res. 21:94–101.

Solkoff, N., Yaffe, S., Weintraub, D., and Blase, B. 1969. Effects of handling on the subsequent development of premature infants. Dev. Psychol. 1:765–768.

Speidel, B. D. 1978. Adverse effects of routine procedures on preterm infants. Lancet 1:864–865.

Wachs, T. D., and Gruen, G. E. 1982. Early Experience and Human Development. Plenum Press, New York.

Wallace-Lande, P., Sherman-Brown, S., Bagrash, F., and Gottfried, A. W. 1981. Vibratory environmental phenomena: Interactive influences on growth and behavior of mammalian neonates. Unpublished manuscript. California State University, Fullerton.

White, J. L., and LaBarbara, R. C. 1976. The effects of tactile and kinesthetic stimulation on neonatal development in the premature infant. Dev. Psychol. 9:569–577.

Wurtman, R. J. 1975. The effects of light on the human body. Sci. Am. 233:68–77.

Wurtman, R. J., and Weisel, J. 1969. Environmental lighting and neuroendocrine function: Relationship between spectrum of light source and gonadal growth. Endocrinology 85:1218–1221.

4

Nursery Environments
The Behavior and Caregiving Experiences of Full-Term and Preterm Newborns

Juarlyn L. Gaiter

Methods of studying infancy change over time as a result of a particular Zeitgeist, economic considerations, and interest in research. A major research topic in the 1980s is the effect of environmental risks upon infant development. Specific interest in the effects of hospital nursery environments on the subsequent development of infants grew out of the last decade when scientists introduced a plethora of interventions for preterm babies (Barnard, 1972; Kramer and Pierpont, 1974; Powell, 1974; Scarr-Salapatek and Williams, 1973; Wright, 1971). Three major factors have contributed to and sustained the momentum of these technological developments:

1. The recognition accorded the newborn as a competent organism, capable of shaping the caregiving environment and thereby ensuring the newborn's own developmental progress (Bell, 1974; Brazelton et al., 1974).

Support for this research was provided in part by Social and Behavioral Sciences Grant #12–24 from the March of Dimes Birth Defects Foundation and Grant #81–5 from Children's Hospital National Medical Center.

2. A shift in conceptualization of the infant's caregiving environment from that of a static system from which emerge individualized patterns of behavior to a transactional model that proposes that reciprocal and dynamic interaction occurs between the caregiving environment and the newborn (Sameroff and Chandler, 1975).
3. Collaborative research of behavioral and medical scientists in dissecting the complexity of biosocial risk factors in early development.

Prevention of developmental disfunction and follow-up monitoring of the neurobehavioral progress of vulnerable infants are the primary foci of this new research collaboration.

The modification of nursery environments and treatment regimens to minimize adverse effects of the later development of babies has largely been the research activity of behavioral scientists. A growing awareness of the potential iatrogenic risks inherent in highly technical medical care has occurred within the medical profession. Sufficient evidence has been provided by social scientists to point to sociobehavioral factors as far more enduring and critical to later infant developmental functioning than birth trauma and neonatal complications. Taken together, these developments have focused efforts toward *change* of hospital nursery environments rather than *study* of inherent aspects of nursery care (i.e., constant monitoring, handling, etc.) that may have enduring sociopsychological consequences for caregiver-infant interaction. As a result of dramatically increased survival rates of very low birth weight babies, medical technology has surpassed psychological predictions of growth and subsequent functioning of this vulnerable infant population. The paucity of descriptive data and systematic investigation of hospital nursery environments have been major hindrances to theoretical and practical gains in behavioral science research.

Rationale for Observational Research

This chapter presents research that documents the early life support experiences of term and preterm newborns in hospital nursery environments. The purposes of this study were to:

1. Provide an objective description of stimulation that is potentially functional for newborns in hospital nurseries.
2. Document the pattern of nursery staff and infant interaction that is peculiar to the care of term and preterm newborns.
3. Compare the behavior and early caregiving experiences of sick preterm, healthy preterm, and term newborns.

Nursery staff and infant interactions can be regarded as congruent with an early parenting model. Observations of these interactions may advance understanding of the initial social communication experiences of hospitalized babies. An ever-expanding literature attests to the impact of early infant-caregiver interactions in shaping the infant's sensory environment, caregiving experience, and subsequent developmental outcome (Field, 1977; Goldberg, 1978).

The normal term newborn is preadapted with a range of signaling behaviors that serve to ensure special care and developmental organization. However, preterm infants are physiologically vulnerable because of attendant complications of prematurity, and are also at risk for failure to adapt in any environment. Consequently, preterm infants and their parents often have problems in establishing the early synchronous patterns of interaction and communication that characterize the caregiving experiences of the term infant (Goldberg et al., 1980; Leifer et al., 1972). Sander (1980) and Luce (1970) described the prototypical newborn as possessing semi-independent physiologic subsystems that gradually organize their functions to control infant waking, sleeping, and feeding rhythms. Caregiver and infant interactions result in the harmonious regulation of this organizational process. Progressive competent behavioral functioning enables infant behavior to be synchronous with the activity of a particular caregiving environment. Thus, joint negotiation of these complex tasks is accomplished through the variously competent interactions between the newborn and the caregiver. Consequently the successful regulation of infant developmental and caregiver tasks is the major accomplishment of the early months of postnatal life.

Each of the three groups of infants in this investigation (sick preterm, healthy preterm, and term newborns) has a unique set of adaptive-regulatory characteristics determined by their functional maturity and the degree of perinatal stress they have endured. Because of birth complications, the preterm infant's requirements for highly technical medical therapy often necessitate a lengthy separation from parents. The prolonged course of hospitalization is frequently punctuated by recurrent setbacks that require the resumption of intense medical procedures. In contrast, healthy term babies are more likely to room in with their mothers and be discharged with them 3 to 4 days after birth.

Observational Study Hypotheses

Caregiver Effects

The following hypotheses are based on methodology and findings from a pilot study (Gaiter et al., 1981) that described the frequency and pattern of caregiving stimulation experienced by hospitalized, sick preterm infants:

1. Caregivers will have more physical contact (handling) with ill preterm newborns in intensive care than with the healthy preterm and normal term infants.
2. Caregivers will engage in more social handling of term babies (rocking and cuddling) than both groups of preterm newborns.
3. Nursery personnel will speak more frequently to term infants than to preterm infants.

Infant Effects

The variables of physiologic immaturity and illness were expected to adversely affect the responsivity of preterm infants to caregiver stimulation. Consequently, it was hypothesized that lower levels of activity, alertness, irritability, and vocalizations would be highly characteristic of the behavior of hospitalized preterm infants compared to that of term infants.

The following hypotheses were derived for infant effects:

1. Preterm newborns (critically ill and healthy) will exhibit less limb and body activity than term infants.
2. Preterm newborns (critically ill and healthy) will display significantly less eye opening (looking) behavior than term infants.
3. Term infants will engage in more mouthing and sucking behavior than both preterm groups.
4. Term infants will exhibit more fussing/crying behavior during the course of nursery care than the preterm infants.

Observation Methodology

A structured observation system designed and used in the pilot study (Gaiter et al., 1981) allowed observers to record caregiver and infant behavior at the infant's bedside. Trained observers coded the frequency of 33 behavioral variables in 5-second intervals. The variables were divided into four categories of nursery care activity—caregiving, social, medical, and inanimate stimulation. A fifth category consisted of 10 frequently occurring infant behaviors—eye opening, vegetative sounds, smiling, sucking, vocalizing, fussing/crying, limb movement, body movement, activation of monitoring alarms, and absence of infant activity.

Infants were observed for a total of 6 hours, which were divided into 30-minute segments across a 3-day period. Each half-hour of observation yielded 30 precoded observation forms consisting of twelve 5-second rows, with frequency columns representing 1 minute of recording time per form. A tape delivered an auditory signal to the observer, who wore earphones, at 5-second intervals for 30 minutes. At the sound of the auditory signal the observer recorded precoded behaviors that were observed during the previous 5-second interval. Thus, by continuous recording, 360 frequency counts for each of the 33 behavioral events were generated during every 30-minute observation.

A total of 60 newborns were observed for 30 minutes on 12 different occasions during a 3-day period. For each infant, a total of 4320 frequency counts of behavioral data were generated. Each of four observers independently recorded data on one-half of the 60 infants; on subsequent sessions, the observers observed the same infant. Interobserver reliability was established and checked periodically during the observations. It was never less than .89.

The decision to observe the newborns on three separate days was based on two factors:

1. The term infants were routinely discharged after the third day of birth.
2. The preterm infants experienced three levels of care (intensive, intermediate, and predischarge), which generally corresponded with their gradual recuperation from birth complications and less need for medical interventions.

On the second day following admission to intensive care, the 40 preterm infants were observed four times. Critically ill infants were receiving ventilatory assistance and were minimally clothed to facilitate handling and medical management as they lay under radiant warmers. The second set of four observations occurred during the intermediate care period. For these observations the criteria for the critically ill preterm sample were that they: 1) no longer required assisted ventilation; 2) were housed in closed isolettes; and 3) had been in the nursery for at least 1 week. This phase of medical treatment was chosen because it represented a distinct change in the infant's physical environment and could play a role in the mediation of varying types of stimulation, e.g., feedings, holding (see hypothesis 1, caregiver effects).

The third and final set of observations occurred 1 week prior to the infant's discharge from the nursery. During this time, preterm infant care is typically characterized as that of the "growing preterm baby." Swaddled in open cribs and without respiration and heart rate monitors, the infants could be easily handled by parents and nursery staff. The four initial (intensive care) observations for the healthy preterm sample occurred on their second day in the term nursery at the George Washington University Hospital. Intermediate care observations occurred following at least 7 days of hospitalization, and the final observations were done a few days before discharge from the nursery (approximately 2 weeks after nursery admission). The healthy preterm babies were housed in traditional nursery cribs throughout all phases of nursery care. None of them required medical procedures except vital sign checks and heelsticks for blood tests. Six of these newborns experienced 1 to 3 days of phototherapy for hyperbilirubinemia.

The 20 term babies were observed four times on each of the 3 consecutive days that they were in the normal term nursery. Their day of birth corresponded to the intensive care phase. The second day in the nursery was their intermediate care period, and the third day (eve of discharge from the nursery) was the predischarge care observation period.

In summary, all 60 babies were observed for a total of 12 times (30 minutes each) on three separate days corresponding to designated phases of intensive, intermediate, and predischarge care.

The pilot phase for this investigation revealed that technological advances continuously change the nature of the preterm nursery environment. Consequently, infants experience novel stimulations and treatment regimens. Pilot observations also showed that the routine feeding situations provided the best opportunities to document caregiver-infant interactions and other stimulating events in the nursery environment (Thoman et al., 1971, 1972). During feedings, holding, talking to the infant, and cuddling activities may provide opportunities for the infant to discriminate these stimulations. The four 30-minute observations were conducted during the 12, 2, 4, and 6 PM periods. Representative infant activity during scheduled feedings occurred at the 12 and 6 PM periods. Relative increase in infant activity prior to feedings was expected near 2 PM, followed by a decrease in infant activity after a feeding (3 PM), at 4 PM.

Pilot study observations showed that preterm babies often needed to be awakened for feedings. Also, these infants were likely to have poorly organized sucking and swallowing behaviors. Therefore, many preterm infants required stimulation from nurses during feedings for the adequate ingestion of formula. Initially, the sick babies were fed intravenously; commensurate with recovery from acute illness, they were fed by gavage feedings (directly to the stomach), then later were introduced to bottle feeding.

Observational Settings

Newborn observations took place at two nursery sites: the Children's Hospital National Medical Center Neonatal Intensive Care Nursery (a

Level III facility—tertiary care) and the George Washington University nurseries—a Level I facility for normal newborns and a Level III facility for the care of critically ill newborns.

The Children's Hospital nursery has five modules with a total of 36 newborn beds. Twelve beds are designated for intensive care patients and 24 for intermediate care. A staff of 87 nurses is specially trained for either intensive or intermediate care management. In the intensive care unit the nurse-infant ratios are 1:1 and 1:2. In intermediate care the ratios are 1:3 and 1:4. The critically ill preterm babies in this study were observed in the special care nursery at the Children's Hospital.

Although the George Washington University has a term nursery and an intensive care nursery, for this study only the term nursery was used. This unit has four modules and 28 beds. The healthy preterm and term babies in the study were observed at this nursery.

Subjects

Sixty newborns comprised the study sample. The following criteria were used for infant recruitment to the study:

Group A—Critically ill preterm newborns ($N = 20$) were less than 37 weeks gestation and weighed less than 2500 grams at birth. Within 4 hours of birth they had been clinically diagnosed as having hyaline membrane disease (defined as respiratory illness), which was confirmed by x-ray and required assisted ventilation.

Group B—Preterm healthy newborns ($N = 20$) were less than 37 weeks gestation, weighed less than 2500 grams, and were products of uncomplicated births.

Group C—Term healthy newborns ($N = 20$) were between 38 and 40 weeks gestation, weighed 2500 grams, and were singleton births.

None of the 60 newborns had congenital anomalies, any other identifiable genetic disorders, or the need for major surgery (see Table 4.1 for a summary of newborn data for the 60 study subjects). Parents signed informed consent statements that allowed permission for the investigating staff to observe the recruited subjects.

Data Analysis Plan

The study used a 3×3 factorial repeated measures analysis. The *between*-subjects effect was Type of Baby (critically ill preterm, healthy preterm, or term); the *within*-subjects effect was Period of Care (intensive,

Table 4.1. Characteristics of newborn sample.

	Type of baby		
Characteristic	Term ($N = 20$)	Sick preterm ($N = 20$)	Healthy preterm ($N = 20$)
Mean birth weight (grams)	4491.85	1193.50	1755.85
	(1403.60)[a]	(231.92)	(295.12)
Mean gestation (weeks)	40	30	33
	(0)	(2.16)	(1.74)
Days in hospital	3	64	17
	(0)	(36)	(6)
Number of males	8	12	13
Number of females	12	8	7

[a]The figures in parentheses represent the standard deviation.

intermediate, or predischarge). The data comprised four categories of dependent variables (infant behavior, caregiving, social stimulation, and medical stimulation), representing 33 behavioral events.

The data (frequency counts of behavioral events) were coded in 5-second intervals and pooled over the three 2-hour periods of observation. Univariate repeated measures analyses of variance were used to analyze frequencies for each of the behavioral events. To assess whether the computed value of the F ratio for each effect was significant at the 0.05 level, Box's conservative testing strategem was applied (Dayton, 1970). In addition, the Newman-Keuls test was used to assess significant interaction effects between type of baby and period of care. Zero-order correlations were calculated, which resulted in two matrices. In the first matrix, seven infant behavioral variables (Looking, Smiling, Inactivity, Sucking and Mouthing, Limb Movement, Body Movement, Fussing/Crying, and Activation of Monitoring Alarms) were intercorrelated with a selected group of the caregiver stimulation variables (Handling, Feeding, Vocalization to Baby, Staff Conversations, Social Handling, Rocking, Vital Sign Checks, Check Baby, and Special Medical Procedures). The second matrix consisted of the intercorrelations between the grouping variable (the three types of babies) and the nine caregiver stimulation variables.

Observational Findings

The data discussed in the following sections are presented in Tables 4.2 through 4.6. Table 4.2 presents the percentage of observational periods during which selected newborn and caregiver interactions were observed. A listing of infant behaviors that were observed is found in Table 4.6. Tables 4.3 through 4.5 present only significant correlational findings for term, healthy preterm, and sick preterm babies, respectively.

Newborn and Caregiver Interactions

Handling Term newborns were handled (positioned and bathed) significantly more often during hospitalization than both groups of preterm newborns ($F_{2,57} = 37.81$, $p < .00001$) (Table 4.2). There was a nonsignificant decrease in the amount of times that caregivers handled term newborns from the second (intermediate observations) to the third (predischarge observations) day of life. Correlational data showed that during the second day in the nursery caregiver handling of term newborns was significantly correlated ($p < .05$) with talking to and rocking the babies (Table 4.4).

Table 4.2. Percentage of time during periods of care when selected newborn and caregiver interactions were observed.

Interaction and type of baby	Intensive care period	Intermediate care period	Predischarge care period
Handling			
Term	32	33	26
Healthy preterm	16	14	16
Sick preterm	4	17	25
Social Handling			
Term	4	3	1
Healthy preterm	1	1	1
Sick preterm	1	4	3
Feeding			
Term	11	14	13
Healthy preterm	5	10	12
Sick preterm	—	18	12
Staff Vocalizations to Babies			
Term	11	12	9
Healthy preterm	6	5	5
Sick preterm	2	7	9
Staff Conversations			
Term	12	12	13
Healthy preterm	7	7	10
Sick preterm	9	8	6
Rocking			
Term	3	6	3
Healthy preterm	3	4	8
Sick preterm	—	2	6
Vital Sign Checks			
Term	1	1	1
Healthy preterm	7	1	1
Sick preterm	7	1	1
Special Medical Procedures			
Term	—	—	—
Healthy preterm	1	—	—
Sick preterm	60	1	—
Check Baby			
Term	<1	<1	<1
Healthy preterm	<1	<1	<1
Sick preterm	2	1	<1

[a] Each period of care is represented by 2 hours of observation time. Each infant was observed for 6 hours total time.

Table 4.3. Significant correlations for term newborns.

Variables	Correlation[a]
Intensive care	
Social Handling × Vocalization to Baby	.45
Vital Sign Checks × Looking	−.56
Sucking and Mouthing × Smiling	.77
Fussing/Crying × Limb Movement	.61
Limb Movement × Smiling	.49
Inactivity × Feeding	.45
Limb Movement × Feeding	−.57
Body Movement × Feeding	−.50
Check Baby × Inactivity	.46
Intermediate care	
Handling × Vocalization to Baby	.50
Handling × Rocking	.60
Social Handling × Special Medical Procedures	.66
Rocking × Vocalization to Baby	.45
Handling × Limb Movement	.52
Feeding × Inactivity	.48
Feeding × Limb Movement	−.47
Inactivity × Looking	−.47
Sucking and Mouthing × Inactivity	−.45
Predischarge care	
Vocalization to Baby × Smiling	.59
Vocalization to Baby × Rocking	.50
Feeding × Rocking	.52
Limb Movement × Fussing/Crying	.51
Sucking and Mouthing × Looking	.63
Staff Conversations × Looking	.55
Staff Conversations × Feeding	.73
Special Medical Procedures × Fussing/Crying	.50

[a] r of .45 required for $p < .05$ level of significance.

A significant Type of Baby × Period of Care interaction ($F_{2,57} = 3.08, p < .05$) indicated an increase in the frequency of caregiver handling of the critically ill preterm babies during the intermediate and predischarge care periods. Critically ill preterm newborns were handled somewhat less frequently than the preterm healthy babies, but at rates equal to term infants at predischarge care. The frequency of caregiver handling of the healthy preterm babies was consistent across care periods.

During intensive care, handling of the sick preterm newborns was significantly related to the sounding of monitoring alarms, an indication of infant distress (Table 4.6). This measure excluded alarms caused by electrodes being dislodged from the infant's skin. Intermediate care handling of these babies by nursery staff was significantly correlated with rocking them.

Table 4.4. Significant correlations for healthy preterm newborns.

Variables	Correlation[a]
Intensive Care	
Handling × Sucking	.66
Handling × Vocalization to Baby	.57
Social Handling × Sucking	.87
Social Handling × Activation of Monitoring Alarms	.84
Handling × Activation of Monitoring Alarms	.67
Social Handling × Feeding	.46
Feeding × Vocalization to Baby	.66
Vocalization to Baby × Fussing/Crying	−.57
Vocalization to Baby × Sucking	.77
Vocalization to Baby × Inactivity	.47
Inactivity × Feeding	.54
Looking × Feeding	.52
Looking × Sucking	.52
Sucking × Body Movement	.64
Special Medical Procedures × Looking	−.50
Body Movement × Special Medical Procedures	.58
Vocalizations to Baby × Special Medical Procedures	.62
Limb Movement × Special Medical Procedures	.47
Staff Conversations × Special Medical Procedures	−.57
Intermediate care	
Handling × Rocking	.68
Social Handling × Sucking	.50
Social Handling × Smiling	.48
Handling × Limb Movement	.46
Limb Movement × Special Medical Procedures	.58
Body Movement × Sucking	.49
Fussing/Crying × Activity	−.70
Inactivity × Looking	−.67
Sucking × Smiling	.55
Vocalizations to Baby × Sucking	.73
Check Baby × Looking	−.61
Check Baby × Activation of Monitoring Alarms	.76
Predischarge care	
Social Handling × Fussing/Crying	.48
Rocking × Fussing/Crying	.54
Rocking × Feeding	.50
Fussing/Crying × Inactivity	−.50
Looking × Inactivity	−.82
Vital Sign Checks × Sucking	.54
Check Baby × Sucking	.51
Check Baby × Vital Sign Checks	.46

[a] r of .45 required for $p < .05$ level of significance.

Table 4.5. Significant correlations for sick preterm newborns.

Variables	Correlation[a]
Intensive care	
Handling × Activation of Monitoring Alarms	.56
Handling × Staff Conversations	.49
Activation of Monitoring Alarms × Fussing/Crying	.66
Social Handling × Fussing/Crying	.58
Body Movement × Sucking	.50
Body Movement × Special Medical Procedures	−.45
Sucking × Limb Movement	−.49
Intermediate Care	
Handling × Vocalization to Baby	.51
Handling × Smiling	.46
Handling × Rocking	.63
Social Handling × Feeding	.55
Check Baby × Activation of Monitoring Alarms	.72
Predischarge care	
Handling × Rocking	.67
Social Handling × Vocalization to Baby	.55
Social Handling × Body Movement	.47
Social Handling × Looking	.45
Feeding × Sucking	.47
Body Movement × Limb Movement	.55
Body Movement × Smiling	.47
Body Movement × Looking	.55
Limb Movement × Smiling	.59
Inactivity × Looking	−.79

[a] r of .45 required for $p < .05$ level of significance.

Social Handling Very little social handling (cuddling and stroking of infants) was observed. However, healthy preterm infants experienced significantly less of this caregiver contact than the critically ill preterm and term newborns ($F_{2,57} = 3.52$, $p < .03$). The data indicate that there were no significant differences between care periods in the amount of social handling observed. However, there was a significant Type of Baby × Period of Care interaction ($F_{4,114} = 4.23$, $p < .003$). Term infants received significantly more social handling during their first day in the hospital than either of the two groups of preterm infants received during intensive care.

The critically ill preterm newborns experienced significantly more social handling contact during intermediate care than the healthy preterm babies but not more than the term infants. At predischarge care, however, these preterm sick babies experienced three times as much social handling as the preterm healthy and term infants (Table 4.2).

The social handling of term infants was significantly correlated with instances of staff speaking to the babies during their first day in the nursery

(Table 4.3). Blood sampling (special procedures) for term babies was significantly correlated with social handling during intermediate care (on their second day of life). During intermediate care, social handling was significantly related to feeding interactions for the sick preterm babies. At predischarge, social contact also related significantly to instances of staff speaking to these babies (Table 4.5). Intensive care correlations for the healthy preterm group showed that social handling was significantly related to feeding interactions (Table 4.4).

Caregiver Checking of Infants Preterm infants experienced significantly more momentary physical contact with nursery caregivers who were servicing or adjusting equipment (Check Baby) in or around infants (e.g., connecting nasal prongs for oxygen delivery) than the healthy preterm or term newborns ($F_{2,57} = 27.60$, $p < .0001$) (Table 4.2). Also found was a highly significant Period of Care effect, an indication that this type of infant monitoring occurred more frequently during intensive care management ($F_{2,57} = 10.32$, $p < .0002$). The Type of Baby × Period of Care interaction ($F_{4,114} = 8.63$, $p < .0001$) revealed that during intensive care preterm sick babies were significantly more likely to be touched when equipment was checked. This activity represented approximately 1% of the observations during intensive care and was negligible thereafter.

Feeding of Infants A highly significant Period of Care effect for feeding indicated that feeding was less likely to occur during intensive care ($F_{2,57} = 33.30$, $p < .00001$). However, the interaction of Type of Baby with Feeding was highly significant ($F_{4,114} = 10.42$, $p < .0001$) from intensive to intermediate care. For the sick preterm infants intermediate care marked the beginning of gavage and bottle feedings.

For the term and healthy preterm newborns, feeding was significantly correlated with instances of infants remaining still (Inactivity) during intensive and intermediate care observations. Feeding was also significantly related to social handling and staff vocalizations during intensive care for preterm healthy babies. At predischarge care, feeding interactions were significantly related to rocking for term and preterm healthy infants.

Nursery Staff Vocalizations to Newborns The nursery staff spoke significantly more often to term infants ($F_{2,57} = 7.62$, $p < .001$) than to either of the two preterm groups. Staff vocalizations showed a significant increase from intensive to predischarge care ($F_{2,57} = 3.35$, $p < .04$). No significant differences were found in the amount of talking during the intermediate and predischarge care periods (Table 4.2). However, there was a significant Type of Baby × Period of Care interaction ($F_{4,114} = 5.53$, $p < .001$). This effect was carried by the preterm sick group, who were spoken to significantly less frequently compared to the healthy preterm and term infants during intensive care. Thereafter, there were significant increases in the frequency at which staff spoke to the sick preterm infants. During predischarge care, these babies were spoken to as frequently as the term babies and significantly more often than the preterm healthy babies.

The correlational analyses revealed that, for term newborns, staff vocalizations significantly related to handling and rocking on the second day. On the third day, just before discharge from the nursery, staff vocalizations were significantly related to the rocking of babies and to infant smiling behavior. Staff conversations to healthy preterm infants were significantly correlated with handling, feeding, special medical procedures, babies' fussing/crying, sucking, and inactivity during intensive care. During intermediate care, staff vocalizations correlated significantly to infant smiling. For the critically ill preterm babies, staff vocalizations related significantly to handling, infant smiling, and inactivity during intermediate care and to social handling at predischarge care.

Staff Conversations at Infant's Bedside The staff spoke to each other significantly more often in close proximity to the term infants than either of the preterm groups ($F_{2,57} = 4.52$, $p < .01$). No significant interaction effects were found.

Staff conversations were significantly related to feeding and infant looking behavior at predischarge care. For the healthy preterm babies, staff conversations correlated significantly with special medical procedures during intensive care. Staff conversations related significantly to handling during intensive care and to special medical procedures during intermediate care for the sick preterm group.

Rocking No significant group effects for the amount of rocking were observed. Significantly more rocking occurred during predischarge care than during intensive care ($F_{2,57} = 5.30$, $p < .01$). For the intermediate and predischarge care periods, there were no significant differences in rocking rates. During intermediate care, the rocking of babies was significantly related to handling for all three groups of babies. At predischarge, rocking was significantly correlated with handling of the sick preterm babies and to the feeding of and the fussing/crying behavior of healthy preterm newborns. Rocking was significantly related to the feeding of term babies during predischarge care.

Medical Interventions

Vital Signs All three groups differed significantly from each other on the frequency of vital sign measurements (pulse, temperature, and heart rate) taken by nursery staff ($F_{2,57} = 13.00$, $p < .0001$). Vital sign monitoring occurred during approximately 1% of the observations for any given period. For term infants, observations of vital sign monitoring were negligible. Vital sign monitoring occurred significantly more frequently ($F_{4,114} = 30.1$, $p < .02$) during intensive care than during either the intermediate or predischarge care periods. At predischarge care for healthy preterm babies, vital sign monitoring correlated significantly with infant sucking.

Special Medical Procedures Preterm sick babies experienced significantly more medical interventions (e.g., transfusions, injections, and x-rays) than the healthy preterm and term infants ($F_{2,57} = 47.00$, $p < .00001$). The latter two groups did not differ significantly from each other on this variable at intermediate care. Special medical interventions were significantly more likely to occur during intensive care management ($F_{2,57} = 45.51$, $p < .00001$). The sick preterm group experienced a dramatic decrease in the frequency of special medical procedures ($F_{4,114} = 44.13$, $p < .00001$) from intensive to predischarge care. For term infants, special medical procedures (e.g., heelsticks) were significantly related to infant fussing/crying behavior at predischarge. For the healthy preterm babies, special medical procedures during intensive care correlated significantly with staff conversations, infant limb movement, staff vocalizations, and infant body movement. Special medical procedures during intensive care for the sick babies correlated significantly with infant body movement.

Infant Behavior

Infant Activity During hospitalization, preterm sick infants were significantly more immobile than term infants, but not significantly less mobile than healthy preterm infants ($F_{2,57} = 4.01$, $p < .02$) (Table 4.6). No significant differences in inactivity were observed for preterm healthy and term newborns. All three groups of infants became increasingly more active over time ($F_{2,57} = 29.00$, $p < .00001$). During intensive care, significantly more infant inactivity was observed, but between intermediate and predischarge care no significant differences occurred in rates of infant inactivity. The sick preterm babies were less active than either of the other two groups during intensive care ($F_{4,114} = 7.58$, $p < .0001$).

For the term babies, inactivity during their first and second days in the nursery was significantly correlated with feedings. On the second day, inactivity was also related to infant looking and sucking behaviors. Inactivity for the healthy preterm babies in intensive care was significantly related to staff vocalizations and to feedings. During intermediate and predischarge care, inactivity was related negatively to infant looking and fussing/crying behavior. For the preterm sick babies in intermediate care,

Table 4.6. Percentage of time during periods of care when selected infant behaviors were observed.

	Percentage of period interaction was observed[a]		
Interaction and type of baby	Intensive care period	Intermediate care period	Predischarge care period
Inactivity			
Term	58	46	48
Healthy preterm	56	55	50
Sick preterm	73	55	45
Looking			
Term	12	19	18
Healthy preterm	5	15	23
Sick preterm	<1	15	21
Sucking and Mouthing			
Term	11	12	12
Healthy preterm	9	7	7
Sick preterm	7	12	22
Fussing/Crying			
Term	4	6	7
Healthy preterm	8	2	2
Sick preterm	3	2	2
Limb Movement			
Term	20	32	21
Healthy preterm	27	24	24
Sick preterm	20	23	21
Body Movement			
Term	2	4	5
Healthy preterm	5	4	2
Sick preterm	2	2	<1

[a] Each period of care is represented by 2 hours of observation time. Each infant was observed for 6 hours total time.

inactivity correlated negatively, but significantly, to infant looking, sucking behavior, and staff vocalizations. At predischarge, inactivity was negatively related to infant looking behavior.

Infant Looking Behavior No significant differences were found in eye opening behavior for the three infant groups (Table 4.6). Infant looking behavior, however, significantly increased from intensive through predischarge care ($F_{2,57} = 42.00$, $p < .00001$). Preterm sick babies dramatically increased their eye opening behavior from intensive to predischarge care ($F_{4,114} = 4.03, p < .005$). The healthy and sick preterm babies evidenced significant increases in looking behavior throughout hospitalization; term infants showed only modest increases in their looking behavior over the course of the 3-day nursery stay.

Looking behavior for term babies during their first day in the nursery was significantly correlated with the monitoring of their vital signs by nursery staff. At predischarge, looking behavior related significantly to staff conversations in close proximity to the babies and to sucking and monitoring behaviors. For the preterm healthy infants, looking behavior during intensive care observations significantly related to infant sucking and feeding behaviors and to special medical procedures. At predischarge, infant looking behavior related significantly to social handling and body movement for the sick babies.

Smiling Smiling behavior was rarely observed (less than 1% of observations at any given time period). There were no significant differences in the amount of smiling observed among the three groups of newborns. However, significantly less smiling occurred during the intensive care observations ($F_{2,57} = 8.24$, $p < .001$) compared with the intermediate and the predischarge periods. For the sick preterm babies, significant increases in smiling behavior occurred from intermediate to predischarge care ($F_{4,114} = 4.88$, $p < .001$). Term infants smiled significantly more often (on their first day in the nursery) than both preterm groups during intensive care. The preterm sick infants smiled more often than the preterm healthy and term babies during the intermediate period. At predischarge, both preterm groups smiled slightly more often than the term infants.

On the first nursery day, term infant smiling was significantly related to sucking and mouthing. At predischarge, their smiling correlated significantly with the frequency at which they were spoken to by nursery staff. At intermediate care, smiling was significantly correlated with social handling, staff vocalizations, body movement, and sucking. For the preterm sick infants, smiling during intermediate care was significantly related to caregiver handling and staff vocalizations. At predischarge, smiling related significantly to infant limb and body movements.

Mouthing Preterm sick newborns engaged in significantly more mouthing behavior during observations than the preterm healthy newborns ($F_{2,57} = 8.32$, $p < .001$) (Table 4.6). Preterm sick babies did not differ from the term babies in mouthing behavior. Preterm healthy infants mouthed the least, significantly less than the term and sick preterm babies. A significant Period of Care effect showed that less mouthing occurred during intensive care compared to intermediate and predischarge care. Mouthing rates did not differ for intermediate and predischarge care. Preterm sick babies significantly increased their mouthing behavior at each care period ($F_{4,114} = 13.10$, $p < .00001$). Mouthing activity for preterm healthy babies significantly decreased in frequency from intensive to intermediate care but did not change significantly from intermediate to predischarge. Term infants increased mouthing activity from intensive to intermediate care, but their mouthing rates at intermediate and predischarge care were not different.

The correlational data revealed that the mouthing by term infants related significantly to smiling, inactivity, and looking on the first, second, and third nursery days, respectively. For the healthy preterms in intensive care, mouthing related significantly to handling, social handling, staff vocalizations, infant looking, and body movement. At intermediate care, mouthing behavior was significantly correlated with social handling, body movement, and smiling. At predischarge, vital sign monitoring and checking technical equipment near infants related significantly to mouthing behavior. For sick preterm babies, mouthing activity was significantly related to body movement during intensive care, inactivity during intermediate care, and feeding interactions during predischarge.

Fussing/Crying Preterm sick babies evidenced significantly less fussing/crying behavior compared to healthy preterm and term infants ($F_{2,57} = 9.13$, $p < .001$). There were differences in irritability for the healthy preterm and term groups. However, preterm healthy infants had a significant decrease in irritable fussing/crying behavior from intensive to intermediate care. No significant changes occurred in the frequency of irritable behavior from intermediate to predischarge care. Term infants were increasingly irritable from intensive to intermediate care, but did not change during predischarge care observations.

For term newborns on their first and third days in the hospital, fussing/crying behavior was significantly related to limb movements; on the third day, fussing/crying behavior correlated significantly with special medical procedures (e.g., heelsticks). During intensive care, the irritable behavior of healthy preterm babies correlated significantly with staff vocalizations; irritability related negatively to inactivity during intermediate and predischarge care and to social handling and rocking at predischarge. Observations during intensive and intermediate care showed that fussing/crying behavior related significantly with the activation of monitoring alarms for the sick babies.

Limb Movement Preterm sick babies displayed significantly less limb activity than did term babies ($F_{2,57} = 4.71$, $p < .01$). The healthy preterm infants did not differ significantly from the term and sick preterm infants in limb movements. The first-day observations of term babies showed that limb movement was significantly related to fussing/crying behavior, smiling, and feeding interactions. On the second day, limb movement continued to relate to feeding interactions and to caregiver handling. On the third day, limb movement related significantly to fussing/crying behaviors. For the healthy preterm group, limb movement during intensive and intermediate care was significantly related to special medical procedures and to handling during intermediate care. Intensive care observations of preterm sick infants revealed that limb movement related significantly to suctioning (special medical procedures). At predischarge, limb movement was related to smiling.

Body Movement Preterm sick newborns evidenced significantly fewer body movements than preterm well and term babies ($F_{2,57} = 7.56$, $p < .002$). Preterm sick and healthy babies evidenced little change in the frequency of body movement from intensive to intermediate care but showed a decrease during predischarge. However, term infants showed moderate but steady increases in body activity across the 3 days of hospitalization.

On their first day in the nursery, body movements for the term newborns were significantly related to feeding interactions. For the healthy preterm group, body movements during intensive and intermediate care were significantly related to sucking behavior. During intensive care, the body movements of sick preterm babies were significantly related to sucking behavior and special medical procedures.

Activation of Monitoring Alarms Because of distress, preterm sick infants activated monitoring alarm equipment significantly more often than the other two groups of babies ($F_{2,57} = 11.00$, $p < .0002$). During intensive and intermediate care for preterm sick babies, activation of alarms correlated highly with fussing/crying behavior. For the healthy preterm babies, activation of monitoring alarms during intensive care was significantly related to social and caregiver handling.

Discussion

Caregiver Effects on Infants

A most significant finding revealed by this investigation is that the nursery staff adjusted the frequency with which they handled and stimulated infants to the degree of infant behavioral organization. The social and caregiving experiences of preterm infants differed most from those of term infants during the intensive period of hospitalization. On their first day in the hospital, term infants were handled, cuddled, talked to, and rocked by caregivers. In contrast, the experience of the preterm babies was characterized by significantly less handling, affectionate contact, vocalizations, and vestibular stimulation. Given the consistent reports from other studies that a relationship exists between caregiver handling and infant distress, this finding about preterm and caregiver contact is encouraging. However, whether infant distress elicits handling or whether the caregiver response generates negative reactivity is a conundrum. This intricate problem is further exacerbated by the lack of current knowledge about the effects of routine handling on the physiologic stability of sick preterm babies (Marton et al., 1980).

Long et al. (1980) investigated the effects of nursery caregiver handling of sick babies and the incidence of abnormalities in oxygenation of these infants as measured by conventional methods (such as intermittent arterial blood gas sampling and cardiorespirographic monitoring) and by continuous transcutaneous oxygen monitoring. Handling disturbances were found to be a significant cause of poor oxygenation in babies who received routine handling for medical management of respiratory disease. Caregivers who could see the disturbing handling effects that were apparent from the use of continuous transcutaneous oxygen monitoring equipment modified the frequency and the quality of their physical contact with sick babies. Long et al. (1980) therefore advocated the use of continuous transcutaneous oxygen monitoring in the nursery to guide medical interventions. They estimated that hypoxemia and hyperoxemia, intensified by routine caregiver handling, could be reduced by as much as 80%. The findings of the present observational study indicated that, although sick preterm babies receive less caregiving stimulation than term infants, they still may be especially vulnerable to routine handling contact during hospitalization.

Infant Effects on Caregivers

During intensive care, when behavioral organization of the three groups was compared, a pattern of initial behavioral disorganization emerged for the term and sick preterm babies, indicated by lower levels of activity and responsivity. However, this effect was not as apparent for the healthy preterm group. It is not clear what factors accounted for these findings.

The pattern of affectionate handling of babies and nursery staff vocalizations in this study revealed caregiver sensitivity to evidence of developing newborn behavioral organization. On their first day in the nursery, as predicted, term infants received much more cuddling, stroking, kissing, and conversation from caregivers than either group of preterm infants. During intensive care, term and healthy preterm infants were rocked in the arms of caregivers, but the preterm sick babies did not experience comparable levels of vestibular stimulation. However, at intermediate and predischarge care, social contact (cuddling and staff vocalizations) for term and preterm sick babies were comparable. Adaptive interactions that signaled the coordination of caregiver behaviors with infant behaviors were the hallmarks of intermediate care, especially for the sick babies. A gradual increase in the amounts of stimulation for the preterm sick infants was especially apparent at this time. This "phasing in" of stimulation may be interpreted as a result of "infant effects" on caregivers. Although all three groups of infants became more active, alert, and responsive over time, significant changes in responsive activity even occurred for term infants. However, dramatic changes were evident for the preterm sick babies. This result probably reflected their progressive behavioral organization that was concurrent with improved medical status of the preterm babies. Further indication of progressive physiologic and behavioral organization of the sick babies was the significant relationship found between the activation of monitoring alarms and infant irritability.

During intermediate care, feedings were begun for the sick babies. Along with feedings, caregivers also talked more often to the infants. By the time the preterm babies were ready for discharge from the nursery, their improved behavioral competence elicited caregiver handling comparable to that of the term infants.

In contrast to the handling experience of the sick babies, the frequency of caregiver handling of the healthy preterm babies remained the same throughout their hospitalization. Because these newborns were not sick on admission to the nursery, they received routine "growing premie care" to ensure the adequate weight gain required for nursery discharge. Progress in their developmental functioning, therefore, was probably less conspicuous than that of either the term or sick preterm infants. Thus, their influence on caregiver behavior was less apparent.

Infant Activity During Nursery Care

The hypothesis that the term infants would be significantly more active than the preterm babies during intensive care was not confirmed. In fact, when sucking and irritable fussing/crying behaviors were compared for the three groups, the term and sick infants had similar low levels. The healthy preterm babies were the most active of the three groups. The distinguishing behavior of the term infants was that during intensive care they exhibited more visual alertness than the other infants.

The hypothesis that preterm babies would exhibit less limb and body movement than term babies was not confirmed by this study. The data revealed two important behavioral characteristics of the preterm groups:

1. They were much more likely than term babies to be immobile during the intensive care observations.

2. When they were active, especially the sick ones, their limb activity was high and equaled that of the term infants.

Of interest here is Korones' (1976) report that infants handled as often as 9 minutes per hour became highly disturbed. The finding in this study that high rates of limb activity occurred during the most acute phase of medical care may indicate the preterm infant's reaction to overwhelming and disturbing stimulation. This conclusion may be valid despite the finding that caregivers handled preterm infants less often than term infants.

Barnard (see Chapter 6) and Brazelton et al. (1974) argued that, in the early adaptive interactions of infants and caregivers, a primary function of the caregiver is to assist the infant in regulating levels of arousal. Caregivers also learn to provide the baby with soothing stimulations, which inhibit external and internal disturbing stimuli. Barnard noted the special vulnerability of preterm infants who may not be capable of shutting out disturbing stimulation even after a medical intervention has ceased. Without external assistance, the preterm infant may restimulate himself or herself (by recurrent limb activity and sucking responses) and remain highly aroused. The impact of continued arousal frequently generates cardiorespiratory distress (activation of monitoring alarms). Thus, this study's findings of high levels of sucking and mouthing responses of the sick babies (behaviors often associated with caregiving handling) have important medical and neurobehavioral ramifications.

The high rates of infant inactivity documented by this study suggest that, even for term infants, undisturbed rest with no movement may be self-protective for the newborn. An inactive infant does not spontaneously invite caregiver handling and stimulation. Periods of complete shutdown of motoric responses may function to insulate the infant from disruptive stimulation. Moreover, minimal physical contact (Handling) during these inactive periods may allow the infant the opportunity to learn how to regulate arousal and establish self-imposed schedules of necessary rest.

Environmental Change—Transition to Simulated Home Environment

Change in medical status for the sick babies was highly evident by their "graduation" from being unclothed and housed under radiant warmers to supervision in closed isolettes (during intermediate care) in a different location in the nursery. Perhaps an even more important contributor to the increased alertness and responsivity of the sick infants was that they were no longer intubated for intensive management of their respiratory disease. Freedom from intubation allowed a greater range of movement, less discomfort, and an opportunity for increased responsivity to caregiver stimulation. Consequently, intermediate care therapy for the sick babies effected a twofold change, in the environment and in the nursery staff (from intensive to intermediate care specialists). In contrast, the term and healthy preterm infants did not experience new environments or different levels of nursing care.

Prior to discharge from the nursery, the preterm babies began to experience caregiving interactions that resembled those expected with parents at home. Sick infants were handled, talked to, and affectionately cuddled at rates nearly equal to those for the term infants. Further investigation is needed, however, to understand the effects of increased levels of stimulation at predischarge for sick preterm infants. Field (1977) demonstrated that parents of preterm babies, in their attempts to elicit infant responsivity, may overload their infants with highly arousing interactions. Researchers (Holmes et al., 1982; Brazelton et al., 1974) using the Brazelton Neonatal Assessment Scale (Brazelton, 1973) have shown that, despite phenomenal recovery from critical illness, the preterm infant still retains some of the adverse effects of prolonged hospitalization and constant bombardment by sound, light, and medical interventions (Gottfried et al., 1981). They have also indicated that, upon discharge from the nursery to a home environment, preterm infants are not functionally equivalent to term infants.

In this study, infant recovery from the birth experience and progressive physiologic stability occurred at significantly different points in time. Term infants were observed in the hospital nursery on each of the three successive days following birth. In contrast, preterm sick infants were first observed on the day of their birth but during the most acute period of their illness. They were at least 2 weeks old when their intermediate care observations were completed; at that time, improved behavioral organization was evident. Most were about 2 months old when the predischarge observations occurred. Similarly, the preterm healthy infants were initially observed on their day of birth but were at least 7 days old during intermediate care and about 2 weeks old at the time of the predischarge observations. Chronologically older than the full term sample, the preterm babies showed remarkable recovery of behavioral organization, despite physiologic vulnerability. This evidence of infant recovery was perceived by caregivers who gradually increased their levels of handling and general physical stimulation of the babies.

Even though preterm infant behavior may indicate improved adaptive and behavioral functioning, it is often clear to nursery staff that preterm babies have varying boundaries of tolerance for physical contact and handling. Continuation of earlier sensitive contact (intensive care management) and interactions is a more obvious need for some infants than for others. As predischarge approaches, the careful monitoring of the responsivity of individual infants to routine caregiving contact may give important clues to the special needs and adjustments some babies require. In addition, parents could be instructed in infant behavioral monitoring so that their contact during visits and later at home will provide continuity with the level of infant stimulation provided by the nursery staff. A smooth transition from hospital nursery care to home care may therefore be more efficiently accomplished by synchronizing nursery staff and parent behaviors.

Behavioral scientists, together with neonatologists and pediatricians, have observed the marvelous adaptive capacities of fragile newborns surviving in the highly technical environment of the intensive care nursery. On discharge from this specialized world, vulnerable infants still require care; this is an obvious fact. However, the emphasis shifts to the receiving environment—one adequately prepared to nurture and protect the competence of the newborn.

Acknowledgments

The author wishes to thank Dr. Gordon B. Avery, Director of the Division of Neonatology, Dr. Anne B. Fletcher, Director of Nurseries at Children's Hospital National Medical Center, and Dr. Maureen Edwards, Director of Nurseries at George Washington University Hospital for their assistance in carrying out this research. A special thanks goes to the following persons who collected data for this study: Alix A. S. Johnson, Ph.D.; Cassandra J. Jackson, Ph.D.; and Linda Terrell. Dr. Norman Leung provided statistical and computer analysis of the data. Dr. Lettie Austin, Professor of English at Howard University, was gracious and kind in reading and critiquing several earlier drafts of this manuscript.

References

Barnard, K. E. 1972. The effect of stimulation on the duration and amount of sleep and wakefulness in the premature infant. Unpublished doctoral dissertation, University of Washington, Seattle.
Bell, R. Q. 1974. Contributions of human infants to caregiving and social interaction. In: M. Lewis and L. A. Rosenblum (eds.), The Effect of the Infant on Its Caregiver. Wiley, New York.
Brazelton, T. B. 1973. Neonatal Behavioral Assessment Scale. Lippincott, Philadelphia.
Brazelton, T. B., Koslowski, B., and Main, M. 1974. The origins of reciprocity: The early mother-infant interaction. In: M. Lewis and L. A. Rosenblum (eds.), The Effect of the Infant on Its Caregiver. Wiley, New York.
Dayton, C. M. 1970. The Design of Educational Experiments. McGraw-Hill, New York.

Field, T. M. 1977. Effects of early separation, interactive deficits, and experimental manipulations on mother-infant interaction. Child Dev. 48:763–771.
Gaiter, J. L., Avery, G. B., Temple, C. J., Johnson, A. A. S., and White, N. B. 1981. Stimulation characteristics of nursery environments for critically ill preterm infants and infant behavior. In: L. Stern, W. Oh, and B. Friishanson (eds.), Intensive Care of the Newborn. Masson Publishing Company, New York.
Goldberg, S. 1978. Prematurity: Effects on parent-infant interaction. J. Pediatr. Psychol. 3:137–144.
Goldberg, S., Brachfield, S., and DiVitto, B. 1980. Feeding, fussing and play: Parent-infant interaction in the first year as a function of prematurity and perinatal medical factors. In: T. M. Field, S. Goldberg, and A. M. Stern (eds.), High-Risk Infants and Children. Academic Press, New York.
Gottfried, A. W., Wallace-Lande, O., Sherman-Brown, S., King, J., Coen, C., and Hodgman, J. E. 1981. Physical and social environment of newborn infants in special care units. Science 214:673–675.
Holmes, D. L., Nagy, J. N., Slaymaker, F., Sosnowski, R. J., Prinz, S. M., and Pasternak, J.F. 1982. Early influences of prematurity, illness, and prolonged hospitalization on infant behavior. Dev. Psychol. 18:744–750.
Korones, S. B. 1976. Disturbance and infants' rest. In: T. Moore (ed.), Iatrogenic Problems in Neonatal Intensive Care. Report of the 69th Press Conference on Pediatric Research, pp. 129–132. Ross Laboratories, Columbus, OH.
Kramer, L., and Pierpont, M. E. 1976. Rocking waterbeds and auditory stimuli to enhance growth of premature infants. J. Pediatr. 88:297–299.
Leifer, A. D., Leiderman, P. H., Barnett, C. R., and Williams, J. 1972. Effects of mother-infant separation on maternal attachment behavior. Child Dev. 43:1203–1218.
Long, J. G., Alistar, G. S., Phillip, M. B., and Lucey, J. F. 1980. Excessive handling as a cause of hypoxemia. Pediatrics 65:203–207.
Luce, G. G. 1970. PHS Publication No. 2088. U.S. Government Printing Office, Washington, DC.
Marton, P. L., Dawson, H., and Minde, K. 1980. The interaction of ward personnel with infants in the premature nursery. Infant Behav. Dev. 3:307–313.
Powell, L. F. 1974. The effect of extra stimulation and maternal involvement on the development of low birthweight infants and on maternal behavior. Child Dev. 45:106–113.
Sameroff, A., and Chandler, M. 1975. Reproductive risk and the continuum of caretaking casualty. In: F. D. Horowitz, M. Heatherington, S. Scarr-Salapatek, and G. Siegel (eds.), Review of Child Development Research, Vol. 4. University of Chicago Press, Chicago.
Sander, L. W. 1980. Investigation of the infant and its caregiving environment as a biological system. In: S. I. Greenspan and G. H. Pollock (eds.), The Course of Life: Psychoanalytic Contributions toward Understanding Personality Development, Vol. 1. Infancy and Early Childhood. National Institute of Mental Health, Washington, DC.
Scarr-Salapatek, S., and Williams, M. L. 1973. The effects of early stimulation on low-birth weight infants. Child Dev. 44:94–101.
Thoman, E. B., Barnett, C. R., and Leiderman, P. H. 1971. Feeding behavior of newborn infants as a function of parity of the mother. Child Dev. 42:1471–1483.

Thoman, E. B., Leiderman, P. M., and Olsen, J. P. 1972. Neonate-mother interaction during breast feeding. Dev. Psychol. 6:110–118.
Wright, L. 1971. The theoretical and research base for programs of early stimulation, care and training of premature infants. In: J. Helmuth (ed.), The Exceptional Infant, Vol. 2. Studies in Abnormality. Brunner/Mazel, New York.

5

An Ecological Description of a Neonatal Intensive Care Unit

Patricia L. Linn, Frances Degen Horowitz, Bonnie Johns Buddin, Janet C. Leake, and Howard A. Fox

Measurement of the environment of premature infants may be especially important for professionals interested in the design of safe, effective interventions in neonatal intensive care nurseries. A rationale for measuring children's environments is presented in this chapter. The research study described here was based on direct observations of prematures hospitalized at the University of Kansas Special Care Nursery. The levels of many aspects of the nursery environment are presented, compared to data on term infants, and discussed in terms of individual differences in preterm medical histories.

Why Measure a Child's Environment?

To understand the conditions necessary for optimal developmental outcome is an important goal for all professionals interested in child health and well-being. In developmental research, one goal is to describe the

---

This research was funded in part by a National Science Foundation Postdoctoral Fellowship to the first author, and a grant from the Bureau of Education for the Handicapped (USOE 300-77-0308).

functional components of good physical and psychological growth so that developmental delay may be prevented and remediated and an optimal developmental outcome for all children may be fostered.

The traditional approach of the developmental researcher has been to study the characteristics of a child and his or her parents from one point in time to another. Recently, another part of "the developmental equation" has begun to receive the attention it deserves: *the child's environment*. For years, the importance of a child's physical and social environment has been acknowledged in a general way, with home and hospital environments described as "deprived" or "enriched," labeled according to "social class" or, more recently, "socioeconomic status." Researchers reported significant relationships between these global descriptions of child environments and various outcome measures (see Caldwell and Bradley, 1979, for a relevant review). However, knowing that a certain type of environment relates to developmental outcome is not enough. As Tulkin (1977) stated, such knowledge explains little about the *process* by which a particular environment might affect a child's development. This process should be understood before interventions can be designed to change a child's experiences. A process-oriented research question might be stated as follows: How do specific characteristics of a particular environment interact with specific characteristics of an individual to influence developmental outcome?

How to Study a Child's Environment

The description of a child's environment is a difficult task considering the large number of objects, people, sounds, and smells that comprise a hospital or home setting. Barker and his colleagues (Barker and Wright, 1954; Gump and Kounin, 1960) proposed a theory and methodology to describe the interactions between children and their environments. How that work influenced the research reported in this chapter is reflected in the authors' efforts:

1. To preserve the ongoing "stream" of the child-environment interplay (versus an arbitrary sampling of time)
2. To directly observe the child in a naturally occurring setting (versus using a parent's report or bringing the child into a laboratory)
3. To observe interactions as unobtrusively as possible (versus manipulating the situation)
4. To record both animate and inanimate sources of environmental stimulation (versus recording only social interaction)

The authors used these techniques to quantify specifics of the early environment for a group of high-risk infants. This was the first step in a research program designed to describe the environmental determinants of developmental outcome.

The Neonatal Intensive Care Unit— A Unique Environment

Infants who are born prematurely provide a unique opportunity to study the manner in which the environment and the individual interact to influence developmental outcome. Because of advances in neonatology, an increasing number of premature and low birth weight infants are able to survive a rocky neonatal course. With the decline of mortality figures and as neonatal intensive care unit (NICU) survivors reach school age, questions as to the quality of the premature infants' survival have been posed. Follow-up data on these infants indicate that they are at a higher risk than term infants for neurologic problems (Davies and Tizard, 1975; Heimer et al., 1964) intellectual deficits (Eisert et al., 1980), respiratory problems (Fitzhardinge et al., 1976), blindness (Pape et al., 1978), and hearing loss (Dayal et al., 1971).

The environmental contribution to developmental outcome may be especially important for the premature infant, whose early birth necessitates a setting that differs markedly from both the in utero environment and the postnatal hospital and home environments of term infants. The NICU setting is designed to provide medical support for the infants' immature physiologic systems; yet this environment is also the context for social, emotional, and cognitive growth during the 1 or 2 months that most premature infants spend hospitalized. Medical interventions are based on well-documented biologic risks to the premature infants, but most environmental interventions are based on undocumented assumptions of stimulus deprivation in NICU settings (Cornell and Gottfried, 1976).

Interventions designed to modify the NICU environment and thereby facilitate the preterm infant's development have been implemented nationwide. Researchers have tried to benefit the "stimulus-deprived" premature baby by introducing stimulation appropriate for term infants in home settings or by mimicking the stimulation thought to be salient in utero. Some study designs have incorporated the premature infant's mother into the intervention procedures, hoping to facilitate early interactional exchanges (Powell, 1974).

Increased handling of the premature infant has been introduced in several studies. Short-term increments in weight gain (Solkoff et al., 1969), higher Bayley scores at 4 months (Powell, 1974), appropriate loss of primitive reflexes (Rice, 1977), and higher Brazelton scores (Scarr-Salapatek and Williams, 1973) were found in these studies, and these gains were attributed to handling.

More complex interventions have involved the provision of cross-modal stimulation thought to be present in utero. Both Kramer and Pierpont (1976) and Barnard (1973, 1980) supplied waterbeds, rocking, and a recorded heartbeat sound to enhance development in premature infants. Kramer and Pierpont found significant gains in weight and head circumference for their experimental group, and Barnard (1973) noted improved sleep cycling.

Many other intervention strategies have been attempted, each of which was designed to supplement an assumed lack of stimulation. Cornell and Gottfried (1976) provided a comprehensive review of these studies. *They were unable to find a single study* in which the ecology of the premature infant was assessed prior to the intervention, nor were there any attempts to match stimulation levels to individual differences in sensory thresholds. Charlesworth (1977) stated an objection to this intervention approach in strong terms:

> Assumptions must underlie most human deprivation/enrichment research, but the nature and degree of variation characterizing behavior and the environment in which it takes place have not been defined and spelled out in sufficient detail, and maybe never will be, given man's great ability and nouveaumaniacal compulsion to change things at an astounding rate. (p. 12)

The lack of an ecological perspective prior to intervention is not just a theoretical concern. A narrow focus on manipulated variables may permit deleterious side effects to go unnoticed. Especially when this situation is paired with a "package" approach to intervention, when a stimulus set is presented to an experimental group without regard to individual sensory capacities, harmful overstimulation may result (Bromwich, 1977). As Als et al. (1980) described, premature infants of the same gestational age may show a wide range of responses to even low levels of stimulation, varying from physiologic distress (e.g., apnea) to alert attention. Unless the environment at baseline is understood, the introduction of stimulation as an intervention involves arbitrary and unscientific decisions with potentially harmful effects on the immature infant.

Techniques of Describing NICU Environments

Several studies published since Cornell and Gottfried's review cited their suggested mapping of the NICU environment as a goal. Lawson et al. (1977) time-sampled every fifteenth minute in an NICU, recording speech and nonspeech sounds, handling, illumination levels, and sound pressure levels. Although the authors were able to highlight patterns of certain environmental stimuli, the general nature of the categories (e.g., handling was not differentiated as being gentle or aversive), arbitrary sampling of the behavior stream, and lack of infant variables prohibit use of these data as ecological descriptors of an NICU environment.

A continuous-interval recording technique was used by Gaiter et al. (1981) to record the occurrence of a variety of caregiver and infant behaviors and background auditory variables during intensive, intermediate, and predischarge care. Gottfried et al. (1981) recorded whether a set of caregiving and background auditory variables occurred in three 1-minute time intervals for each hour of 3 days. Both Gaiter et al. (1981) and Gottfried et al. (1981) also presented sound level and light meter data to describe these important aspects of the physical environment.

The data presented in all of the studies reviewed here reported the *frequency of intervals* in which at least one occurrence of a behavior was observed. However, many of the behaviors recorded, such as caregiver vocalization, handling, or infant looking, also have *durations*. The interval recording techniques provided neither an accurate frequency count of a behavior's occurrence nor the length of time that behaviors occurred. Data that reflect the durations of events may provide a better picture of a preterm infant's experience in an NICU environment.

Another point to be made about interval recording procedures is that the *sequence* of events within an interval is lost. Does caregiver handling precede or follow an infant's cry? Does a feeding interaction begin before or after an infant awakens? One way to answer these types of questions is to record events continuously in real time. The duration of events can thus be recorded and their sequence preserved.

The study described below was designed to provide some answers to the questions raised by Cornell and Gottfried (1976) regarding the ecology of an NICU. Data on a wide variety of animate and inanimate events were recorded continuously in real time so that the duration of events could be reported. The order of infant, caregiver, and auditory events was preserved so that sequential analyses could be performed to describe infant and environmental events in terms of their contingent responsiveness.

Method

Subjects

The subjects were 35 infants who were hospitalized at the Neonatal Special Care Nursery at the University of Kansas Medical Center, Kansas City, from October, 1979 to April, 1980. This Level III nursery accommodates 20 infants at a time and has about 350 admissions per year. All of the infants had in common the following variables: they weighed less than 2500 grams, were born at less than 37 weeks gestation, and the principle reason for their admission to the nursery was prematurity. No attempt was made to limit the sample with regard to the degree of prematurity, severity of initial illness, or length of critical care. The illness variables were recorded and the relationships between them and the observed environmental parameters were analyzed (this is described later). The mean birth weight of the sample was 1648 grams ($SD = 601$ grams). The mean gestational age was 31 weeks ($SD = 3$ weeks), and they averaged 21 days of age ($SD = 17$ days) at the time they were observed.

The infants were observed during the intermediate care phase of their hospital stay, meaning that they were no longer receiving mechanical ventilatory assistance or extra oxygen in the isolette and had not yet been moved to a crib in the "graduate care" side of the nursery. This decision about the timing of the observations was made for two reasons. First, the authors were interested in coding observable behavioral responses of the infant to environmental stimuli. Infants in intermediate care are less likely to have their eyes covered for phototherapy and are more likely to be alert and behaviorally responsive to their surroundings than infants in critical condition. Second, this intermediate care period is generally the longest phase of a premature infant's hospital stay.

Procedures

Staff Education The goals of the study required unobtrusive observations of infant and staff behavior in a busy clinical facility. In order to accomplish this task, it was necessary to educate the nurses, doctors, and parents about the purposes and procedures of the study. The nonjudgmental, descriptive nature of the study was stressed, and the staff and parents were shown the electronic data collector in informal discussions and staff meetings. The importance of this staff education phase of the study cannot be overemphasized.

The Observation Code A large number of infant, caregiver, and background environmental variables were recorded continuously by an observer standing near the infant's isolette (see Table 5.1). The observation code consists of 10 categories, within which the codes are mutually exclusive and exhaustive. This code has been used in studies of term infants from the newborn period (Linn and Horowitz, 1983) through 1 month of age (Buddin, 1982), but was developed to be applicable also for use in an intensive care setting. Six categories were coded continuously throughout the hour-long sessions: infant state,[1] infant visual and vocal behavior, proximity of a caregiver to the infant, two categories describing the type of background sounds available, and a category descriptive of the mobiles and toys at which the infant might look. Then, when an interaction began, the observer also recorded the type of caregiver attention, the identity of the caregiver, and the nature of the caregiver's tactile, visual, and vocal stimulation of the infant.

Observer Training and Reliability Extensive observer training was required. Two observers were trained for approximately 75 hours each until two reliable sessions were achieved for each observer. An agreement was counted when an event was coded by both observers within 4 seconds of each other. This criterion for agreement was determined empirically during the observer training sessions as the minimum discrepancy that the observers could consistently achieve. Disagreements included all jointly coded events in which times were more discrepant than 4 seconds plus all coding omissions from either record. The formula used to calculate percentage of agreement was to double the number of agreements, divide it by the total number of codes entered by both observers, and multiply that figure by 100. The criterion level of agreement established for observer reliability in this "live" coding situation was an 80% agreement across all categories, with no single category falling below 70% agreement. (Table 5.1 shows the mean reliabilities for each category.) Observer agreement was rechecked three times during the data collection period.

---

[1] An attempt was made to use the six states from the Neonatal Behavioral Assessment Scale (Brazelton, 1973), but the premature infants tended to present ambiguous state cues, depending on whether the eyes or body activity were monitored (e.g., crying with no body activity or quiet sleep with partially opened eyes) so that these dimensions were separated in Code Category 1.

Table 5.1. The observation code[a].

1 Infant State (82%)[b]	2 Infant Behavior (85%)	3 Proximal Stimulation (92%)
11 Eyes closed/no activity	21 Vocalize	31 Vestibular
12 Eyes closed/activity	22 Look at caregiver	32 Touch gentle
13 Eyes drowsy/no activity	23 Vocalize/look	33 Vigorous-aversive
14 Eyes drowsy/activity	24 Distress vocalize	34 Vestibular/touch gentle
15 Eyes open/no activity	25 Distress/look at caregiver	35 Vestibular/aversive
16 Eyes open/activity	26 Reject nipple	36 Touch/aversive
	27 Reject nipple/vocalize	37 Vestibular/touch gentle/aversive
	28 Reject nipple/distress	3H None
	29 Look at toy	
	20 Look at toy/positive vocalization	
	2* Look at toy/distress vocalization	
	2H None	

4 Animate Auditory (87%)	5 Inanimate Auditory (91%)	6 Toys (100%)
41 Person speaking	51 Activity pattern	61 Toy/mobile
42 Infant crying	52 Mechanical	62 Toy—mobile moving
43 Person speaking/infant crying	53 Short	63 Toy—mobile sound
4H None	54 Musical	64 Toy—mobile moving/sound
	55 Activity/mechanical	6* New toy
	56 Activity/music	6H None
	57 Mechanical/music	
	58 Mechanical/music/activity	
	5H None	

C Caregiver (96%)

C1	Mother
C2	Father
C3	Nurse
C4	Doctor
C5	Therapist or technician
C6	Sibling
C7	Other adult
C8	Multiple
C*	New person
CH	None

7 Setting (85%)

71	Cradle/fondle/soothe/induce sleep
72	Nipple feeding
73	Burp/break/relax from feeding
74	Groom/diaper/dress
75	Medical—vital signs
76	Non-care attention
77	Interruption
78	Gavage feeding
79	Peripheral attention
70	Suctioning
7*	Needle/heelstick
7H	None

8 Proximity of Caregiver (95%)

81	Cuddle
82	Hold
83	Cuddle/enface
84	Hold/enface
85	In arm's reach
86	In room
87	In arm's reach/enface
8H	None

9 Distal Stimulation (80%)

91	Vocalize
92	Look
94	Vocalize/look
9H	None

[a] Linn, P. L, Daily, D. K., and Johns, B. J. 1978. Code for naturalistic observations of newborn environments. Manual available from the Infant Laboratory, Haworth Hall, University of Kansas, Lawrence, KA 66045.
[b] Percentage of agreement within each category; mean of eight reliability sessions.

Data Collection Period Each of the 35 infants was observed for the 8 daytime hours between 9 AM and 5 PM. These 8 observation hours were spread across 3 consecutive days, with no observer coding for more than 1 hour without a break. For each observation hour, the observer would stand quietly, out of the infant's visual field and as close to the infant's isolette as possible without interfering with the infant's care. Four of the code categories were entered first in a simultaneous manner (Infant State, Identity of Caregiver, Setting, and Proximity of Caregiver), and then the observer began 60 minutes of sequentially coding the onset and offset of the behaviors and events listed in Table 5.1 by punching their numeric equivalents into the keyboard of a Datamyte (Electro/General Corporation) electronic data collector. For example:

> An observer watches through the portals of the isolette as a nurse nipple-feeds a drowsy infant. The observer records the sequence C3–72–13–85. As the nurse speaks to the baby and the baby looks at her, the sequence 94–22 is added. The Datamyte stores each code and the elapsed time associated with it, resolved to 0.6 seconds. Following the observation session, the observer connects the Datamyte to a computer terminal and transmits the timed, sequential record of the session directly to the computer for storage and data analysis.

The timed, sequential coding procedure permitted two general types of data to be analyzed. Since the onset and offset of each code were recorded, the total *durations* of each of the events listed in Table 5.1 could be derived. These data reflect how time was filled with the various events in question during the daytime hours in the NICU. Descriptive graphs, a preterm/term comparison, analyses comparing two different nurseries, analyses of staff size, and infant individual differences all utilize the duration data. The continuously coded, timed data also allow a *sequential* analysis of events based on the conditional probability that one event will follow another within a certain time frame. This sequential analysis resulted in descriptions of nurse and infant responsivity during their interactions in the nursery.

Results and Discussion

Descriptive Data

A visual presentation of the durations of the coded behaviors and events is shown in Figure 5.1. All categories are shown except for Infant Visual and

Vocal Behavior and Setting; the average durations of the individual codes in these two categories were all low and could not be represented clearly as graphs. The data shown are the percentages of each observation hour that each code was turned "on," based on the mean durations across all 35 infants.

Within each code category, two sources of variability can be observed, just as in a repeated measures ANOVA design. First, the amounts of the specific codes in the category vary. Note that the relative order of the code durations is often maintained, regardless of the time of the observation. For example, in Figure 5.1A, Eyes Closed/Quiet Activity was the most common infant state observed across all daytime hours, while the Open Eyes/Active state was rarely observed at any time of the day.

Second, hour-to-hour variability in the durations of specific codes can also be observed. Some knowledge of the daily schedule in the nursery is helpful in interpreting this source of variability. For example, the duration of painful stimulation (Figure 5.1D) was highest between 9 AM and 10 AM, when the heelsticks for laboratory analysis of blood samples were done. Most of the hour-to-hour variability of all the codes occurred between 9 AM and 10 AM when the laboratory work was done on the infants and teaching rounds occurred, at 12 noon when staffing patterns changed to accommodate the noon meal, and between 3 PM and 4 PM when the nursing shift changed.

The descriptive data were surprising in some respects and confirmed current assumptions about an NICU environment in other respects. Surprising results included the findings that, although toys were usually placed in the infant's isolettes, the infants were usually positioned so that the toys were not visible (see Figure 5.1F); and that the amount of painful/aversive tactile stimulation was actually quite low (see Figure 5.1D), although the observer's judgment about what is painful or aversive may not equal the infant's perceptions. The small amount of caregiver interaction time (Figure 5.1B and C), touching and vestibular contact (Figure 5.1D), and talking to the infant (Figure 5.1E) and the large number of mechanical sounds in the environment (Figure 5.1H) supported popular notions about the ecology of an NICU.

Ecological data such as these provide insights into the patterns of stimulation available to the premature infants in an NICU. They serve as baseline measurements of the levels of various environmental parameters and are necessary starting points for individuals interested in designing NICU interventions. For example, if an intervention in the University of Kansas Special Care Nursery were instituted, an individual might decide

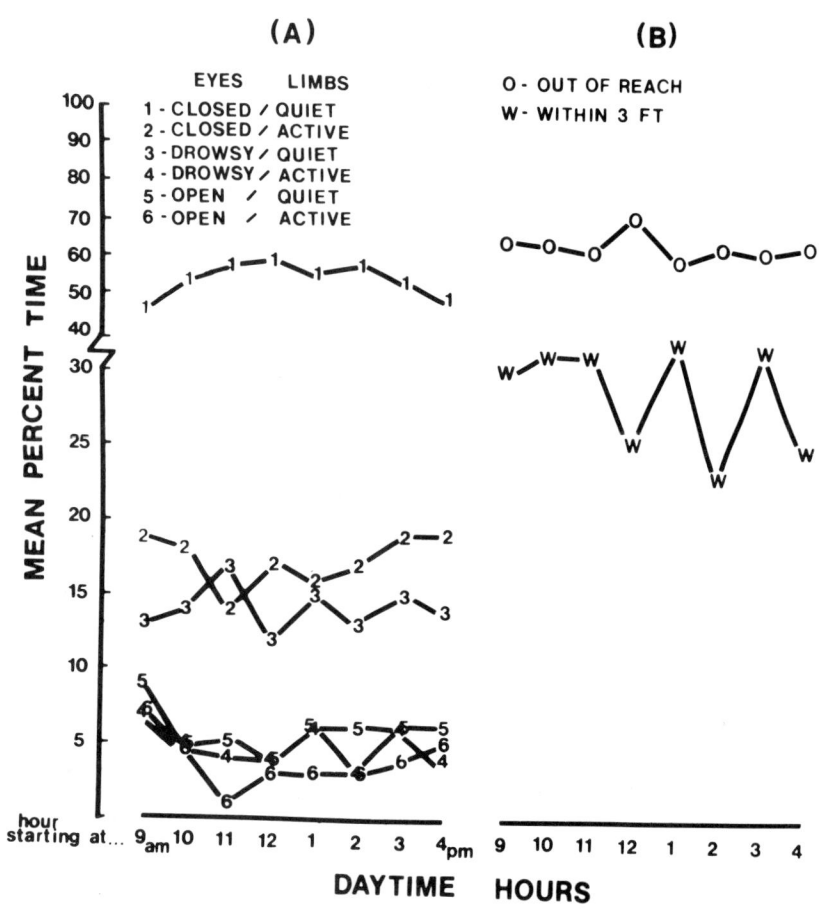

Figure 5.1A-B. Mean percentage of 8 hour-long observation sessions during which Infant State (A) and Caregiver Proximity (B) (see Table 5.1) were recorded and averaged across 35 infants.

against the addition of tape-recorded language stimulation, given the large number of speech sounds already available in the nursery. The provision of toys and mobiles in the infant's isolette should be accompanied by instructions to the staff to maintain them within the infant's visual field. Infants' isolettes might be rotated away from another isolette with a respirator in order to reduce the high level of repetitive mechanical sounds in the environment.

However, the ecological data presented here are limited in several important aspects. First, it is not known how the measurements of these events might vary from one NICU to the next (although some insight into

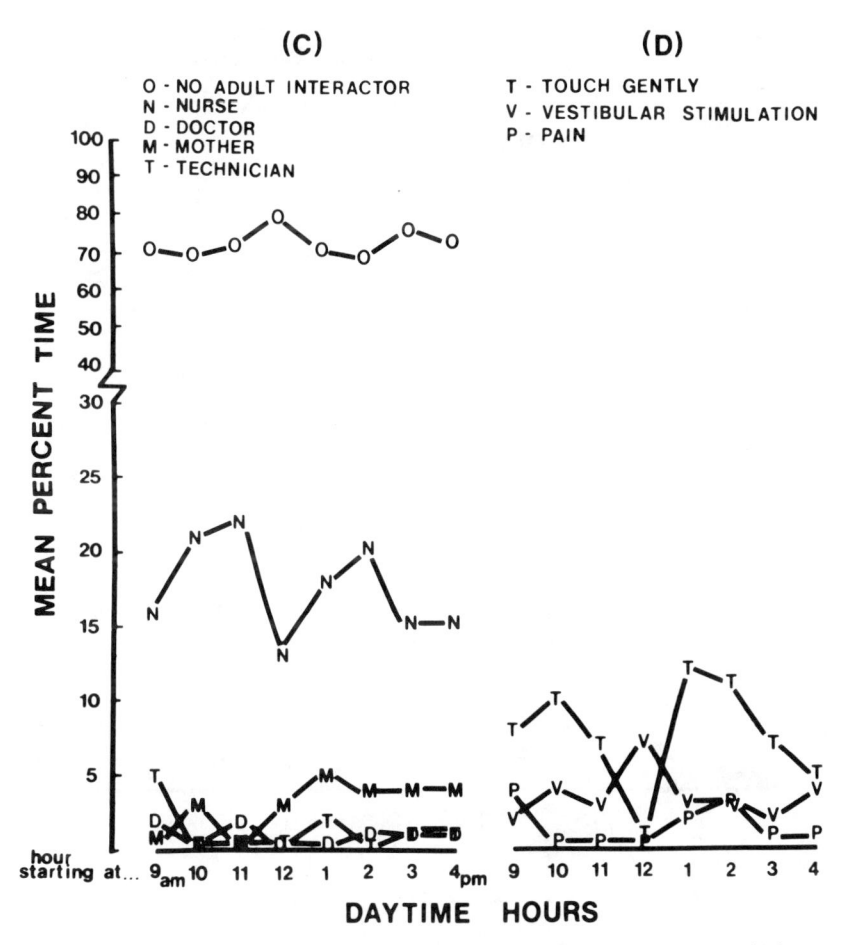

Figure 5.1C-D. Mean percentage of 8 hour-long observation sessions during which Caregiver Identity (C) and Proximal Stimulation (D) (see Table 5.1) were recorded and averaged across 35 infants.

this question is provided in the next section). Second, the data were collected during the daytime hours, while evening and nighttime hours (when many parents visit) were not sampled. Third, although the coding scheme is comprehensive, it does not include other possibly important aspects of environmental input, such as changes in illumination levels, and other visual stimuli. Finally, the data were collected only during the intermediate care phase of the infants' stay. Gaiter et al. (1981) found significant differences in environmental events and infant behaviors occurring in critical, intermediate, and predischarge care.

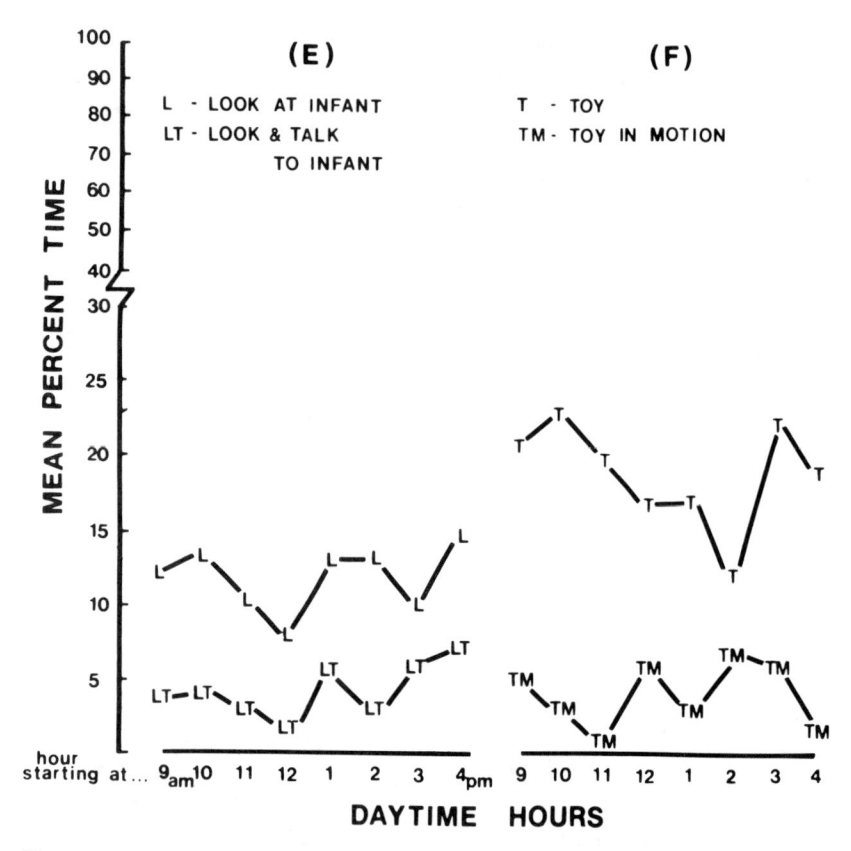

Figure 5.1E-F. Mean percentage of 8 hour-long observation sessions during which Distal Stimulation (E) and Toy in Visual Field (F) (see Table 5.1) were recorded and averaged across 35 infants.

Comparison across Two Physical Settings

One of the major concerns about the usefulness of environmental measurements as presented here is the degree to which the data might be generalized across different NICU settings. Intensive care facilities for young infants differ along a variety of dimensions that may affect the levels of environmental variables. These variables include: 1) the physical layout of the unit; 2) the characteristics of the staff (size, level of training, or the degree to which certain medical or developmental issues are stressed); 3) characteristics of the infant population served by the unit (e.g., transported versus in-born or types of illness treated); and 4)

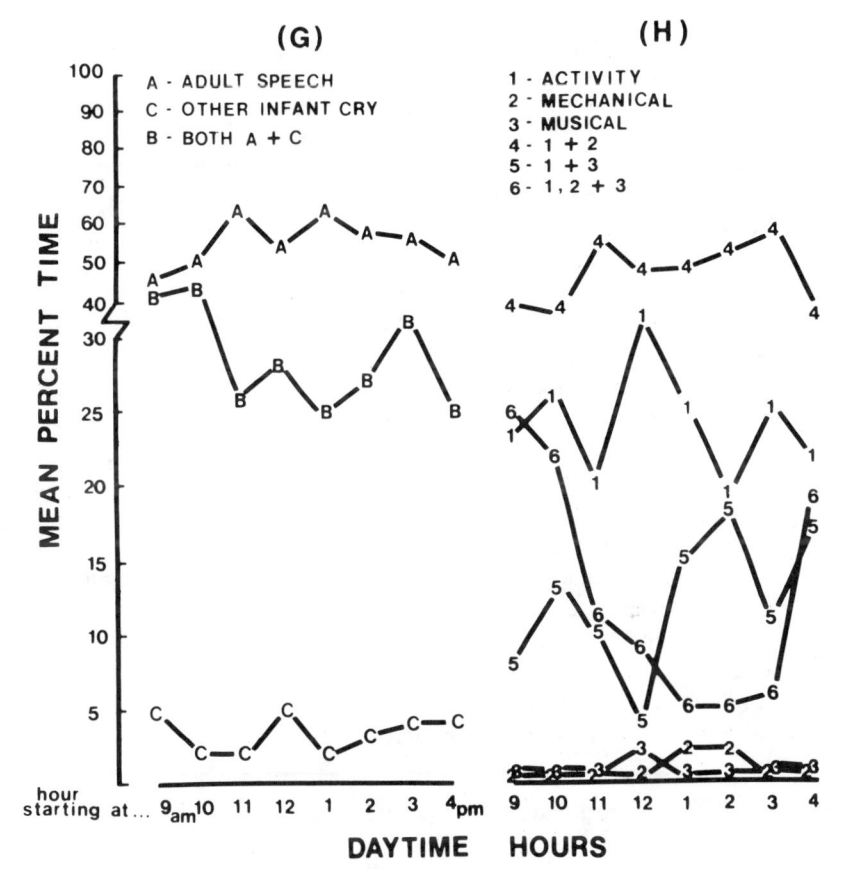

Figure 5.1G-H. Mean percentage of 8 hour-long observation sessions during which Background Sounds—Animate (G) and Background Sounds—Inanimate (H) (see Table 5.1) were recorded and averaged across 35 infants.

preferred techniques of treatment as they vary from one institution to another (e.g., use of enclosed incubators versus open radiant heaters). Most NICUs differ from one another along *all* of these dimensions, complicating any comparisons across facilities.

In the study of the NICU reported here, a unique opportunity became available that permitted the study of changes in the physical layout of the unit, with no change in staff or infant population characteristics. After data collection had begun, the University of Kansas Special Care Nursery moved from small, cramped quarters to a spacious unit in a new hospital building. In the old nursery, the intensive and intermediate care unit was L-shaped, approximately 753 square feet, with the graduate care nursery across the hall. The new facility combined three levels of care in one large, rectangular room, covering approximately 3024 square feet.

Eight hours of observations were completed on each of 6 infants in the old nursery before the move took place. The 6 infants observed in the new nursery who best matched the first 6 infants in terms of birth weight, gestational age, and age at observation were selected for comparison. The total durations of each of the coded variables, summed across 8 hours of observation, were compared across the two sets of observations using analyses of variance with nursery location as the independent variable. Staff and general characteristics of the infant population were identical for both sets of observations. It was hypothesized that because of the increase in space (which resulted in a greater separation between isolettes and a different arrangement of them), variables such as Proximity of Caregiver might differ in the two settings, perhaps influencing caregiver looking at the infants (Distal Stimulation) and Infant State.

The results of this analysis were surprising in that *no* significant differences between the two NICU locations were found for any of the codes. From this fortuitous opportunity, it was concluded that behavioral differences in the medical staff and the nature of the patient population served by the unit are more likely than physical characteristics of NICU facilities to contribute to variability across NICU settings.

Staffing Patterns and Social Interactions

It may be that in many NICUs the amount of *social* interaction between the staff and the infants (looking, talking, and touching that are not directly related to medical or other caregiving procedures) is influenced by the number of staff available per infant.

Two variables that were recorded during each of the 280 observation sessions were: 1) the number of staff (doctors and nurses) available during that hour of that day; and 2) the number of infants receiving care. A staff-infant ratio was derived for each observation hour, and that ratio was correlated with the total duration of social attention (see Table 5.1, Observation Code 76) recorded during that hour. It was predicted that the correlation would be positive and significant; the higher the staff-infant ratio, the more time each staff member would have to engage the infants in social interactions.

The Pearson *r* resulting from this analysis was $-.06$, a nonsignificant result. Contrary to the authors' intuitive feelings, it seems that in the NICU studied here the amount of time that the staff spent in social interactions with the infants was not related to staff-infant ratios. In a chronically understaffed nursery, when the number of infants in the unit drops and the pressure of patient needs relents somewhat, the personnel may tend to withdraw. As suggested below, variables other than staff-infant ratio, such as infant characteristics or staff perception of the importance of social contact, may play a more important role in regulating social interactions with infants in an NICU.

Preterm/Term Comparison

The descriptive data presented to this point involve percentages of observed time that several variables occurred in the NICU environment. The levels of each of the variables may be difficult to interpret without a reference point, such as "How much painful stimulation is a 'small amount'?" or "How often do mechanical sounds need to be recorded to consider that sound source 'excessive'?" One problem is the lack of a suitable group to compare with hospitalized premature infants. With few exceptions, there are no healthy infants of a similar gestational and chronologic age available for comparison with the hospitalized premature infant.

As part of an ongoing study of infants and environments, data were collected using the same Observation Codes as in Table 5.1 during the same 8 daytime hours in the homes of 20 term lower-class infants (Hollingshead's two lowest classes from Myers et al., 1968) when they were 1 month old. A lower-class home environment may not provide an ideal comparison to the NICU situation, yet this is one type of term infant environment to which many NICU graduates go and in which comparable data have been collected and analyzed.

Although a comparison between NICU and term environments can be useful, caution should be used in interpreting this analysis. On the one hand, *both* postnatal environments should be expected to provide developmentally facilitative opportunities for the infants who experience them. However, those committed to interventions in preterm environments should be cautious about duplicating term levels of stimulation in the NICU without regard to individual differences in infants. As is evident from the descriptions of preterm behavioral organization presented by Als and her colleagues (e.g., Als et al., 1980), many preterm infants cannot handle levels of stimulation that are appropriate for term infants. Therefore, these term data are presented to provide points of comparison rather than as goals to achieve in NICU interventions.

In order to provide the preterm/term comparison, the durations of each code were first totaled for the 8 observation hours for each infant. The means were derived for the preterm and the term infants, and simple *t*-tests were used to determine whether the means were significantly different. Four of the code categories were selected to demonstrate this comparison, and the means were transformed to percentages of the 8 observation hours, as shown in Figures 5.2 to 5.5. Figure 5.2 contrasts the three types of animate background sounds that were coded in the preterm NICU environment (PT) and the full-term home environment (FT). The mean percentage of the 8 observation hours in which adult speech was salient to the observer standing near the infant was significantly greater ($t = 4.27, p < .001$) in the NICU environment than in the term homes. The amount of time in which the sound of another infant's crying was recorded was also significantly different in the two settings ($t = 2.51, p < .05$), as was the combination of adult speech and infant cries ($t = 15.28, p < .001$). It may be that some of these sounds do not reach the preterm infants because they are attenuated by the walls of the isolette, although Gottfried et al. (1981) found nearly identical sound levels both inside and outside isolettes.

The types of inanimate background sounds also contrast the two environments. As shown in Figure 5.3, the most prevalent sound pattern in the NICU environment was a combination of nonspecific activity sounds and the repetitious, invariant mechanical sounds of the respirator and monitoring equipment (Activity + Mechanical) ($t = 9.50, p < .001$). Lower-class homes typically provided a background of nonspecific activity and musical or other patterned sounds, such as a radio or TV (Activity + Musical) ($t = 8.49, p < .001$). Nonspecific activity sounds were more likely to occur alone in the NICU than in the homes ($t = 4.00, p < .001$), and musical sounds occurred more in the homes than in the NICU ($t = 7.40, p < .001$). Only the mean percentages of mechanical sounds occurring alone were low in both settings, and the difference between the settings was nonsignificant ($t = 1.74$, NS).

The type and amount of tactile stimulation provided by caregivers in the two environments are shown in Figure 5.4. Although the amounts of gentle touching of the infants were almost equal in the two environments ($t = 0.03$, NS), term infants received significantly more vestibular stimulation ($t = 5.77, p < .001$), and the combination of vestibular and touching stimulation ($t = 3.54, p < .001$). Given the large amount of vestibular stimulation to which the fetus is subjected in utero, it is interesting to speculate on the possible effects of the low levels of vestibular movement on the premature infant in this NICU environment.

Differences in environmental stimulation of preterm and term infants may be attributable in part to differences in infant behavior that tend to "signal" a need or otherwise instigate or perpetuate an interaction with the caregiver. Figure 5.5 shows that term infants were found to vocalize ($t = 9.76, p < .001$), look at the caregiver ($t = 5.74, p < .001$), and cry ($t = 2.17, p < .05$) more than the preterm infants. These data clearly

Ecological Description   **101**

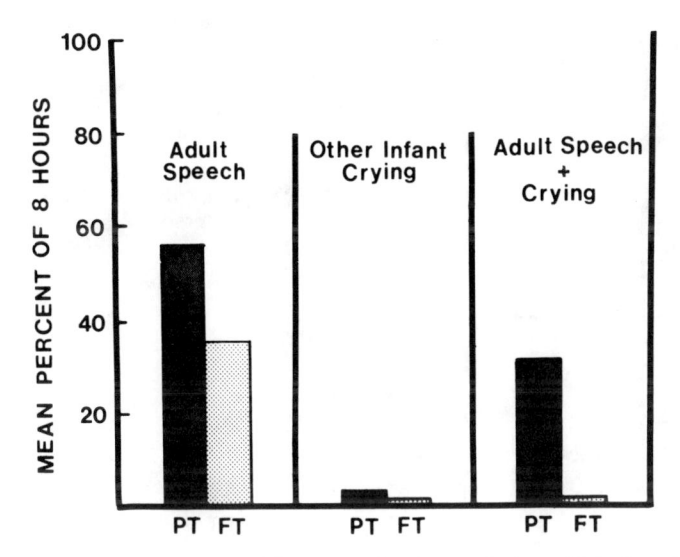

Figure 5.2. Mean percentages of 8 observation hours during which three kinds of animate background sounds were recorded, averaged across 35 preterm infants (PT) in an NICU environment and 20 full-term (FT) infants in home environments.

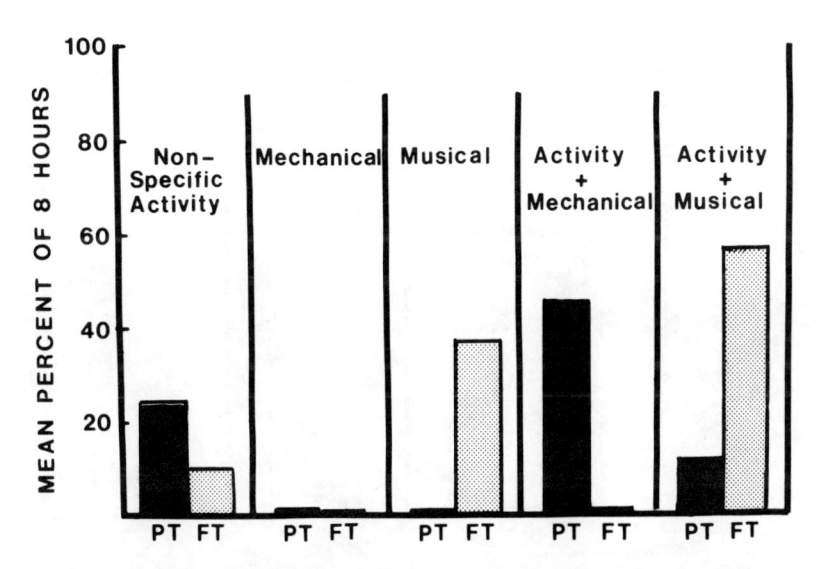

Figure 5.3. Mean percentages of 8 observation hours during which five kinds of inanimate background sounds were recorded and averaged across 35 preterm infants (PT) in an NICU environment and 20 full-term (FT) infants in home environments.

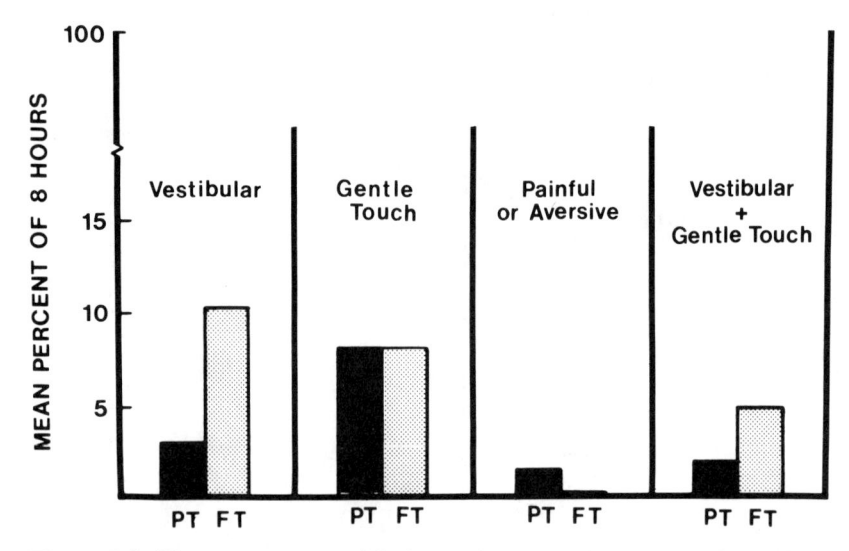

Figure 5.4. Mean percentages of 8 observation hours during which four kinds of tactile stimulation were recorded and averaged across 35 preterm infants (PT) in an NICU environment and 20 full-term (FT) infants in home environments.

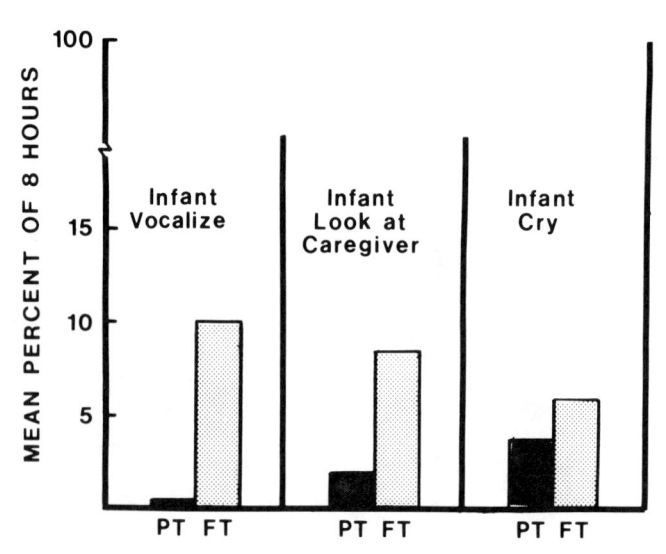

Figure 5.5. Mean percentages of 8 observation hours during which three infant behaviors were recorded and averaged across 35 preterm infants (PT) in an NICU environment and 20 full-term (FT) infants in home environments.

show the differences between preterm and term infants in the occurrence of behaviors that typically elicit social and caregiving responses from adults, and may be useful in teaching both NICU staff members and parents what they can expect from preterm infants.

Individual Differences

The data described so far are based on means across the 35 preterm infants in the sample. Because the preterm sample represented a heterogeneous group with respect to medical and physical histories it might be asked whether the observed levels of environmental events and caregiver and infant behaviors were related to the medical and physical characteristics of the infant. The next analysis was designed to address these questions of individual differences. Estimated gestational age (EGA), birth weight, age at observation, and degree of illness were selected as predictors of the total durations (summed across the 8 observation hours) of a subset of coded variables. A stepwise multiple regression technique was chosen to: 1) assess the added contribution of each predictor; and 2) allow the predictor variables to enter the regression equation based on the amount of variance they explained.

In order to categorize the infants by their degree of illness, two neonatologists who were familiar with the medical histories of the infants independently categorized each of the 35 preterms into one of the four illness classifications, based on their clinical judgment of the severity of the infant's initial disease. The categories were: 1) least ill, 2) intermediate degree of illness, 3) critically ill—good chance of survival, 4) critically ill—chance of survival questioned. The agreement between the physicians for exact placement of the 35 infants in the illness categories was 74%.

Rather than try to predict the durations of all of the coded events from the medical background variables, only 17 codes were chosen. These codes were significantly related to the illness groups (by an analysis of variance) or significantly correlated with EGA, birth weight, or age at observation. It is important to note that the selection of criterion (code) variables was based on a significant relationship to one or more predictors. The regression analysis reported here serves to evaluate the relative importance of the predictors to each other. The durations of these 17 coded events were each used as the criterion in separate regression analyses. Table 5.2 lists the best predictors of the coded variables as judged by a significant increase in explained variance attributable to that predictor.

The neonatologists' judgment about whether or not the infant was in the Least Ill category (ILL 1) was the best predictor of seven of the coded

Table 5.2. Significant first predictors of coded events.

ILL 1[a]	Age at observation	EGA
Eyes closed/no activity (11[b]/ILL 2[c])	Eyes open/no activity (15/Birth weight)	Vestibular (31)
Eyes drowsy/no activity (13)	Eyes open/activity (16/Birth weight)	Vestibular/touch gentle (34)
Eyes drowsy/activity (14/ILL 2)	Toy—mobile moving/sound (64/EGA)	Nipple feeding (72/ILL 2)
Vigorous-aversive (33)	Gavage feeding (78)	Burp/break/relax from feeding (73)
Peripheral attention (79)		Doctor (C4)
Heelstick (7*)		
Nurse (C3)		

[a] The illness categories (ILL 1, ILL 2, and ILL 3) were entered as three "dummy variables" (i.e., subjects were coded as either in or not in that category). ILL 4 was the "reference category," i.e., it was not entered as a predictor per se because it was explained by the other three variables.
[b] Code number of observed event (see Table 5.1).
[c] Variable that was a second significant predictor in the regression equation.

events, ranging from closed eye and drowsy states to the likelihood of specific medical procedures (Heelstick) and the attention of the nurse. The infant's EGA predicted five of the coded events, and the infant's age at observation predicted four events. Birth weight and placement in the "intermediate" illness category (ILL 2) were significant secondary predictors in some cases. It should be noted that the classifications of the infants according to degree of illness were arrived at by "clinical gestalt" rather than objective risk scoring. Further analyses are planned to compare the usefulness of objective risk scoring systems versus clinical categories in differentiating preterms infants' NICU experiences and subsequent developmental outcomes. However, at this point it can be stated that, although the infants were over their critical illness by the time the observations were made, there seemed to be "carryover" effects of factors such as the infant's initial medical complications and degree of prematurity on the infant's subsequent level of arousal and on the patterns of staff attention to the infant.

Contingent Responsivity of Caregivers and Infants

Because the data reported in this study were recorded continuously in real time, the sequences of behaviors could be described, and questions about the contingent responsiveness of the caregivers to the infants and the infants to their caregivers could be addressed. In order to describe and evaluate this mutual responsivity, a method was used to plot the probability of one variable following another (a *conditional probability*) across a series of time intervals, called *time lags* (Sackett, 1979). For example, one behavior such as Infant Cry can be selected as the criterion behavior, and the probability that a matching behavior, such as Caregiver Talking, will follow any instance of the criterion can be assessed. This conditional probability of "caregiver talking, given infant crying" can be considered significantly different from chance if it exceeds or falls below a confidence interval. The confidence interval is based on the simple probability that caregiver talking will occur at any point during the session.

An example of a graph in which a caregiver tends to provide contingent vocal responses to an infant's cries is shown in Figure 5.6. On the ordinate are the conditional probabilities, ranging from 0.0 to 1.0. The abscissa specifies the time lags (which are simply sequential intervals of time following the onset of the criterion behavior), each lasting 5 seconds in this case. The band across the middle of the graph is the .05 confidence interval of caregiver speech that occurs regardless of infant cries. Given that the infant cries at time lag 0, the caregiver represented in Figure 5.6

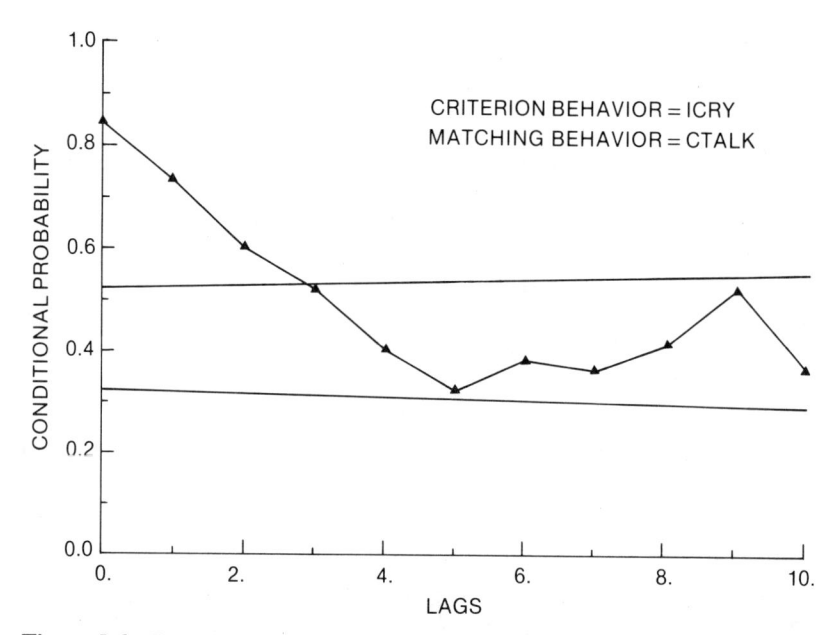

Figure 5.6. Conditional probability of caregiver talk, given infant cry, for ten 5-second time lags. The band across the middle of the graph (between solid lines) represents the .05 confidence interval of caregiver talk occurring regardless of infant cries. The probability that the caregiver will talk falls above the confidence interval, indicating a contingent response.

shows a heightened probability of talking within the same time lag and the two following lags. In other words, this caregiver showed a significant tendency to speak within about 10 seconds (two time lags) of the infant's cry. The probabilities fall within the chance range in subsequent lags. An example of a graph in which the caregiver does not respond above or below chance levels is shown in Figure 5.7. In this case, the caregiver did not have a greater tendency to speak following the infant's cry.

In order to determine if the caregivers in the NICU were contingently responsive to the infants, graphs such as those in Figures 5.6 and 5.7 were plotted for each of the 35 preterm infants in the sample. First, from the 8 hour-long sessions, the observation session that included the longest interaction was selected. Three infant behaviors were chosen (Infant Positive Vocalizations, Looks at the Caregiver, and Distress Vocalizations) that often cue an adult to interact with an infant. These were the *criterion behaviors*. Caregiver Vocalizations to, Looking at, and Touching the infant were selected as likely responses, or *matching behaviors*.

Ecological Description 107

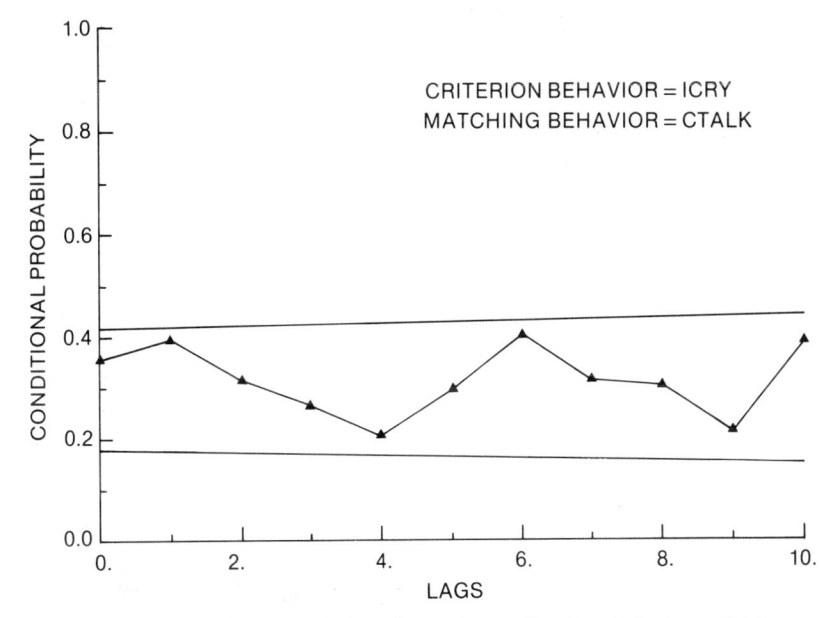

Figure 5.7. Conditional probability of caregiver talk, given infant cry, for ten 5-second time lags. The band across the middle of the graph (between solid lines) represents the .05 confidence interval of caregiver talk occurring regardless of infant cries. The probability that the caregiver will talk does not extend outside the confidence interval, indicating no contingent response.

One conclusion from this analysis was that the rates of these infant behaviors in the preterm sample were very low. Indeed, 49% of the infants never vocalized, 37% never looked at the caregiver, and 29% never cried during these selected observations. These premature infants, who averaged 3 weeks of age, rarely gave the caregivers a chance to respond contingently. For those infants who did display these vocal and visual behaviors, 80% to 100% (depending on the criterion behavior selected) were responded to contingently by the caregivers.

Another question to ask of these NICU interactions was how responsive the *infants* were to their caregivers. In this case Caregiver Vocalizations, Looking, and Touching were the criterion behaviors, and the probability that the infant would look at the caregiver was assessed. Inspection of the probability graphs revealed that 63% of the infants responded visually to at least one of the three caregiver criterion behaviors. The remaining 37% of the infants never looked at their caregivers above the chance level, despite the caregivers' looking, talking, and touching. Although nurses in this study provided social stimulation to the infants, many of the infants did not respond. A consistent lack of reinforcement for nurses combined with high stress levels in intensive care settings may provide important clues to nurse burnout (Marshall and Kasman, 1980).

Summary and Conclusions

This observation study of preterm infants in one NICU has provided a large amount of data descriptive of the quantity of social, auditory, and visual stimulation available during 8 daytime hours. These descriptive data, especially when compared with similar data collected on a term sample, confirm a point made by Cornell and Gottfried in their 1976 review: the NICU environment cannot be globally described as either "deprived" or "overstimulating" when compared to a term environment. For some variables, such as the amount of noncontingent adult speech in the background, the NICU environment greatly exceeded the home environment observed. Other variables, such as touching or vestibular stimulation, were equal in the two settings or were observed at a lower level in the NICU than in the homes.

One subgroup of the coded variables, including infant state, vestibular stimulation, nurse versus doctor attention, and specific caregiving actions, was related to individual clinical characteristics, including degree of illness, age at observation, and EGA. Clearly, different preterm infants are subject to different levels of stimulation within one NICU and show different levels of arousal and responsivity to that environment. However, an important question that remains unanswered is whether these differences in caregiver attention and infant behavior are functional in determining preterm infant developmental outcome. A subsequent study must combine NICU environmental measurements with a longitudinal design to answer these questions.

The method of coding infant and caregiver behaviors in their proper order in "real time" was necessary in order to describe the contingent responsiveness of the caregivers to the infants and the infants to their caregivers. Durations of events in an NICU environment are important descriptors of "a day in the life" of the premature infant.

From the descriptive data, it is clear that the NICU environment is very different from the home environment observed. This was expected. The term infant does not "time share" the caregiver's attention with so many other infants, and the preterm infant is in an environment designed for medical intervention. A term infant in a home, even when fed according to a schedule, tends to run the show, at least for the first couple of months, but from the hourly patterns in Figure 5.1 it is clear that the preterm infant's day depends on the nursery schedule that the adults impose. Care of the preterm baby is individualized to some extent, as the Degree of Illness analysis showed, but, in general, a schedule of feeding, lab work, bathing, and play-time dictate the day. Other NICUs may differ in this regard—the "old nursery-new nursery" analysis seemed to indicate that differences across nurseries may be attributable to the staff, not the physical layout. The extent to which the staff facilitate social and cognitive development of the babies depends on many factors (e.g., knowledge, time). The fact that the nurses did not increase their social attention to the infants when they had fewer infants assigned to them indicates that other pressures on them, their "self-preservation" from emotional investments in these babies, and the priority they give, or are allowed to give, to social attention may be critical factors.

From the sequential analysis it was clear that the contingent responsiveness of the nurses was high if and when the infants were looking or vocalizing. However, these latter instances were few. Training nurses to use information from Als and her colleagues (1980) (detailing a hierarchy of adult behavior that facilitates the preterm infant's social response, and likely approach or withdrawal responses from the preterm infant) may be a way to intervene in an NICU environment.

If human development is partially influenced by the functional aspects of infant-environment interactions and if the premature infant is particularly vulnerable to the effects of environmental stimulation, then a relatively microanalytic strategy may prove to be especially fruitful in fostering an understanding of early development in normal and high-risk infants.

Acknowledgments

The authors wish to thank Drs. Valya Visser and Donnal Walter, Mary McCue, R.N., Vicki Czernicki, Wayne Mitchell, James Sturiano, and Mary Buckett. The study could not have been completed without the cooperation of the parents of the infants in the Newborn Special Care Unit.

References

Als, H., Lester, B. M., Tronick, E. C., and Brazelton, T. B. 1980. Towards a research instrument for the assessment of preterm infant's behavior (A.P.I.B.).

In: H. E. Fitzgerald, B. M. Lester, and M. W. Yogman (eds.), Theory and Research in Behavioral Pediatrics, Vol. 1. Plenum Press, New York.

Barker, R., and Wright, N. 1954. Midwest and its Children. Row, Peterson, and Co., Evanston, IL.

Barnard, K. 1973. A program of stimulation for infants born prematurely. Paper presented at the biennial meeting of the Society for Research in Child Development, March, Philadelphia.

Barnard, K. 1980. Sleep organization and motor development in premature infants. In: E. J. Sell (ed.), Follow-Up of the High Risk Newborn—A Practical Approach, pp. 92–100. Charles C Thomas, Springfield, IL.

Brazelton, T. B. 1973. Neonatal Behavioral Assessment Scale. Lippincott, Philadelphia.

Bromwich, R.M. 1977. Stimulation in the first year of life? A perspective on infant development. Young Child., January, p. 71.

Buddin, B. J. 1982. Neonatal behavior and mother-infant interaction at one month. Unpublished master's thesis, University of Kansas, Lawrence.

Caldwell, B. M., and Bradley, R. H. 1979. Home observation for measurement of the environment. Center for Child Development and Education, University of Arkansas, Little Rock.

Charlesworth, W. R. 1977. Ethology: Its relevance for observational studies of human adaptation. In: G. P. Sackett (ed.), Observing Behavior, Vol. 1, pp. 7–32. University Park Press, Baltimore, MD.

Cornell, E. H., and Gottfried, A. W. 1976. Intervention with premature human infants. Child Dev. 47:32–39.

Davies, P. A., and Tizard, J. P. M. 1975. Very low birthweight and subsequent neurological defect. Dev. Med. Child. Neurol. 17:3–17.

Dayal, V. S., Kokshanian, A., and Mitchell, D. P. 1971. Combined effects of noise and Kanamycin. Ann. Otol. Rhinol. Laryngol. 80:897–901.

Eisert, D. C., Spector, S., Shankaran, S., Faigenbaum, D., and Szego, E. 1980. Mothers' reports of their low birthweight infants' subsequent development on the Minnesota Child Development Inventory. J. Pediatr. Psychol. 5(4):353–364.

Fitzhardinge, P. M., Pape, K., Arstikaitis, M., Boyle, M., Ashby, S., Rowly, A., Netley, C., and Swyer, P. R. 1976. Mechanical ventilation of infants of less than 1501 grams birthweight: Health, growth, and neurological sequelae. J. Pediatr. 88:531–541.

Gaiter, J. L., Avery, G. B., Temple, C. J., Johnson, A. A. S., and White, N. B. 1981. Stimulation characteristics of nursery environments for critically ill preterm infants and infant behavior. In: L. Stern (ed.), Intensive Care in the Newborn, pp. 389–410. Masson Publishing Co., New York.

Gottfried, A. W., Wallace-Lande, P., Sherman-Brown, S., King, J., Coen, C., and Hodgman, J. E. 1981. Physical and social environment of newborn infants in special care units. Science 214:673–675.

Gump, P. V., and Kounin, J. S. 1960. Issues raised by ecological and "classical" research efforts. Merrill-Palmer Q. 6:145–152.

Heimer, C. B., Cutler, R., and Freedman, A. M. 1964. Neurological sequelae of premature birth. Am. J. Dis. Child. 108:122–133.

Kramer, L. I., and Pierpont, M. E. 1976. Rocking waterbeds and auditory stimuli to enhance growth of premature infants. J. Pediatr. 88:297–299.

Lawson, K., Daum, C., and Turkewitz, G. 1977. Environmental characteristics of a neonatal intensive care unit. Child Dev. 48:1633–1639.

Linn, P. L., Daily, D. K., and Johns, B. J. 1978. Code for naturalistic observations of newborn environment. University of Kansas, Lawrence.

Linn, P. L., and Horowitz, F. D. 1983. The relationship between infant individual differences and mother-infant interaction during the neonatal period. Infant Behav. Dev. 6:415–427.

Marshall, R. E., and Kasman, C. 1980. Burnout in the neonatal intensive care unit. Pediatrics 65:1161–1165.

Myers, J. K., Bean, L. L., and Pepper, M. R. 1968. A decade later: A follow-up study of social class and mental illness. John Wiley, New York.

Pape, K. E., Buncic, R. J., Ashby, S., and Fitzhardinge, P. M. 1978. The status at two years of low-birth-weight infants born in 1974 with birthweights of less than 1001 gm. J. Pediatr. 92:253–260.

Powell, L. F. 1974. The effect of extra stimulation and maternal involvement on the development of low birth weight infants and on maternal behavior. Child Dev. 45:106–113.

Rice, R.D. 1977. Neurophysiological development in premature infants following stimulation. Dev. Psychol. 13:69–76.

Sackett, G. P. 1979. The lag sequential analysis of contingency and cyclicity in behavioral interaction research. In: J. D. Osofsky (ed.), Handbook of Infant Development, pp. 623–649. John Wiley, New York.

Scarr-Salapatek, S., and Williams, M. L. 1973. The effects of early stimulation on low-birth-weight infants. Child Dev. 44:94–101.

Solkoff, N., Yaffe, S., Weintraub, S., and Blase, B. 1969. Effects of handling on the subsequent development of premature infants. Dev. Psychol. 1:765–768.

Tulkin, S. R. 1977. Social class differences in maternal and infant behavior. In: P. H. Leiderman, S. R. Tulkin, and A. Rosenfeld (eds.), Culture and Infancy: Variations in the Human Experience, pp. 495–537. Academic Press, New York.

6

Analysis of Caregiving Events Relating to Preterm Infants in the Special Care Unit

Susan T. Blackburn and Kathryn E. Barnard

The care of newborns born prematurely and the influence of their early environment are of concern to health professionals responsible for these vulnerable infants. The preterm infant differs in two major ways from the term infant: 1) the preterm infant is born early and must deal with the extrauterine world with an immature nervous system; and 2) he or she spends the last weeks or months of gestation in the incubator and the intensive care nursery, environments that are quite different from the uterus. The premature infant is dependent on these environments for the maintenence of vital functions and the promotion of growth and development.

With few exceptions, the uterine environment offers an optimal environment for the normal growth and development of the fetus. The uterine environment provides a rich variety of stimuli with continuous modulation of intensity levels. These stimuli include:

1. Auditory stimuli from the maternal heartbeat and bowel sounds
2. Vestibular, tactile, and kinesthetic stimuli from maternal and fetal movements

---

Supported by Maternal and Child Health and Crippled Children's Services, DHHS, Grant # MC–R–530348.

3. Rhythmic and cyclic stimuli from the maternal heartbeat, maternal sleep/activity patterns, and neurohormonal cycles (Barnard, 1973; Grimwade et al., 1970; Korner, 1974; Payne and Bach, 1965; Sander et al., 1979).

In striking contrast to this intrauterine environment are the constant bright lights, sudden loud noises, and temperature changes of the neonatal intensive care unit (NICU). Removed from the containment and movement of the uterus, the premature infant is poked and prodded on a variable and unpredictable schedule. The infant is deprived of the influence of the maternal sleep cycle, periods of activity and quiescence, and other aspects of maternal rhythms, such as the patterned sensory input of the maternal heartbeat and rhythmic secretion of neurohormonal regulatory substances. In addition, there is often an irregular pattern of handling in response to the infant's emerging behavioral organization (Barnard, 1973; Dreyfus-Brisac, 1974).

After birth the infant has to organize his or her endogenous rhythms, physiologic functions, and behavior to respond appropriately to the extrauterine environment. The caregiving that the infant receives influences behavioral differentiation and organization and may nurture or hinder early adaptations.

Yarrow (1968) conceptualized a distinction between the *animate* and the *inanimate* or physical environment, which includes the variety, responsiveness, and complexity of objects and stimuli available to the infant for exploration and manipulation. The animate environment involves interactions with other people, especially the caregiver, who influences the amount and variety of stimulation the infant receives, alters sensory thresholds, and modulates the infant's arousal. Shaping the interaction between the infant and the caregiver are the infant's physiologic, maturational, and behavioral characteristics and the caregiver's timing, sensitivity to cues, and contingency acts.

Sander et al. (1972) suggested that the initial adaptation of the infant depends on *phase synchrony*, or contingency beween periodicities in infant state, and the periodic recurrence of caregiving events. The occurrence of repetitive sequences between these two elements over the first weeks of life may be important in establishing specific caretaking cues around which the 24-hour regulation of infant state becomes stabilized.

One factor that contributes to the initial temporal coordination of caregiver and infant is the ability of the caregiver to perceive and respond to infant state fluctuations. Sander and his associates studied early infant-caregiver environments with three groups of term infants: 1) those infants experiencing regular newborn nursery care; 2) those rooming in with their mothers; and 3) those rooming in with a consistent nurse caregiver. The usual newborn nursery care was characterized by marked asynchrony between behavioral changes in the infant and caregiver response. These infants had longer, more intense crying, more feeding distress (such as spitting up and poor feeding), an absence of day/night differentiation, and a persistently poorer 24-hour state organization. In the rooming-in situations, caregiving was characterized by greater attention to infant behavioral cues and response to these cues, an early form of contingency perception (Sander, 1975; Sander et al., 1975).

No clear-cut evidence exists that documents whether intensive care nurseries promote stability and growth of preterms or defines what the relationship of environmental events is for infant behavior, i.e., contingency perception. Studies have shown that most caregiving is related to medical or nursing interventions and that social interactions occur much less frequently. Feedback between the infant and the caregiver is minimal until near discharge. Integrated sensory experience and rhythmic diurnal variation of animate and inanimate aspects of the intensive care nursery environment for the most part are lacking (Gaiter et al., 1981; Gottfried et al., 1981; Lawson et al., 1977). In comparison with term infants, preterm infants spent more time alone, received less directed adult speech, and were more often asleep during social interactions (Linn et al., 1981). When social stimulation was available, the infant often is not in the appropriate state to benefit optimally from the stimuli.

Investigators disagree regarding the level, amount, and type of sensory stimulation that promotes optimal development of the preterm infant. Likewise there is no agreement about the roles of a particular stimulus and its effect on state modulation.

Premature Infant Refocus Project

The Premature Infant Refocus Project was designed to test the influence of a rocking-heartbeat stimulation experiment on the immediate and long-term behavior of premature infants. Three experimental variations of temporally organized stimulation were tested: fixed interval stimulation, self-activating stimulation, and quasi–self-activating stimulation. Infants were placed in the stimulation program during the first 14 days after birth and received additional stimulation until they were transferred from the incubator to a bassinette prior to discharge. A control group received normal hospital care with no additional rocking-heartbeat stimulation.

All subjects in the study were born at or prior to 33.1 weeks gestation, as determined by maternal history and Dubowitz Gestational

Age Assessment. They were admitted to a tertiary NICU between September, 1975 and June, 1978. Infants were excluded who had known central nervous system or chromosomal anomalies, required assisted ventilation for more than 2 weeks (which was not compatible with use of the rocking bed), came from families living more than 50 miles from Seattle, or were born to mothers with late pregnancy drug addiction.

Study infants were assigned to treatment groups according to a balanced, permuted block design, with strata defined by four levels of gestational age, two levels of initial health status, and two levels of previous maternal caregiving experience. One hundred twenty-six infants began the study, and 88 completed it.

The general hypothesis of the study was that the provision of temporally patterned stimulation to prematurely born infants will facilitate organization of their sleep/wake behavior, mature responses to sensory stimuli, and interactive behavior with parents. Data were collected during the infant's hospitalization and after discharge at 1, 4, 8, and 24 months of chronological age. The dependent measures were sleep/wake activity; neurologic, motor, and mental development; and parent-infant interaction (Barnard and Bee, 1983).

Methods

Data on caregiving activities and infant activity were obtained from 24-hour time-lapse video recordings at six time points: baseline; at 4, 8, and 12 days of treatment; at 34 weeks gestational age; and 24 hours after transfer to crib. The time-lapse video recording was a modification of a system developed by Anders and Sostek (1976) and allowed nonintrusive, longitudinal monitoring of infant behavior in the incubator and bassinette. A Sony model AVC-3260 camera with a 300-mm zoom lens mounted on a tripod (at a distance of approximately 2 feet) focused on the infant through the front or top of the Plexiglas incubator or the bassinette. The video signals were recorded on a GYYR odetics time-lapse video recorder model DAS 300. A 13.1 reduction used on the time-lapse recorder resulted in 13 hours of recorded behavior per 1-hour videotape. Every 4.5 seconds of time-lapse recording equaled 1 minute of actual time.

The time-lapse videotapes were coded for infant activity level, caregiving events, and stimulation program (Table 6.1 contains a summary of variables). Coding, done every 4.5 seconds of playback time, was equivalent to 1 minute of actual time. Intrascorer and interscorer reliability remained above .80.

Table 6.1. Time-lapse video recording coding system.

Motor activity[a]	Intervention[b]	Stimulation
	0. None	0. Bed on
1. No motor activity	1. Social stroking	
2. Low motor activity	2. Miscellaneous (shot, apnea stimulation, bath, etc.)	
3. High motor activity	3. Not used	
	4. Diaper change, vital signs	
	5. Blood gases	
	6. Bagging	
	7. Feeding	
	8. View obstruction	
	9. Nonvisible (out of incubator or crib)	

[a] The highest level of activity in an epoch was recorded.
[b] The last intervention in an epoch was recorded if multiple interventions occurred.

Using data from the Premature Infant Refocus Project, Blackburn (1979) categorized the following caregiving activities:

1. Diaper/Feeding (including routine vital signs visually obtained with feeding)
2. Miscellaneous/Technical Procedures (including injections, blood drawing, suctioning, stimulation for apnea, bath, other technical/ medical procedures)
3. Nonvisible/Out of Incubator or Crib (infant removed from crib or incubator)
4. Social Stroking (caressing, patting)

Description of the Sample

The sample consisted of 102 of the 126 infants who participated in the Premature Infant Refocus Project. All infants were in incubators in the NICU. Their mean postbirth age was 6.8 days (SD, 0.37); mean gestational age at birth, 32.26 weeks (SD, 1.46); and mean birth weight, 1309 grams (SD = 309.7). Most of the infants were being gavage fed on a 2-hour feeding schedule, and experienced apneic-bradycardic episodes. Table 6.2 contains neonatal and clinical data.

Table 6.2. Description of neonatal and clinical data on the sample ($N = 102$).

Variable	Data
Gestational age	
Mean	32.26 weeks
SD	1.46 weeks
Range	27.34–34.29 weeks
Postbirth age	
Mean	6.8 days
SD	3.7 days
Range	2–15 days
Sex	
Male	47 infants (46%)
Female	55 infants (54%)
Weight	
Mean	1309 grams
SD	309.7 grams
Range	580–2200 grams
Weight trend (over past 5 days)	
Gaining	36 infants (35%)
Losing	66 infants (67%)
Required oxygen	
Yes	14 infants (14%)
No	88 infants (86%)
Intravenous/intraarterial line	
Yes	33 infants (32%)
No	69 infants (68%)
Phototherapy	
Yes	15 infants (15%)
No	87 infants (85%)
Type of feeding	
Drip	4 infants (4%)
Gavage	86 infants (84%)
Alternate	10 infants (10%)
Nipple	2 infants (2%)
Interfeeding interval	
Continuous/1 hour	10 infants (10%)
2 hours	60 infants (59%)
3 hours	27 infants (26%)
4 hours	5 infants (5%)
Apneic-bradycardic episodes	
Yes	74 infants (73%)
No	28 infants (27%)
Median	4.5 episodes
Range	1–37 episodes

Results

Amount and Frequency of Caregiving

Caregiving activity occurred during 14.4% of the 24-hour period. Table 6.3 lists the frequency, length, and duration for each type of caregiving. The most frequent type of caregiving was handling related to miscellaneous/technical procedures ($\bar{x} = 22.4$ episodes, with a range of 1.0 to 61.0); the least frequent was social stroking ($\bar{x} = 5.2$ episodes, with a range of 1.0 to 31.0). In terms of duration or total amount of caregiving each day, care of infants out-of-incubator had the greatest number of minutes ($\bar{x} = 86.0$ minutes, range 1.0 to 437.0), followed by diapering/feeding ($\bar{x} = 56.7$ minutes, range 5.0 to 133.0) and miscellaneous/technical ($\bar{x} = 47.4$ minutes, range 6.0 to 135.0). Social stroking occurred for the least amount of time ($\bar{x} = 18.6$ minutes, range 1.0 to 100.0). Some infants ($N = 25$) experienced no social stroking in the incubator. Each episode of social stroking, diaper/feeding, or caregiving was relatively short (3.6 minutes or less) except for care out of the incubator or crib, which averaged 8.5 minutes. Considerable variation for individual infants was found; some were handled as little as 5.4% of the 24-hour day, while others averaged 38.1%.

Relationships between Caregiving Activities and Infant Activity Levels

Activity Pre- and Postcaregiving The infant activity levels were summed and averaged over the 1440 1-minute epochs in 24 hours. Means for the 5 minutes prior to and after each caregiving episode were also calculated. Table 6.4 compares the 24-hour activity with the pre- and postcaregiving means. There were significantly high levels of motor activity prior to diapering/feeding, miscellaneous/technical procedures, and time out of the incubator or crib ($p < .02$). In addition, the mean activity level prior to diapering/feeding was significantly higher than the activity level after diapering/feeding ($p < .001$). Decreases in activity were observed with out-of-incubator or crib episodes ($p < .06$). Table 6.5 and Figure 6.1 present data relative to the question of differences in infant activity levels immediately prior to and after caregiving events.

Activity levels tended to be high prior to episodes of miscellaneous/technical procedures and to remain high following the caregiving episode. Because this caregiving type involved activities with a high stimulus input and arousal potential for the infant, it is reasonable that the infant's

Table 6.3. Frequency, length, and duration of four types of caregiving ($N = 102$).

	Mean	Minimum	Maximum	SD	Median	Mode
Social Stroking						
Frequency[a]	5.2	1.0	31.0	5.5	3.3	1.0
Length[b]	3.6	1.0	25.7	4.1	2.0	1.0
Duration[c]	18.6	1.0	100.0	2.7	10.0	1.0
Miscellaneous/Technical Procedures						
Frequency	22.4	4.0	61.0	12.6	17.8	17.0
Length	2.2	1.0	4.4	0.7	2.0	1.5
Duration	47.4	6.0	135.0	29.9	37.5	31.0
Diapering/Feeding						
Frequency	18.2	5.0	34.0	6.0	17.8	16.0
Length	3.2	1.0	6.0	0.9	3.0	2.5
Duration	56.7	5.0	133.0	22.6	56.1	58.0
Nonvisible/Out of Incubator or Crib						
Frequency	10.0	1.0	39.0	6.4	9.8	5.0
Length	8.5	1.0	42.0	8.1	5.4	2.8
Duration	86.0	1.0	437.0	94.6	43.5	34.0

[a] Number of episodes per 24 hours.
[b] Length of individual episodes (in minutes).
[c] Total minutes per 24 hours.

Table 6.4. Comparison of mean activity level for 24-hour period with mean activity before and after caregiving episodes.

Activity	n	Mean activity level for 24-hr period	Time	Mean activity level	t^a	d.f.	p
Diapering/	98	1.90	Before	2.05	−5.86	97	.001
Feeding		1.90	After	1.91	−0.58	97	n.s.
Miscellaneous/	96	1.90	Before	1.99	−2.61	95	.01
Technical		1.90	After	1.98	−2.44	95	.01
Out of	73	1.91	Before	2.06	−2.39	72	.02
incubator or		1.91	After	1.97	−1.55	72	n.s.
crib							
Social stroking	30	1.95	Before	1.96	−0.17	29	n.s.
		1.95	After	1.96	−0.14	29	n.s.

[a] 1-tailed test of significance.

activity level remained elevated. The increase in activity prior to miscellaneous/technical events may relate to regular scheduling of some events (e.g., injections, baths, and certain blood drawings); hence, the infant was programmed to be more active at this time.

Similar relationships between infant motor activity level and stroking were not observed. Activity level tended to increase or remain the same after stroking, although the findings were not statistically significant. It may be that stroking occurred too infrequently and/or irregularly and for too short a duration to provide enough stimulus for state modulation. Significant correlations between stroking and out-of-incubator events with miscellaneous/technical activities ($p < .001$) suggest that caregivers were stroking infants who had undergone more technical procedures.

24-Hour Activity Patterns Infant activity level and caregiving events were also analyzed by 2-hour segments over the 24 hours. Figure 6.2 shows the relationships between caregiving and infant activity during this period. There was less infant activity and caregiving activity between midnight and 6:00 AM. From 6:00 AM to 8:00 AM both caregiving frequency and infant activity level increased. These changes are possibly related to the organization of nursing and medical activities on the unit. During the daytime hours, caregiving tended to occur in peaks, with the highest frequencies at 8:00 AM, 2:00 PM, and 8:00 PM and the lowest frequencies at 10:00 AM and 4:00 PM. Infant activity tended to remain at

Table 6.5. Comparison of mean activity levels before and after caregiving.

Time	n	Mean activity Level	t^a	df	p
Prior to Diapering/Feeding	98	2.04	5.67	97	0.00
After Diapering/Feeding		1.91			
Prior to Miscellaneous/Technical procedures	96	1.98	0.36	95	0.36
After Miscellaneous/Technical procedures		1.97			
Prior to Out of Incubator or Crib	73	2.06	1.51	72	0.06
After Our of Incubator or Crib		1.96			
Prior to Loving/Stroking	29	1.96	0.04	28	0.48
After Loving/Stroking		1.94			

[a] 1-tailed test of significance.

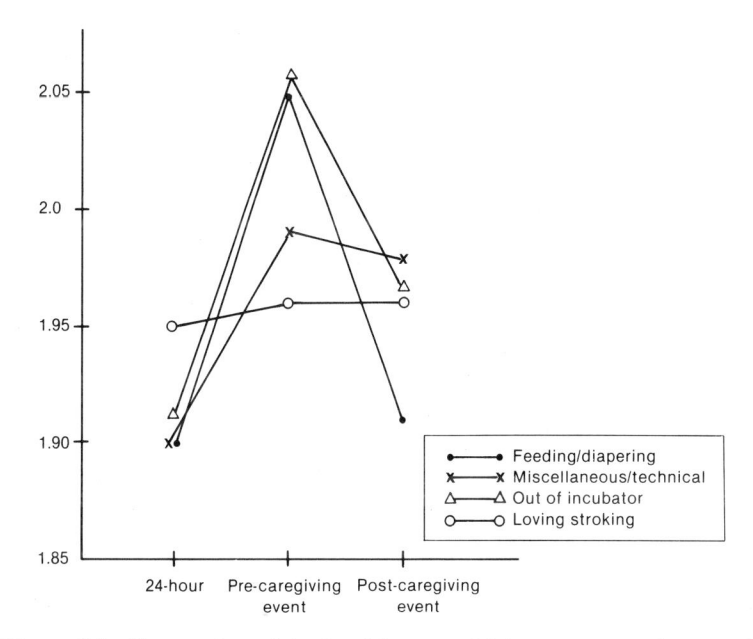

Figure 6.1. Changes in activity level between 24-hour means and pre- and postcaregiving.

peak levels between 8:00 AM and 6:00 PM, regardless of the intensity of caregiving events.

Discussion

The results demonstrate that early caregiver-infant interactions are associated with the infant's behavioral organization. The ability of the infant to organize behavioral and physiologic rhythms after birth is crucial in allowing the infant to respond appropriately to his or her environment and in providing his or her parents with clearer, more consistent cues.

One of the primary functions of the caregiver in early life is thought to be modulation of levels of arousal in the infant. The present findings raise two important questions:

1. Should infant arousal and/or soothing be promoted?
2. What types of stimuli should be used to intervene to arouse and/or soothe infants in the NICU?

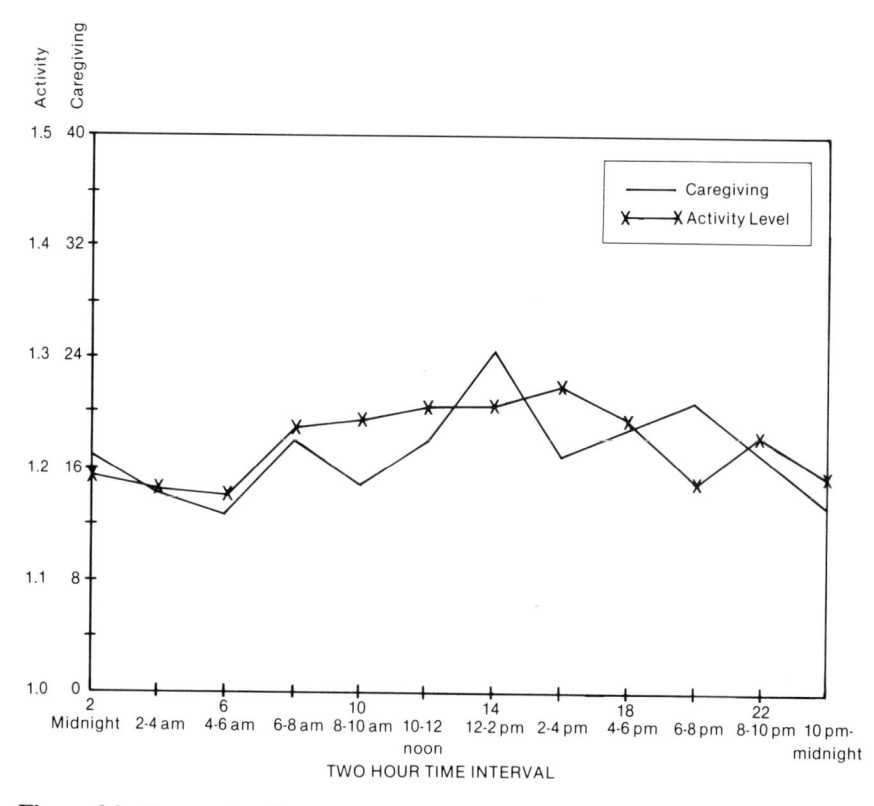

Figure 6.2. Twenty-four hour patterns of infant activity and caregiving activities.

Incorporation of State Modulation Concepts

In the data of this study, two dimensions of synchrony (the relationship of the infant's 24-hour activity pattern to the 24-hour pattern of caregiving activities, and the immediate changes in infant activity state to specific caregiving events) suggested that the initial phase synchronization between infant activity level and caregiving activities can be demonstrated in preterm infants after 6 days in an intensive care nursery. How the phasing between the infant and his or her environment changes over time is not presently known, but should be examined in light of Sander's findings regarding the lack of synchrony in the usual newborn nursery and its disruptive influence on infant 24-hour state regulation (Sander et al., 1972, 1975).

In general, infant activity levels seemed to rise during periods of high caregiving activity and fall during periods of less intense caregiving activity. These results suggest phase synchrony. However, during the night, infant activity level and caregiving decreased. These findings differ from those of Gaiter et al. (1981), who reported that infant limb movement increased significantly late at night and that a possible relationship exists between limb movement and increased stimuli from adult speech. The differences between the two studies may be related to or confounded by other factors in the environment, in particular by the level of environmental noise from both animate (caregiver vocalizations) and inanimate (equipment noises) sources.

State modulation did not occur after caregiving associated with miscellaneous/technical procedures. The infant's activity levels remained elevated. A possible explanation for this finding is that many miscellaneous/technical activities (e.g., baths, injections, blood drawings) tend to reoccur in the intensive care nursery on a relatively fixed schedule and may have an excitatory influence on preterm infant behavior. Examination of these data supported by Sander et al. (1972, 1975, 1979), Watson (1979), and others suggests, then, that infant state modulation should be promoted and that activities by the caregiver to facilitate the ability of the preterm infant to move from an aroused to a nonaroused state provide an important regulatory framework for the infant.

Regarding changes in infant activity levels prior to and after caregiving, the findings showed that infant state changes also occurred on a micro level. Infant activity levels (5-minute averages) were higher than baseline levels prior to diapering/feeding and out-of-incubator or crib events. Activity levels remained elevated after miscellaneous/technical procedures. Social stroking showed no relationship to changes in infant activity level.

A specific constellation of recurring behaviors (increase in gross body and limb movements; neck stretching, rooting, and non-nutritive sucking movements; and oral orientation of arm movement, including mouth swipes and increased contact of hands with facial area) was identified. Further definition, along with documentation, of these infant behaviors may enable caregivers to use these cues for synchronizing their caregiving activities with infant state changes (Blackburn, 1979).

Among individual infants, considerable variation within each type of caregiving was found. The greatest variation occurred with social stroking and out-of-incubator or crib episodes (activities that make up the infant's social animate environment), whereas the other types of caregiving (miscellaneous/technical procedures and diapering/feeding) involved physical aspects of the environment. These variations may represent important individual differences in infant receptivity to social stimulation. It will be useful to examine the effect of different levels of social stimulation on infant behavior.

Promotion of Arousal and/or Soothing

Although caregiving activities occur frequently in an NICU, few episodes are organized to decrease infant arousal. In contrast, caregiver actions with term infants are more often designed to comfort or soothe the infant and to regulate sensory inputs and motor responses. As a consequence, a shield or external stimulus barrier is created (Korner, 1974).

Infants need to experience a variety of state experiences. Schaefer et al. (1980) noted that "stimulation" takes place through the activation of any sensory modality and achieves its beneficial effects by rousing or by quieting. Activities that arouse or alert bring the infant to more focused attention on the environment. Activities that soothe allow the processing of environmental input. Infants need to experience an even balance between experiences that raise and lower their behavioral states.

In this study, infants tended to remain aroused after miscellaneous/technical events (the most frequent type of caregiving). Once aroused, the preterm infant may have difficulty in modulating his or her level of arousal, even after the stimulus (i.e., caregiving intervention) is removed. In the absence of environmental restraints, the preterm infant may be vulnerable to his or her own behavior, restimulating himself or herself and remaining aroused. The impact of continued arousal on the infant's functional status and behavior may have adverse physiologic results (e.g., cardiorespiratory irregularities, color changes, and more irregular motoric responses, such as tremors, startles, and jerky movements). An important goal of caregiving in the intensive care nursery, therefore, may be to promote soothing stimulation that lowers the preterm infant's state after highly arousing caregiving episodes.

There were few episodes of animate social stimulation in the NICU; therefore it seems that the preterm infant experiences few opportunities for interaction with the caregiver during alert "play" periods. Another important goal of caregiving in the intensive care nursery, then, is to promote periods of arousal in conjunction with animate stimulation when medically appropriate.

Types of Caregiving and Stimulation

Finally, the question of appropriate caregiving activities and types of stimulation for preterm infants in the ICN is greatly in need of study. Optimum levels, types, and complexity of stimulation that enhance an infant's behavioral development during hospitalization have yet to be established. However, the data of this study suggest that the role of animate social stimulation, particularly tactile stimulation, should be examined. The premature infant experiences very little social stimulation apart from a functional caregiving event. Of the four types of caregiving studied, social stroking was the least frequent event, had the shortest mean duration for the group as a whole, and was not observed in nearly one-fourth of the sample. The finding that little social stimulation occurs in comparison with caregiving associated with medical/nursing interventions for preterm infants in an intensive care nursery is consistent with reports from other studies. The traditional medical literature discourages handling of the immature infant and suggests that handling may exact a physiologic cost from the infant. Gaiter et al. (1980), for example, found that handling was associated with negative changes in infant medical status.

Very few studies have examined tactile stimulation, which tends to create quiet states in young infants and may be a source of tension reduction in addition to providing circulatory, muscular, and sensory stimulation. Recently, Rausch (1981) reported that tactile stimulation improved gastrointestinal function in preterm infants. Further research may demonstrate that various types of tactile contact with preterm infants unrelated to medical/nursing interventions may have therapeutic value in activating body systems and promoting system regulation.

Wachs (1984) questioned the assumption that "good" environmental stimulation uniformly enhances all aspects of cognitive development at all ages for all children and that "bad" environmental stimulation has the opposite effect. He proposed a bifactor environmental model (BEAM) and hypothesized that: 1) specific aspects of the environment are age related to child development (*age specificity*); 2) different aspects of the environment will influence different aspects of child development (*environmental specificity*); and 3) the impact of the environment on the child will be mediated by individual characteristics (*organismic specificity*).

After the birth of a child, the ability of the caregiver to perceive and respond to infant state changes may be one of the more important environmental parameters that enable an infant to organize his or her biologic and behavioral processes (age specificity). Dimensions of the early caregiving environment (such as different types of animate versus inanimate stimulation, state modulation activities, and contingency of responses by the caregiver) may create an expectancy by the infant that he or she can affect his or her environment and thereby enhance the infant's neurobehavioral and physical development. By providing opportunities for the infant to explore, to learn about environmental predictability, and to relate behavior to environmental events (environmental specificity), the caregiver contributes to the infant's development. Moreover, different types of handling and tactile stimulation in the intensive care nursery may be an important dimension of the environment for the preterm infant's functional status. Infant physiologic, maturational, and behavioral differences may mediate differential responses to the caregiving environment (organismic specificity). Although appropriateness of any given caregiving environment may vary with different infants, the exact parameters that describe these individual response differences are unclear and need to be defined for preterm infants.

In the formulation of future designs to investigate the NICU environment and its impact on the later development of the preterm infant, Wach's environmental stimulation model may prove to be of great value.

References

Anders, T. F., and Sostek, A. M. 1976. The use of time-lapse video recording of sleep wake behavior in human infant. Psychophysiology 13:155–158.

Barnard, K. E. 1973. The effect of stimulation on the sleep behavior of the premature infant. Commun. Nurs. Res. 6:12–40.

Barnard, K. E., and Bee, H. 1983. The impact of temporally-patterned stimulation on the development of preterm infants. Child Dev. 54:1156–1167.

Blackburn, S. 1979. The effects of caregiving activities in the neonatal intensive care unit on the behavior and development of premature infants. Unpublished doctoral dissertation, University of Washington, Seattle.

Dreyfus-Brisac, C. 1974. Organization of sleep in prematures: Implications for caregiving. In: M. Lewis and L. A. Rosenblum (eds.), The Effect of the Infant on Its Caregiver, pp. 123–140. John Wiley, New York.

Gaiter, J., Avery, G. G., Temple, C., Johnson, A., and White, N. 1981. Stimulation characteristics of nursery environments for critically ill preterm infants and infant behavior. In: L. Stern, B. Salle, and B. Friis-Hansen (eds.), Intensive Care in the Newborn III, pp. 389–410. Masson Publishing Company, New York.

Gottfried, A. W., Wallace-Lande, P., Sherman-Brown, S., King, J., Coen, C., and Hodgman, J. E. 1981. Physical and social environment of newborn infants in special care units. Science 214:673–675.

Grimwade, J. C., Walker, D., and Wood, C. 1970. Sensory stimulation of the human fetus. Aust. J. Ment. Retard. 2:63–64.

Korner, A. F. 1974. The effect of the infant's state, level of arousal, sex, and ontogenetic stage on the caregiver. In: M. Lewis and L. A. Rosenblum (eds.), The Effect of the Infant on Its Caregiver, pp. 105–121. John Wiley, New York.

Lawson, K., Daum, C., and Turkewitz, G. 1977. Environmental characteristics of a neonatal intensive care unit. Child Dev. 48:1633–1639.

Linn, P., Horowitz, F. D., Buddin, B., Leake, J., and Fox, H. 1981. A description of a neonatal intensive care unit. Paper presented at the meeting of the Society for Research in Child Development, Boston. MA.

Payne, G. S., and Bach, L. M. 1965. Perinatal sleep-wake cycles. Biol. Neonate 8:308–320.

Rausch, P. B. 1981. Effects of tactile and kinesthetic stimulation on premature infants. JOGN 10(1):34–37.

Sander, L. W. 1975. Infant and caretaking environment: Investigation and conceptualization of adaptive behavior in a system of increasing complexity. In: E. J. Anthony (ed.), Explorations in Child Psychiatry. Plenum Press, New York.

Sander, L. W., Julia, H. L., Stechler, G., and Burns, P. 1972. Continuous 24-hour interactional monitoring in infants reared in two caretaking environments. Psychosom. Med. 34:270–282.

Sander, L. W., Chappell, P. F., and Snyder, P. 1975. An investigation of change in the infant-caretaker system over the first week of life. Unpublished paper.

Sander, L. W., Stechler, G., Burns, P., and Lee, A. 1979. Changes in infant and caregiver variables over the first two months of life: Regulation and adaptation in the organization of the infant-caregiver system. In: E. Thoman (ed.), Origins of the Infant's Social Responsiveness, pp. 349–407. Erlbaum, Hillsdale, NJ.

Schaefer, M., Hatcher, R. P., and Barglow, P. 1980. Prematurity and infant stimulation. Child Psychiatry Hum. Dev. 10:199–212.

Wachs, T. D. 1984. Proximal experience and early cognitive intellectual development: The social environment. In: A. Gottfried (ed.), Home Environment and Early Cognitive Development. Academic Press, New York.

Watson, J. S. 1979. Perception of contingency as a determinant of social responsiveness. In: E. Thoman (ed.), Origins of the Infant's Social Responsiveness, pp. 33–64. Erlbaum, Hillsdale, NJ.

Yarrow, L. 1968. Conceptualizing the early environment. In: L. Dittman (ed.), Early Child Care, pp. 15–27. Atherton Press, New York.

7

Recording Environmental Influences on Infant Development in the Intensive Care Nursery

Womb for Improvement

Pamela C. High and Peter A. Gorski

Advances in neonatal medicine have contributed enormously to the successful management of acute cardiopulmonary, metabolic, and infectious crises in high-risk, prematurely born neonates. However, following rescue and stabilization from acute medical jeopardy, the infant must often endure a prolonged recovery phase of hospitalization, during which he or she often must double in physical size while also developing lasting physiologic stability and neurobehavioral competence. This phase of the preterm infant's hospital course is often fraught with recurrent medical setbacks.

Some of the vulnerabilities of preterm life most likely result from interfacing an immaturely formed central nervous system with an intensive care nursery (ICN) ecology that is sharply contrasted with the intrauterine environment. Unlike the robust term infant who is biologically prepared for extrauterine life, the preterm infant has few neurologic controls available with which he or she can inhibit his or her own exaggerated and costly response to excessive or poorly timed stimulation

(Gorski et al., 1979, 1983). Moreover, the weak or subtle behavioral signals of the prematurely born infant are difficult to read and can cause frustration for caregivers attempting to understand or satisfy the infant's needs. The authors' research attempts to find ways in which caregiving settings and actions may effect and potentially support physiologic and neurobehavioral progress in preterm infants born at risk.

This report first describes a new methodology for recording naturalistic and continuous data in the ICN on the states, behaviors, and various physiologic responses of the preterm infant as well as the nursery caregiving ecology. Second, it describes a new system for categorizing the development of states of consciousness in the preterm infant. The third section of this chapter presents data, derived from the authors' study, on the development of sleep/wake state organization in prematurely born neonates. The fourth section of this chapter presents data on the characteristics and consequences of caregiver interventions upon preterm infants in the ICN.

Computerized System for Observation of the Preterm Neonate and the Surrounding ICN Environment

The major focus of this text is the study of the environment of the intensive care nursery. Researchers agree that, because many events occur simultaneously, the methodology for this type of massive data collection and analysis can be cumbersome. Choosing also to monitor the infant and his or her responsivity to the environment increases the amount of data exponentially. For these reasons, the data in this study were entered directly into a computer at the time of observation. This computerized observational system enabled the monitoring of developmental changes over time in the infant's sleep/wake state organization, activity level, behavioral responsivity, heart and respiratory rates, and transcutaneous oxygen levels while concurrently tracking patterns of caregiver activity. The broad yet detailed nature of the data collection system permits the generation and testing of hypotheses that range from surface-level, practical questions about nursery routines to complex, interactive mappings of environment-infant cycles of activity and rest as they relate to infant health and growth.

The authors' experience and that of others suggest that there are behavioral correlates to physiologic responses in preterm neonates

(Gorski et al., 1979, 1983). These behavioral cues may include states of consciousness, quality and quantity of motor activity, postural shifts, gaze aversion, hiccoughs, grimacing, and vomiting. Changes in these may indicate infant reactions to the environment or to caregiver interactions and may serve as early warnings of infant distress. Understanding these signals might enable caregivers to sensitively time their interventions with a particular baby and to respect the infant's developmental strengths and weaknesses. Therefore this ethological research method was conceived to capture (microscopically as well as macroscopically) an infant's behavior and physiology, the surrounding ICN environment, and interactions between the infant and the caregiver environment.

Infants enrolled in this study were generally observed twice weekly for 3 weeks or until their hospital discharge. The mean duration of each observation period was 6 hours—from morning through early afternoon. Observations were made naturalistically, without alteration of caregiver routine or location. Each observer took a successive 75-minute shift and entered data into a cart-mounted computer collection system at the baby's bedside in the ICN. The computer also stored simultaneous physiologic data on the infant being observed, which were recorded from standard ICN monitoring instruments. Respiratory rate for each second was recorded along with a maximum, minimum, and mean respiratory rate for each 30-second time period. Maximum, minimum, and mean values both for transcutaneous pO_2, as measured by a Litton Oxymonitor, and for heart rate from the Tektronix neonatal monitor were also recorded every 30 seconds.

Raters entered data on the infant's state, skin color, and activity level every 30 seconds by typing abbreviated codes on the computer keyboard. Observers also entered codes for all medical, social, or custodial interventions performed on the infant; the person who performed each intervention; and any behavioral responses the infant expressed. There were 18 different coded medical interventions, 10 social interventions, 22 custodial interventions, 9 environmental interventions, 10 agents, and 41 codes for infant behavioral responses. These responses included nasal flaring, hiccoughs, retractions, seizures, non-nutritive sucking, grimaces, gaze aversion, yawning, and visual searching. Precise timing of starts and stops of interventions (e.g., feeding, diapering), environmental circumstances (e.g., lights on, people talking), or infant behaviors (e.g., arching, sucking) were also entered into the continuously running data file. Interrater reliability was checked every 6 months by scoring representative color videocassette tapes of ICN infants. Reliability was maintained at about .85 (Gorski et al., 1983).

Infant State Classification

An infant's state of consciousness influences the degree, duration, and variety of his or her reactions to a given stimulus and is influenced by his or her general well-being, including the length of time from the last feeding, the amount of external stimulation sustained, and the state of health (Brazelton, 1973; Prechtl, 1977; Wolff, 1966). The authors were interested in observing the development of states in preterm infants with increasing postmenstrual age (PMA) (i.e., age as calculated from mother's last menstrual period). The authors strongly suspected that caregiver attention to state, especially in the convalescing preterm infant, could facilitate successful feeding as well as enhance social interactions, thereby shortening the hospital course. Such early gains could then promote other advances in subsequent physical, cognitive, and social development (Beckwith et al., 1976; Sigman et al., 1981).

The criteria for determining state in preterm infants were observationally derived. Based on the 6-state scale described by Brazelton (1973) for term infants, the classification was expanded into a 10-state system in order to more fully differentiate the waking states experienced by preterm infants.

Like Brazelton (1973), Prechtl and Beintema (1964), and Anders and Sostek (1976), this study defined only two sleep states: quiet sleep (State 1); and active sleep (State 2). Electro-oculogram (EOG), EEG, and EMG were not included in the data base because of their intrusive nature and the known "laboratory effect" that they have on infant sleep/wake organization (Sostek and Anders, 1975). Several investigators (Anders and Sostek, 1976; Fuller et al., 1978) have shown a high correlation between polygraphic state determinations and time-lapse video recordings of sleep/wake states in term and premature infants. Indeed, then, the correlation that might have been obtained between the authors' sleep data and polygraphically determined sleep states would have been even higher than that of a time-lapse observer's sleep/wake determinations because the authors' observer in real time had a much greater opportunity to view the changes in respiratory pattern that Wolff (1966) used as his major defining criterion for depth of sleep state. Also, the observer in this study could move around the child in order to view his or her eye movements.

The eight waking states in the authors' categorization of preterm states of consciousness are an expansion of the four awake states of term infants previously described by Brazelton (1973) and Wolff (1966). The 10-state classification system may be collapsed into a 6-state system analogous to Brazelton's 6-state system or further collapsed into a 4-state system, consisting of sleep, drowsy, awake nonfussing, and irritable states (see Table 7.1).

Table 7.1. Infant state classification systems.

10-state	6-state	4-state
State 1: Quiet Sleep eyes closed, no movement except startles, regular respirations	State 1: Quiet Sleep	State 1: Sleep
State 2: Active Sleep ± rapid eye movements, some motor activity, irregular respirations	State 2: Active Sleep	
State 3A: Transitional Waking eyes open and close, irregular respirations, increasing activity level	State 3: Drowsy	State 2: Drowsy
State 3B: Mild Fussiness same criteria as 3A plus unsustained crying, grimace, ± color change		
State 4A: Lidded Alertness eyes half-open >15 seconds, little spontaneous movement	State 4: Awake Alert	State 3: Awake Nonfussing
State 4B: Bright Alertness eyes wide open >15 seconds, regular respirations, no body movement		
State 4C: Hyperalertness eyes bulging open, poor motor tone, no movement		
State 5A: Active Awake eyes open, much spontaneous activity, irregular respirations	State 5: Active Awake	State 4: Irritable
State 5B: Active Fuss with Cry irritable and active, cry sustained ≤15 seconds		
State 6: Crying sustained cry >15 seconds	State 6: Crying	

The following is a detailed description of the authors' 10-state classification system of sleeping and waking in preterm infants:

State 1: Quiet Sleep The infant has closed eyes and little or no motor activity, with the exception of occasional startles or jerky movements. No spontaneous rapid eye movements (REMs) are observed under the closed lids. Respirations are of regular rhythm and amplitude. Responses to external stimuli may be delayed. This is the deepest of sleep states.

State 2: Active Sleep The infant's eyes are closed, but REMs may be observed under them. Activity level is low, consisting of smooth limb movements, occasional stirring, or grimacing. Sucking movements and minor color changes may occur randomly. Respirations are irregular in amplitude and rhythm. This is light sleep during which stimulation may evoke startles or awakening.

State 3A: Transitional Waking This is a drowsy state during which eyelids open and close and activity level may vary. Startles may occur, but responses to stimuli are often delayed. Respirations are less erratic than in State 2. No fussing may be present in this state.

State 3B: Mild Fussiness The criteria for this state are identical with State 3A, except unsustained fussing must be present. More grimacing and color changes may also occur in this state.

State 4A: Lidded Alertness In this state, the infant's eyes are half-open for more than 15 seconds. Eyelids seem heavy, with the eyes having an unfocused, glazed appearance. The infant does not seem able to focus his or her attention. There is very little spontaneous motor activity.

State 4B: Bright Alertness The infant's eyes are wide open for more than 15 seconds and he or she seems able to attend to a source of stimulation. The infant may briefly follow a visual object or turn toward an auditory stimulus. He or she seems locked into one stimulus at a time. There is little spontaneous motor activity.

State 4C: Hyperalertness The infant's eyes are bulging open and his or her look is glazed. Muscle tonus is poor and there is no spontaneous motor activity. Color may be dusky, pale, or mottled, and he or she seems totally depleted.

State 5A: Active Awake In this state, the infant has open eyes and frequent spurts of motor activity involving the entire body. Because of this high activity level, he or she does not seem able to attend to a given stimulus, although activity level may increase or decrease in response to stimulation. Color may redden in this state, and respirations are difficult to observe because of this high activity level. No fussing may occur in this state.

State 5B: Active Fuss with Cry The criteria for this state are identical to State 5A, except that the infant is at least as active and certainly more irritable. Fussing must occur in this state, with crying sustained less than 15 seconds.

State 6: Crying This state is defined by intense crying, with vocalizations sustained longer than 15 seconds accompanied by average to high motor tone. Eyes may be open or closed. The crying is often difficult to break through with stimulation.

Sleep/Wake State Maturation in Premature Infants

The differentiation of a wide range of states of consciousness and the ability to maintain states by selectively inhibiting exogenous and endogenous stimulation are fundamental neurologic behaviors of healthy term infants (Brazelton, 1973; Parmelee, 1970; Prechtl, 1977; Wolff, 1966). The organization of sleep and waking states depends upon the maturation of the cerebral cortex and brainstem and the feedback system between them (Parmelee, 1970). Because of this relationship between structure and behavior, sleep/wake state maturation in the developing premature neonate may become an important predictor of the functional integrity of that infant's developing central nervous system.

Studies of extremely immature neonates of 24 to 26 weeks PMA have shown that, even at this early phase of neurodevelopment, a range of states of consciousness exists (Dreyfus-Brisac, 1968). Apparently, however, the concordance of the various criteria for active and for quiet sleep is lower in neonates of 34 weeks PMA than in more mature neonates (Dreyfus-Brisac, 1970; Parmelee et al., 1967; Prechtl et al., 1979). Parmelee et al. (1967) suggested that sleep state maturation is similar for preterm and term infants at term and at 3 months corrected for gestational age; others (Dreyfus-Brisac, 1970; Prechtl et al., 1979) suggested that prematurely born infants have not yet, at 40 weeks PMA, attained a level of state organization equal to that of the full-term newborn. These early reports are limited in their generalizability because of: small numbers of infants at gestational ages below 34 weeks; wide ranges of individual variation of behavior at each age; alteration of physical or caregiving environment during the observation period; and, possibly, more critical medical problems at a given PMA because of revolutionary technologic advances in neonatology that have enabled more fragile neonates to survive.

The results of the authors' study were obtained by applying the computer-linked continuous observation system previously described to access premature infant state organization in a sequential and naturalistic manner in the ICN. Attention was focused on an analysis of developmental change in duration of the various sleep states as well as in awake nonfussing states for preterm infants between 29 and 57 weeks PMA. The authors also attempted to determine whether PMA or chronological ("extrauterine") age (CA) is a better predictor of state distribution in premature infants.

Methods

Sixteen infants born between 26 and 37 weeks PMA were included in this study. Eight infants were free of significant medical complications and were labeled "healthy." Eight babies, labeled "sick," included infants with severe hyaline membrane disease, chronic lung disease, intraventricular hemorrhage, rubella syndrome, and hypoplastic lungs. Two of the eight "sick" babies died suddenly and unexpectedly at home within a month of hospital discharge.

A minimum of one observation and a maximum of nine observations were completed on each infant for a total of 67 observation periods. Forty-one of these observations were on sick premature infants whose mean age at observation was 39.80 weeks PMA, while 26 were on healthy infants whose mean age at observation was 32.73 weeks PMA. The mean duration of each observation was 6 hours.

Developmental trends in sleep/wake state behavior were calculated as follows: percentages of each total observation period spent in each state were averaged among all infants observed at each PMA. Plots were drawn of the percentage of time in each state as a function of PMA in weeks. The mixed longitudinal/cross-sectional nature of the data was ignored, and percentages were pooled over subjects and over days within subjects so that the analysis pertained to "the" infant (Martin et al., 1981).

Results

The total amount of sleep during the 6-hour daytime observation decreased from 71% at 31 weeks to 31% at 56 weeks PMA (see Figure 7.1). This decrement in total sleep time is attributable to a progressive decrease in the amount of active sleep with increasing PMA (see Figure 7.2). Over these same gestational ages, the total amount of quiet sleep remains fairly constant between 12% and 18% of the total observation

Recording Environmental Influences   139

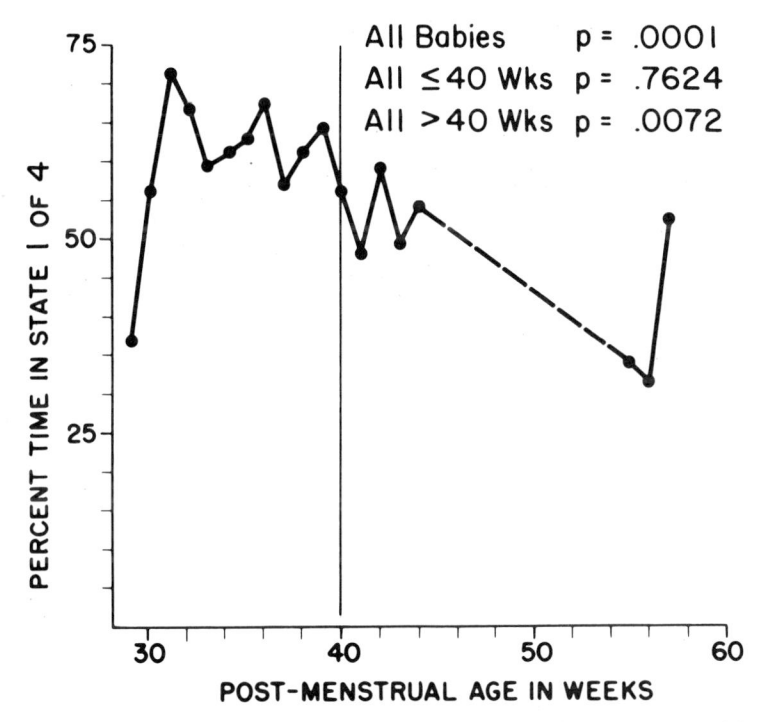

Figure 7.1. Percentage sleep time (state 1 in 4-state classification) during 6-hour daytime observation as a function of PMA.

time, although from 18% of total sleep time at 31 weeks PMA, the amount of quiet sleep doubles to 36% at 56 weeks PMA (Figure 7.3).

A marked increase was found in the amount of time spent by premature infants in awake states over the study period. The total time the subjects spent in awake nonfussing states rose from 10% at 31 weeks PMA to 46% at 56 weeks PMA (see Figure 7.4). This trend was highly significant for all babies ($R^2 = 0.594, p = .0003$) and all babies greater than 40 weeks PMA ($R^2 = 0.595, p = .0004$). With the small sample observed thus far, this trend was not significant prior to 40 weeks PMA ($R^2 = 0.018, p = .2004$). Figure 7.5 demonstrates that this great increase in awake time is primarily a function of the increasing percentage of time spent by the developing premature infants in the bright alert state. This bright alertness is equivalent to the characteristic alert state of which term neonates are capable. The less mature lidded alert state contributes to a

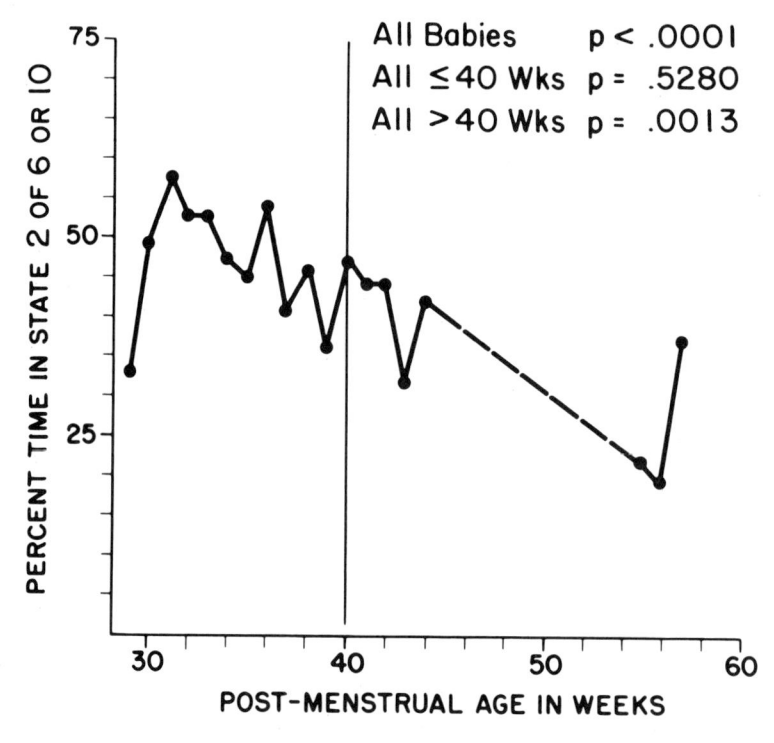

Figure 7.2. Percentage active sleep time (state 2 in 6- or 10-state classification) during 6-hour daytime observation as a function of PMA.

lesser degree to this trend of increasing awake time with increasing PMA (see Figure 7.6).

In order to tease out the differential contributions that maturation (PMA) and experience (CA) make to the above developmental trends in behavioral state organization, PMA and CA were used as predictors in a hierarchical regression model. Both PMA alone ($R^2 = 0.408, p = .0001$) and CA alone ($R^2 = 0.347, p = .0001$) contributed highly significantly to the trend of a decreasing percentage of time spent in active sleep for all babies over the study period. The unique contribution of PMA ($R^2 = 0.066, p = .0091$), however, is far more significant than the unique contribution of CA ($R^2 = 0.005, p = .4286$) to the percentage of time spent by all babies in active sleep. The relative contributions of PMA and CA to the percentages of time the subjects spent in awake, nonfussing states was similarly distributed. For the percentage of time in awake

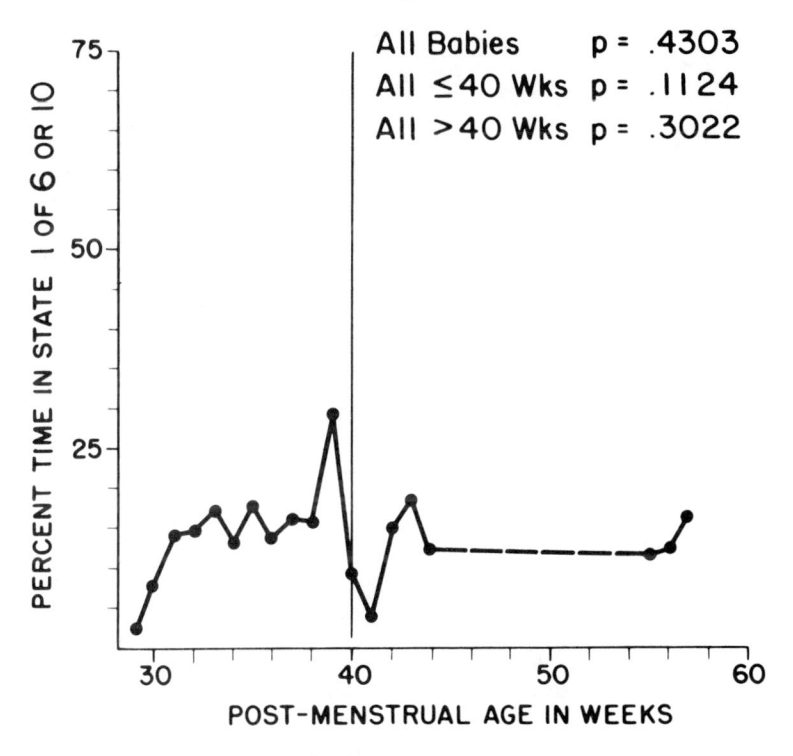

```
                    All Babies      p = .4303
                    All ≤40 Wks   p = .1124
                    All >40 Wks   p = .3022
```

Figure 7.3. Percentage quiet sleep time (state 1 of 6- or 10-state classification) during 6-hour daytime observation as a function of PMA.

nonfussing states, the regression yielded: for PMA alone, $R^2 = 0.594$, $p = .0001$; for CA alone, $R^2 = 0.516, p = .0001$; for the unique contribution of PMA, $R^2 = 0.08, p = .0006$; and for the unique contribution of CA, $R^2 = 0.004, p = .4139$. In these two instances, PMA seemed to be a better predictor of behavioral state maturation than CA.

Discussion

Sleep States

Quantity of Sleep Although other investigators are currently researching in this area, the authors are aware of no other comparative studies of total sleep time in premature infants. Because previous studies of sleep in premature infants were directed toward either discriminating relative amounts of quiet, active, and transitional sleep or determining

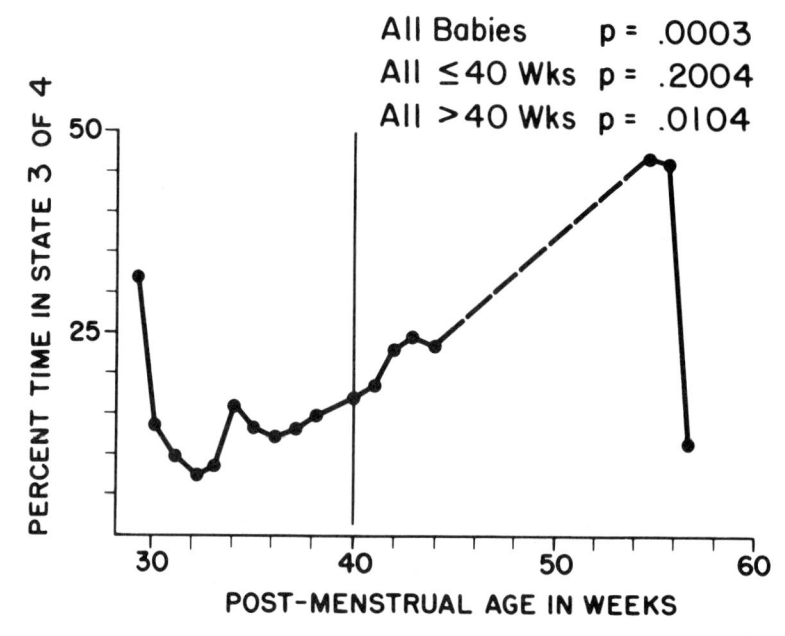

Figure 7.4. Percentage awake nonfussing time (state 3 in 4-state classification) during 6-hour daytime observation as a function of PMA.

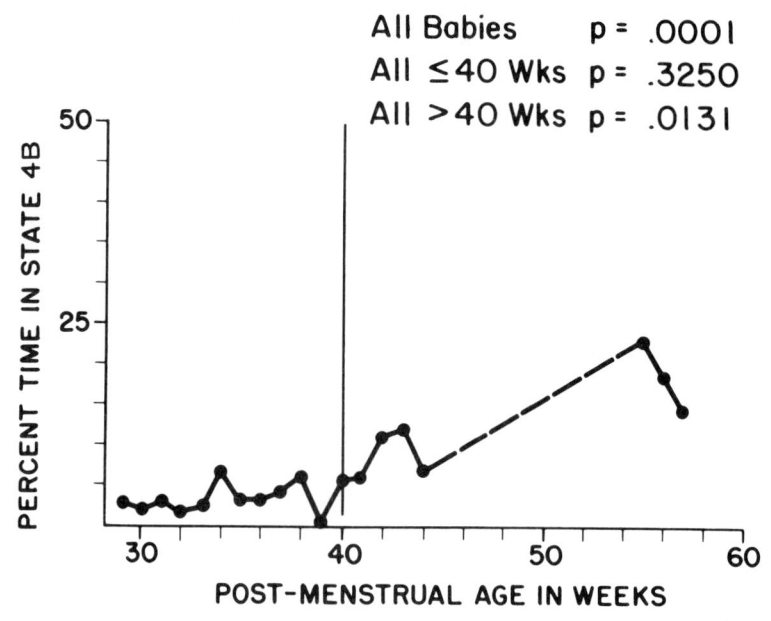

Figure 7.5. Percentage bright alert time (state 4B in 10-state classification) during 6-hour daytime observation as a function of PMA.

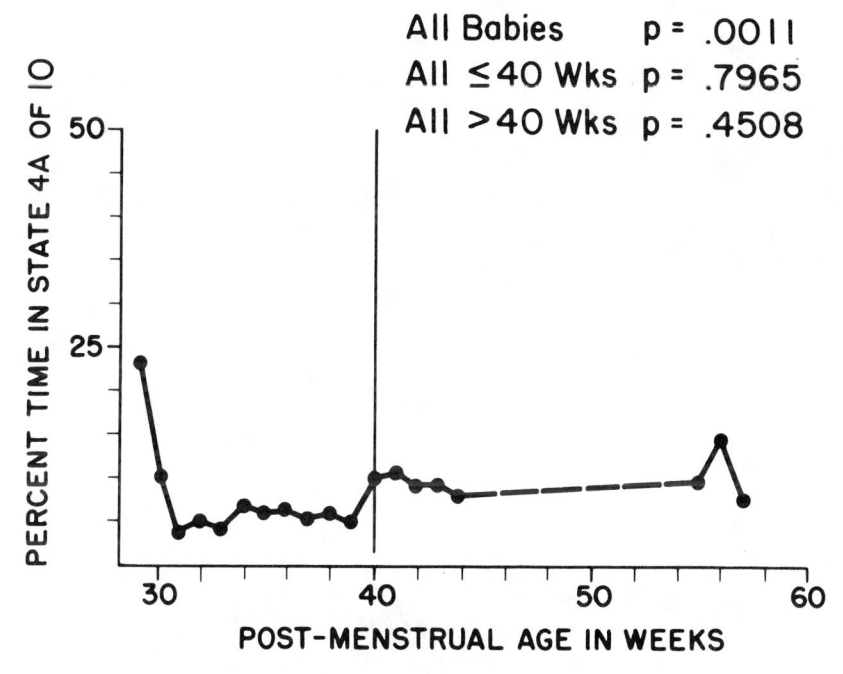

Figure 7.6. Percentage of lidded alert time (state 4A in 10-state classfication) during 6-hour daytime observation as a function of PMA.

sleep cycle length (Parmelee et al., 1967; Stern et al., 1969), these infants were usually observed for periods of less than 3 hours after a feeding while EEG, EMG, EKG, and EOG were monitored. Infants were expected to sleep during these studies and, therefore, the infant's total amount of sleep during recording was not reported.

However, investigators have looked at total sleep time development in term infants. The data from nighttime observations of term infants in naturalistic or adapted conditions show a much greater percentage of sleep than do the daytime data in preterm infants (see Table 7.2). This variance was expected to reflect the predictable influence of a diurnal environment upon state behavior. This hypothesis was substantiated by the much closer correlation between the authors' data and those for daytime sleep in term infants whose ages corresponded with those studied by the authors (see Table 7.2). The authors' data demonstrated that premature infants of 40 to 56 weeks PMA with chronic illness in the ICN have a similar amount of total daytime sleep as do healthy term infants at home. Observations would need to be performed at night in order to determine if

Table 7.2. Total sleep time.

PMA (weeks) (preterm)	Age (weeks) (term)	Nighttime Observations (term)			Daytime observations (term)		Daytime observations (preterm) High and Gorski, this study[f]
		Parmalee et al. (1964)[a]	Sostek et al. (1976)[b]	Anders (1978)[c]	Parmelee et al. (1964)[d]	Sostek et al. (1976)[e]	
32							67%
34							60%
36							67%
38							61%
40	birth						56%
42	2	69%	63%		62%	59%	59%
44	4	71%			56%		54%
46	6						
48	8	76%	75%	84%	49%	55%	
50	10						
52	12	81%			42%		
54	14						
56	16	83%			38%		31%
	9 months			92%			

[a] Maternal report, 7 PM to 7 AM.
[b] Lab videotaping—adapted state, 10 PM to 2 AM.
[c] Home videotaping, 10½-hour night.
[d] Maternal report, 7 AM to 7 PM.
[e] Lab videotaping—adapted state, 6 AM to 10 PM.
[f] ICN continuous 6-hour observation (see text).

these preterm infants demonstrate the same increasing nighttime sleep as do term infants.

Quality of Sleep Many investigators have reported on the difficulty of determining sleep states in premature infants less than 36 weeks PMA because of a lack of concordance of the various criteria used to differentiate active sleep from quiet sleep (Dreyfus-Brisac, 1970; Parmelee et al., 1967; Prechtl et al., 1979). Parmelee et al. (1967) attempted to overcome the difficulty of categorizing asynchronous criteria for sleep states in prematures by defining a third sleep state—transitional sleep. In this classification system, quiet sleep is defined simply as periods with closed eyes, regular or periodic respirations, no gross body movements, and no REMs. Active sleep is defined strictly as periods with eyes closed, irregular respirations, presence of REMs, and gross body movements. All other times when the neonate had closed eyes but did not have the above concordance between respiratory pattern, REMs and body movement were considered transitional sleep. Parmelee et al. (1967) found that transitional (asynchronous) sleep steadily decreased with increasing maturation. For the sake of comparison, the authors combined Parmelee's concepts of transitional sleep and active sleep. In the authors' classification of the active sleep state, which includes but does not require REMs, most of transitional sleep would be classified as active sleep. At all but 54 to 56 weeks PMA the authors' percentages of quiet sleep and active sleep correlated closely with Parmelee's (see Tables 7.3 and 7.4). The data in both tables demonstrate the same trend of increasing sleep time spent in the quiet state and decreasing time spent in the active state. At 56 weeks, the authors' subjects showed considerably less quiet sleep than Parmelee's. It is suspected that the stress or "laboratory effect" of strange environment and intrusive neurologic monitoring led to Parmelee's finding of this great quantity of quiet sleep in prematures. Alternatively, because the authors' data at 56 weeks PMA were obtained from two premature infants with chronic disease, the lower percentage of quiet sleep may reflect neuromaturational delays in ill, fragile subjects. It is also conceivable that the stimulation of the ICN may have caused decreased quiet sleep in these subjects.

Studies of the quality of sleep in term infants have demonstrated an increase in quiet sleep under laboratory conditions (Sostek and Anders, 1975), a diurnal variation in quality of sleep with large amounts of quiet sleep present during afternoon naps (Sostek et al., 1976), and a decreasing percentage of sleep composed of active sleep with maturation producing a reciprocal rise in quiet sleep, as shown in Tables 7.3 and 7.4. The strikingly high proportion of quiet sleep reported by Ellingson and Peters (1980) can probably be explained by a combination of the "lab effect," the afternoon effect, and their less strict criteria for quiet sleep. The

Table 7.3. Percentage of active sleep.

PMA (weeks) (preterm)	Age (weeks) (term)	Term infants				Preterm infants	
		Parmelee et al. (1967)[a]	Sostek et al. (1976)[b]	Anders (1978)[c]	Ellingson and Peters (1980)[d]	Parmelee et al. (1967)[e]	High and Gorski, this study[f]
30						82%	86%
32						90%	78%
34						91%	78%
36						88%	80%
38						75%	75%
40	birth	72%				70%	83%
42	2		62%		70%		75%
44	4				55%		78%
46	6				42%		
48	8		59%	64%			
50	10				35%		
52	12						
54	14	53%			20%	54%	
56	16						61%
9 months				46%			

[a] EMG, EEG, EKG, EOG; 3 hours between feeds; 8 PM to midnight.
[b] Videotape in lab—adapted condition; 6 AM to 10 AM.
[c] Home videotape; 10½-hour night.
[d] Daytime naps in lab; EEG, EMG, EOG, respiratory monitor. Includes transitional or indeterminate sleep for the sake of comparison.
[e] EMG, EEG, EKG, EOG; 3 hours between feeds; 8 PM to midnight.
[f] Six-hour daytime naturalistic observation in ICN.

Table 7.4. Percentage of quiet sleep.

PMA (weeks) (preterm)	Age (weeks) (term)	Term infants				Preterm infants	
		Parmelee et al. (1967)[a]	Sostek et al. (1976)[b]	Anders (1978)[c]	Ellingson and Peters (1980)[d]	Parmelee et al. (1967)[e]	High and Gorski, this study[f]
30						18%	14%
32						10%	21%
34						10%	22%
36						11%	19%
38						24%	25%
40	birth	28%			30%	31%	16%
42	2		38%		45%		24%
44	4				58%		22%
46	6						
48	8		42%	36%	65%		
50	10						
52	12				80%		
54	14	47%				45%	
56	16						36%
	9 months			54%			

[a] EMG, EEG, EKG, EOG; 3 hours between feeds; 8 PM to midnight.
[b] Videotape in lab—adapted condition; 6 AM to 10 AM.
[c] Home videotape; 10½-hour night.
[d] Daytime naps in lab; EEG, EMG, EOG, respiratory monitor.
[e] EMG, EEG, EKG, EOG; 3 hours between feeds; 8 PM to midnight.
[f] Six-hour daytime naturalistic observation in ICN.

premature subjects in the authors' study demonstrated this same trend of increasing proportion of sleep spent in the quiet state with maturation. Comparatively, however, the proportion of quiet sleep was somewhat lower than would have been predicted from extrapolating the data from the term subjects.

It seems from the authors' data that, even in the population of premature infants over 40 weeks PMA with more chronic medical problems, there is a close parallel in both total daytime sleep duration and relative amounts of quiet and active sleep with that of healthy term babies at similar conceptional ages. The one exception to this hypothesis is that, at 56 weeks PMA, the two premature infants with chronic disease exhibited a lesser proportion of quiet sleep than might have been expected. This may subsequently be shown to reflect neuromaturational delays in these subjects, or the stimulation of the ICN environment may have influenced their quality of sleep.

Awake States

Quantity of Wakefulness Previous reports of awake behaviors in premature infants usually have been limited to studies examining behavioral states or visual abilities obtained in response to active neurologic testing (Aylward, 1981; Hack et al., 1981; Lenard et al., 1968; Michaelis et al., 1973; Prechtl, 1977; Prechtl et al., 1967). The authors' study is one of a recent few to record the infants' "natural" state cycles without direct intervention by the observer. The strength as well as the difficulty of analyzing these data on awake state behaviors in premature infants lies in teasing out the effects that the continuous, invasive, noncontingent, stimulating milieu of the modern ICN may have upon maturing state organization. The finding that 41% of the total amount of observation time was spent in awake states at 42 weeks' PMA is almost identical to the 38% of time term 2-week-olds spent awake between 7 AM and 7 PM (Parmelee et al., 1964) and to the 41% of time 2-week-olds spent in wakefulness between 6 AM and 10 AM (Sostek and Anders, 1975). At 16 weeks, normal infants spent 69% of their day awake (Parmelee et al., 1964), whereas the authors' subjects at 56 weeks PMA spent 62% of the observation time awake.

Quality of Wakefulness The primary difference in awake state behavior of the authors' premature subjects from that of term healthy infants lies in the quality rather than the quantity of their wakefulness. At 2 weeks, healthy term babies were alert 63% of their wakeful time, and this rose to 83% by 8 weeks (Sostek and Anders, 1975). In comparison, the premature infants in this study were in awake nonfussing states 55% of their awake time at 42 weeks PMA, and this increased to 67% at 56 weeks PMA. These subjects showed the normal trend of increasing proportion of awake time spent in awake nonfussing states with maturation; however, by 56 weeks PMA greater recovery of alert states approximating term peer abilities was expected. Again, this discrepancy may have resulted from neurodevelopmental lags in the two subjects studied at this PMA. The authors must depend on longitudinal developmental follow-up of their subjects and future studies of more subjects at PMAs beyond term in order to determine if this variation from the expected is clinically significant.

The authors were pleased to find an overall trend toward developing sustained bright alert periods in their premature population. Here, too, the study corroborated earlier theoretical and experimental reporting of distinct but very brief periods of alert behavior in infants before term PMA (Hack et al., 1976, 1981; Miranda, 1970). Because further behavioral and cognitive development depends on reciprocal social and cognitive interaction with the human and inanimate environment (Beckwith, 1980), this increase in alert state behavior may enhance preterm infants' recoveries from initial central nervous system insult.

Effects of Medical Condition Karch et al. (1982) examined sleep/wake behaviors in 10-day-old (CA) prematures of 30 to 37 weeks PMA and in 10-day-old high-risk term infants by using EEG, EOG, EKG, thermistor, and direct observation. They found a decreased proportion of awake time as well as more quiet and indeterminant sleep in their groups of high-risk premature and high-risk term infants as compared to the low-risk premature group. In the few instances between 30 and 35 weeks PMA that the data for sick and healthy infants overlap, the authors did not see any significant group differences. It is suspected that the wide range of individual subject differences in state maturation in the small number of subjects studied to date may obscure any differences attributable to medical condition alone.

Developmental Influences of Gestational and Extrauterine Ages The multiple hierarchical regression analyses used to distinguish the relative contributions of CA and PMA in this report support the concept that absolute neurologic maturation (PMA) rather than extrauterine experience (CA) better predicts sleep/wake state behaviors in developing prematures. The high degree of dependency between CA and PMA is attributed to the homogeneous nature of the subjects studied. The overwhelming majority of subjects studied were between 28 and 32 weeks PMA at birth, therefore displaying little range of CA at each PMA studied. In the future, the continually expanding subject pool should enable the authors to firmly resolve this crucial question of neurodevelopment.

Observations of Caregiver Behavior

Developmental changes in states of consciousness are useful markers of central nervous system organization in premature infants. Similarly, the authors hope to learn whether some sleep/wake states are physiologically more sturdy than others, making the infant at times relatively impervious to or ready for the abundant sensory stimuli of an ICN. Such stimuli arise variously from human and mechanical care. As an entry into the complex nature and consequences of caregiver-infant interaction in this special environment, continuous computer recording is being used to map all of the human contacts with the infants studied. Even before recognizing causal relationships between caregiver interventions and various states of infant consciousness (a subject left to future reports), the possible implications gleaned from current naturalistic data about caregiver behavior toward hospitalized neonates are impressive. Caregiver phenomena addressed in this section include: percentage of time infants are handled or observed by caregivers; comparative time spent intervening versus observing infants; numbers, identity, and consistency of attachment figures; and frequency of positional changes impacting on the child's proprioceptive and vestibular sensory experiences.

Methods

A randomly selected subset of 64 6-hour-long continuous observations from the authors' expansive study included 45 observations of convalescent infants and 19 of more acutely ill infants. Inclusion criteria for "convalescent" comprised all of the following: tolerating nasogastric tube or nipple feedings; extubated more than 24 hours before or 48 hours after surgery; a CA of more than 72 hours; and normal fluid and electrolyte balance. It must be noted that all of the "acute" observations were made on infants free from intensive life-support systems. Therefore, these infants were receiving an intermediate level of ICN care. No observations were made during the most critically ill phase of newborn hospitalization. The mean PMA of infants was 31.5 weeks during acute observations and 33.4 weeks for convalescent observations. These recordings were analyzed so as to describe infants' experience with nursing personnel. These data were records extracted from the previously described study, and all observations were made between 8 AM and 4 PM. Results were calculated by using median rather than mean values. This was done out of respect for the skewed distribution of much of the data so that medians better represented the group's experience.

Results

Percentage of Time Nurse was Present Nurses were present for only 30% of the acute observations and 20% of the convalescent observations.

Percentage of Time No Caregiver Was Present No caregiver of any kind was present for 63% of acute observation periods and 71% of convalescent ones. Implications aside, these statistics may reflect staffing patterns that assign one nurse to several infants at a time when they no longer require critical care.

Interval between Nurse Completing a Caregiving Task and Leaving the Infant's Care Area Nurses spent 85 seconds for acute and 64 seconds for convalescent groups from the time of completing an intervention to the time of leaving the infant's care area.

Percentage of Time in Various Positions Infants spent the majority of time in the prone position (medians = 48% for acute and 59% for convalescent observations). There was little difference between observations in the acute or convalescent stage of recovery. Infants were observed almost no time on their right or left sides. (Supine = 17% of all acute observations, 6% of convalescent; right side = 7% and 1%, respectively, while no observations of acute or chronic infants found them positioned on their left side.)

Amount and Type of Handling Thirteen percent of total observation time included some form of caregiver touching of infants. For acute observations, most touching involved medical procedures (71%), while a nearly equal amount of medical and social touching (54% versus 60%) was experienced by convalescent infants.

Discussion

Several characteristics and implications about modern intensive care are suggested by the current study. Although investigators recognize the abundant sources of sensory stimuli in these environments (Cornell and Gottfried, 1976; Lawson et al., 1977; Lucey, 1977), the authors' continuous observational data revealed that nurses are present at the infant's bedside for minimal amounts of time. In fact, no caregiver was present at all the majority of time observed. Indeed, besides the nurse, all other caregivers combined (including parents, who admittedly visit more consistently during evening hours, physicians, and support staff) were present merely between 6% and 11% of the total time observed.

Interestingly, nurses attended closely to sick infants twice as much of the time as to healthy premature neonates. This phenomenon may reflect the common experience that a nurse is often assigned to care for just one infant when that patient is quite sick, while usually splitting his or her time between two infants if they seem to be in more stable physical condition.

Some of the analyses delineate how nurses tend to use their time when attending to infants. Because the authors were keenly interested in discovering any infant behavioral signals that might herald more serious physiologic irregularities, they looked to determine how available professional caregivers might be for observing and making use of such observations themselves. In fact, a disconcertingly limited time seems to be devoted by staff to observing an infant's responses to caregiving interventions. Convalescent infants were watched about 1 minute following a caregiving procedure of any kind before the nurse left the area. Even relatively ill infants received less than 2 minutes observation time from nurses following interventions. If, as previous research suggests (Gorski et al., 1983), distress signs following and associated with interventions can occur at least 5 minutes after an interaction with caregivers, then nursery staff may be missing opportunities to realize and utilize causal relationships between the timing, content, or manner of interventions and infant behavioral and physiologic responses.

The authors' findings of positions maintained by infants suggest a most asymmetrical proprioceptive experience. Given the occurrence of rapid central nervous system organization during this period of perinatal life, such skewed sensorimotor conditioning might conceivably affect emerging motor patterns and sensory integrative capabilities in this high-risk infant population. Surprisingly, there seemed to be little difference in caregiving approach to sick versus relatively healthy preterm infants with respect to offering them a variety of positions from which to experience their extrauterine world.

Finally, the authors' observations beg comparisons between the nature of interactions for these preterm infants with their caregivers and those of healthy term neonates with their parents at home. Quantitatively, home-reared infants are expected to receive significantly more handling and vocalizing from caregivers during daytime hours than are hospitalized preterm infants. Although both hospitalized and home-reared newborns apparently receive most of their care from one person, that individual changes from shift to shift and day to day for the preterm infant in the nursery. The primary care relationship that term infants enjoy at home is consistently provided by the same person.

Qualitatively, the term infant and parent quickly negotiate an interactive relationship characterized by smooth modulation between periods of close contact and brief rest. The preterm hospitalized infant is often exposed only to an "all or nothing" approach to care, swinging from no human contact to frequently uncomfortable or perhaps painful physical manipulations.

The authors' work cautions against berating the obvious differences in caregiver-infant interactions of hospitalized and home-reared newborns. The control of the immaturely formed nervous system over behavioral and physiologic responses in preterm infants may actually benefit from long rest periods from caregiver interactions. Indeed, the "all or nothing" character of care observed may be ideally tailored to the "all or nothing" responses to stimuli that characterize preterm neurologic behavior (Aylward, 1982). Moreover, parents do console their infants in the nursery just as they might at home. Perhaps just because parents cannot administer the technical care required of many preterm neonates, they remain free to exercise a mutual need for loving contact with their infant during hospitalization. Here, alas, no amount of scientific breakthrough can ever diminish the foremost need for gifted practitioners of the art of medicine who can use their words and manner to help parents tread that fragile bridge from limitless anxiety to realistic faith, loving concern, and hard-earned competence.

References

Anders, T. F. 1978. Home recorded sleep in 2 and 9 month old infants. J. Am. Assoc. Child Psychiatry 17:421–432.

Anders, T. F., and Sostek, A. M. 1976. The use of time lapse video recordings of sleep-wake behavior in human infants. Psychophysiology 13(2):155–158.

Aylward, G. P. 1981. The developmental course of behavioral states in preterm infants: A descriptive study. Child Dev. 52:564–568.

Aylward, G. P. 1982. Forty-week full-term and preterm neurologic differences. In: L. P. Lipsitt and T. M. Field (eds.), Infant Behavior and Development: Perinatal Risk and Newborn Behavior. Ablex Publishing Corp., Norwood, NJ.

Beckwith, L. 1980. The influence of caregiver-infant interaction on development. In: E. J. Sell (ed.), Follow-up of the High Risk Newborn—A Practical Approach. Charles C Thomas, Springfield, IL.

Beckwith, L., Cohen, S. E., Kopp, C. B., Parmelee, A. H., and Marcy, T. G. 1976. Caregiver-infant interaction and early cognitive development in preterm infants. Child Dev. 45:579–587.

Brazelton, T. B. 1973. Neonatal Behavioral Assessment Scale. Clinics in Developmental Medicine, No. 50. Heinemann, London.

Cornell, E. H., and Gottfried, A. W. 1976. Intervention with premature human infants. Child Dev. 47:32–39.

Dreyfus-Brisac, C. 1968. Sleep ontogenesis in early human prematurity from 24 to 27 weeks of conceptional age. Dev. Psychobiol. 1(3):162–169.

Dreyfus-Brisac, C. 1970. Ontogenesis of sleep in human prematures after 32 weeks of conceptional age. Dev. Psychobiol. 3(2):91–121.

Ellingson, R. J., and Peters, J. F. 1980. Development of EEG and daytime sleep patterns in normal full-term infants during the first 3 months of life: Longitudinal observations. EEG Clin. Neurophysiol. 49:112–124.

Fuller, P. W., Wenner, W. H., and Blackburn, S. 1978. Comparison between time-lapse video recordings of behavior and polygraphic state determinations in premature infants. Psychophysiology 15:594–598.

Gorski, P. A., Davison, M. F., and Brazelton, T. B. 1979. Stages of behavioral organization in the high-risk neonate: Theoretical and clinical considerations. Semin. Perinatol. 3(1):61–72.

Gorski, P. A., Hole, W. T., Leonard, C. H., and Martin, J. A. 1983. Direct computer recordings of premature infants and nursery care: Distress following two interventions. Pediatrics 72(2):198–202.

Hack, M., Mostow, A., and Miranda, S. B. 1976. Development of attention in preterm infants. Pediatrics 58(5):669–674.

Hack, M., Muszynski, S. Y., and Miranda, S. B. 1981. State of awakeness during visual fixation in preterm infants. Pediatrics 68(1):87–92.

Karch, D., Rothe, R., Jurisch, R., Heldt-Hildebrandt, R., Lubbesmeier, A., and Lemburg, P. 1982. Behavioral changes and bioelectric brain maturation of preterm and fullterm newborn infants: A polygraphic study. Dev. Med. Child Neurol. 24:30–47.

Lawson, K., Daum, G., and Turkewitz, G. 1977. Environmental characteristics of a neonatal intensive-care unit. Child Dev. 48:1631–1639.

Lenard, H. G., von Bernuth, H., and Prechtl, H. F. R. 1968. Reflexes and their relationship to behavioral state in the newborn. Acta Pediatr. Scand. 57:117–185.

Lucey, J. 1977. Is intensive care becoming too intensive? Pediatrics (Neonatol. Suppl.) 59:1064–1065.

Martin, J. A., Maccoby E. E., Baran, K. W., and Jacklin, C. N. 1981. Sequential analysis of mother-child interaction at 19 months: A comparison of microanalytic methods. Dev. Psychol. 17:146–157.

Michaelis, R., Parmelee, A. H., Stern, E., and Haber, A. 1973. Activity states in premature and term infants. Dev. Psychobiol. 6(3):209–215.

Miranda, S. B. 1970. Visual abilities and pattern preferences of premature infants and full-term neonates. J. Exp. Child Psychol. 10:189–205.

Parmelee, A. H. 1970. Sleep studies for the neurological assessment of the newborn. Neuropediatrics 1(3):351–353.

Parmelee, A. H., Wenner, N. H., and Shultz, M. D. 1964. Infant sleep pattern: From birth to 16 weeks of age. J. Pediatr. 65(4):576–582.

Parmelee, A. H., Wenner, W. H., Akiyama, Y., Schultz, M., and Stern, E. 1967. Sleep states in premature infants. Dev. Med. Child Neurol. 9:70–77.

Prechtl, H. F. R. 1977. The Neurological Examination of the Full Term Newborn Infant, 2nd Ed. Clinics in Developmental Medicine, No. 63. Heinemann, London.

Prechtl, H. F. R., and Beintema, D. 1964. The Neurological Examination of the Full-Term Newborn Infant. Clinics in Developmental Medicine, No. 12. Heinemann, London.

Prechtl, H. F. R., Vlach, V., Lenard, H. G., and Kerr-Grant, D. 1967. Exteroceptive and tendon reflexes in various behavioral states in the newborn. Biol. Neonate 11:159–175.

Prechtl, H. F. R., Fargel, J. W., Weinmann, H. M., and Bakker, H. H. 1979. Postures, motility and respiration of low-risk pre-term infants. Dev. Med. Child Neurol. 21:3–27.

Sigman, M., Cohen, E., Beckwith, L., and Parmelee, A. H. 1981. Social and familial influences on the development of preterm infants. J. Pediatr. Psychol. 6(1):1–3.

Sostek, A. M., and Anders, T. F. 1975. Effects of varying laboratory conditions on behavioral-state organization in two- and eight-week-old infants. Child Dev. 46:871–878.

Sostek, A. M., Anders, T. F., and Sostek, A. J. 1976. Diurnal rhythms in 2- and 8-week-old infants: Sleep-waking state organization as a function of age and stress. Psychosomat. Med. 38(4):250–256.

Stern, E., Parmelee, A. H., Akiyama, Y., Schultz, M. A., and Wenner, W. H. 1969. Sleep cycle characteristics in infants. Pediatrics 43:65–70.

Wolff, P. H. 1966. The causes, controls and organization of behavior in the neonate: Psychol. Issues Monogr. 17, 5(1):1–105.

8

Relationships between the Distribution and Diurnal Periodicities of Infant State and Environment

Katharine Rieke Lawson and Gerald Turkewitz

Almost from their first appearance, many behaviors show regular fluctuations. A prominent example is found in the daily rest activity and sleep-wake behaviors of people (Dreyfus-Brisac, 1974; Parmelee, 1974). Some aspects of these behaviors show cyclicity as early as 21 weeks gestational age (the earliest age examined), and a few show synchronization with each other as early as 28 to 30 weeks (Parmelee and Stern, 1972). Although ultradian periodicity is present very early in life, circadian periodicity (i.e., fluctuations occurring on a basis of approximately 24 hours) becomes recognizable only later, with different circadian rhythms appearing at different ages (Davis, 1981). For example, diurnal rhythms (i.e., fluctuations occurring on a daily basis) for sleep and wakefulness, heart rate, electrical skin resistance, excretion, and body temperature are not evident at birth but emerge at different times during the first few months (Hellbrügge, 1960).

Given its pervasiveness in normal physiologic and behavioral function, circadian periodicity is probably essential for normal growth and

---

Part of this study was carried out while the senior author was a fellow in the Post-Doctoral Training Program in Human Developmental Biology, supported by a National Institute of Health Grant #T32HD07053.

development. A lack of clearly defined circadian periodicity may reflect poor physiologic status and result in physical and behavioral problems. For example, rhythmicity of state is one type of circadian periodicity that would be expected to influence different aspects of development. It is, in itself, a defining characteristic of infant temperament (Thomas et al., 1968). Regulation of infant state provides one basis for synchronization of infant-caretaker behaviors and has obvious ramifications for the development of the mother-infant relationship and for interpersonal relationships in general. Despite its importance, little information is available concerning the establishment of circadian periodicity, particularly its development or maintenance related to diurnal regularities in the environment.

This chapter is devoted to exploring the relationship between environmental events and circadian rhythmicity of state in infants reared in different neonatal intensive care unit (NICU) environments. Prematurely born infants exhibit disturbances of sleep and a variety of other problems that may be related to a lack of clearly defined circadian rhythms. Lack of differentiated circadian rhythms could be a consequence of insufficient or improper development of the nervous or endocrine systems associated with prematurity. Alternatively, the hospital environment of preterm infants may influence the development of circadian rhythms. This chapter considers the effects of different types of early environmental events on term and preterm infants.

Very little information is available regarding the associations between gestational age and circadian rhythmicities. Hellbrügge (1960) suggested that diurnal rhythmicity develops later in preterm than in term infants. It is not clear what role environmental factors play in either the establishment or the disruption of diurnal periodicity. The possibility that environmental events have a guiding or permanent influence on the development of diurnal rhythmicities has not been examined.

NICUs provide a unique opportunity to investigate state-environment relationships. It may be characteristic of NICU environments that events in them occur with less marked periodicity than in the home environment. Lawson et al. (1977) reported a circadian illumination rhythm but pointed out that the distinction between night and day phases of the cycle was greatly reduced in the NICU. Gottfried et al. (1981) reported the absence of circadian rhythmicity for illumination in the NICU. The continuous activity in most NICUs is likely to flatten the amplitude of almost any circadian rhythmicity of events. An understanding of the relationship between environmental periodicity and circadian rhythms of infant state in such units may be particularly useful.

Relationships between Distribution and Diurnal Periodicities 159

Hence, this chapter is concerned with examining the presence of rhythmicities of infant state and of selected environmental events in the NICU. Data collected in two NICUs are presented.

Method

Two NICUs were observed—one located in a municipal hospital center and one located in a private voluntary hospital. Both units housed critically ill infants who required constant surveillance and intermediate care infants who did not require intensive medical supervision. Most of the data presented here pertain only to the intermediate care infants. The municipal hospital unit was observed for four 24-hour periods (a single 24-hour period and, 3 months later, a 72-hour period that included a weekend day). The private hospital unit was observed for three 24-hour periods (a single 72-hour period that included a weekend day).

The municipal hospital unit functioned with five to six nursery rooms (three of which were generally intermediate care rooms). Each nursery room measured 4.8 × 3.4 meters and housed 3 to 7 infants. The nurseries and a separate nurses' station were on either side of a corridor. In each nursery, the wall toward the corridor included a large window and a door; the opposite wall had a window. The municipal hospital unit is referred to as the *corridor unit*. The private hospital unit had two nursery rooms (one of which was generally an intermediate care room). Each measured 5.4 × 5.9 meters and housed 3 to 8 infants. This unit was arranged so that each of the two nursery rooms opened to a central nurses' station, and one wall in each room had a window to the outside. The private hospital unit is referred to as the *open unit*.

Subjects

The data presented here for the corridor unit are based on the 12 babies (five low birth weight premature infants and seven sick term infants) present during the earlier single 24-hour period and the eight babies who were present throughout the later 72-hour period. Of these eight, three were low birth weight premature infants and five were sick term infants. The data presented for the open unit are based on the six babies present for the entire 72-hour period. Of these six, three were low birth weight premature infants, and three were sick term infants.

Procedures

Observations of each of the intermediate care rooms of the corridor unit were made every 15 minutes and required about one minute per room. In each room, an observer: 1) measured light level with a Gossen Lunasix light meter at the position of the baby farthest from the window and facing the window; 2) observed each infant's state and the occurrence of handling at the moment of arrival at that infant's station; and 3) noted the occurrence of audible sound. Infant state was assessed on a 5-point scale:

State 1—Eyes Closed, No Activity (aside from occasional startles or small movements of the extremities)
State 2—Eyes Closed, Activity
State 3—Eyes Open, No Activity
State 4—Eyes Open, Activity
State 5—Eyes Open or Closed, Crying and/or Flailing

Handling was recorded if the infant was being touched by nursery personnel. Speech and nonspeech sounds were recorded separately, and were noted as originating either inside or outside of the nursery room. The procedures used were essentially the same for the open unit, except that the location of the sound was not recorded. The sound level was measured with a Bruel and Kjaer Precision Sound Level Meter.

Data Analysis

Illumination levels in the corridor unit were analyzed by computing a mean illumination level for each of the three intermediate care rooms for each hour and then calculating an hourly mean. For the open unit, hourly means were computed based on the four observations during each hour. The same procedures were used for computing sound levels. Frequency of sound occurrence was analyzed by computing the mean percentage of observations for each room for each hour. To determine whether there was a consistent diurnal rhythm in infant handling and infant state from day to day, the data from each measure were analyzed using Kendall's coefficient of concordance. This entailed assessing the frequency of occurrence of a given event on an hour-by-hour basis, ranking these frequencies, and then testing for the degree of agreement between the hourly ranks across the days of observation.

Data for each unit were analyzed for three general factors: 1) distribution and periodicity of various environmental events[1]; 2) distribution and periodicity of infant state; and 3) the relationships between periodicities of environment and infant state.

Results

Occurrence and Periodicity of Environmental Events

The infants in the two units were exposed to considerably different levels of illumination ($t_{46} = 4.78$, $p < .001$) (Table 8.1). Infants in the corridor unit were exposed to a mean level of 63.2 footcandles, and those in the open unit were exposed to a level of 20.1 footcandles. Despite the fact that each nursery room in both units contained large windows, the ranges of daily means in the two units did not overlap; illumination level ranged from 29.5 to 83.2 footcandles in the corridor unit and from 9.2 to 19.8 footcandles in the open unit. These differences in overall illumination level were accounted for by the following factors: 1) differences in the direction in which the windows to the outside faced; 2) relative size of the windows; and 3) differences in nursery practices (lights were dimmed at night in the open unit but not in the corridor unit).

Both units showed strong diurnal periodicities of illumination level as indicated by Kendall's coefficient of concordance (W) (see Table 8.1). Furthermore, the periodicity in both units was synchronous, as indicated by the significant correlation coefficient between the hourly illumination levels in the two units ($r_{24} = .65$, $p < .01$).

Handling frequency was markedly different for the two units ($t_{46} = 3.68$, $p < .01$). In the corridor unit, handling occurred only half as frequently as in the open unit (Table 8.1). The handling rate exhibited diurnal periodicity in each unit, as indicated by significant Kendall's W values.

In both units, infants were exposed to both speech and nonspeech sounds during a large proportion of the day. In the corridor unit, aspects of this auditory environment were reliably rhythmic, as indicated by significant Kendall's W values for speech in room, speech out of room, and nonspeech out of room. No such evidence of reliable periodicity was obtained for the open unit for speech or nonspeech sounds (Table 8.1).

---

[1] It should be noted that some results for the corridor unit have been published previously (Lawson et al., 1977). However, for some measures, our data base in the current report is different from that of the previous study and results will consequently also be different.

Table 8.1. Environmental events.

	Corridor unit		Open unit	
	Mean across days	Kendall's W^c	Mean across days	Kendall's W^d
Mean percentage of observations				
Speech sounds				
In room	36.1	.51[b]	92.4	.23
Out of room	82.2	.48[b]		
Nonspeech sounds				
In room	65.0	.41[a]	100.00	—
Out of room	96.3	.16		
Handling	11.5	.55[b]	21.4	.66[b]
Illumination level (footcandles)	63.2	.77[b]	20.1	.88[b]

[a] $p < .05$.
[b] $p < .01$.
[c] Based on 4 24-hour periods.
[d] Based on 3 24-hour periods.

Distribution and Periodicity of State

Although infants in both units spent similar amounts of time in State 1 (Eyes Closed, No Activity), they differed in regard to time spent in States 2, 3, 4, and 5. The infants were in State 1 during about two-thirds of the observations (see Table 8.2). They were in States 2 through 5 during 5.8–11.9% of the observations.

In general, the occurrence of the infant states in each unit fluctuated in a reliable pattern from day to day. States 1, 3, and 5 occurred in a recurring 24-hour pattern in both units and State 4 did so on the open unit, as indicated by significant or marginally significant concordances between days; Kendall's W values ranged from .41 to .54 ($p < .10$ to $< .01$) (See Table 8.2). Despite the fact that three of the five states were periodic on both units, the periodicities were not the same in the two units, as indicated by the absence of any significant degree of association between the distribution of their hourly occurrences (r values ranged from .05 to .17).

Relationship between Environmental and Infant State Periodicities

Correlation coefficients of the hourly means of state and environmental events were calculated (see Table 8.3). Such coefficients were computed for each unit for those states and environmental events that showed statistical evidence of regular rhythmicity (that is, significant or marginally significant coefficients of concordance). In addition, because some of the environmental rhythmicities were associated with each other, partial

Table 8.2. Mean percentage of observations during which infants were in each of the five infant states.

	State 1	State 2	State 3	State 4	State 5
Mean across days					
Corridor Unit	66.8	9.0	8.9	5.8	9.2
Open Unit	64.1	11.9	6.1	11.1	6.7
t	0.41	2.52[b]	1.91[a]	3.84[c]	1.73[a]
Kendall's W across days					
Corridor Unit[d]	.52[b]	.17	.43[b]	.27	.41[b]
Open Unit[e]	.54[b]	.44	.49[a]	.54[b]	.47[a]

[a] $p < .10$.
[b] $p < .05$.
[c] $p < .01$.
[d] Based on 4 24-hour periods.
[e] Based on 3 24-hour periods.

Table 8.3. Correlation coefficients of the hourly means of state and environmental events.

	\multicolumn{5}{c	}{Periodic state and environmental events}	\multicolumn{3}{c}{Periodic Environmental Events}
	\multicolumn{5}{c	}{State}	\multicolumn{3}{c}{Environmental Events}
	1	2	3	4	5	Handling	Speech in Room	Speech out of Room
Corridor Unit								
Handling	−.58	—	.71	—	—		.78	.46
Light	—	—	—	—	—		.42	
Speech in Room	−.54	—	.41	—	—			
Nonspeech in Room	−.53	—	.43	—	—			
Speech out of Room	—	—	−.44	—	—			
Open Unit								
Handling	−.51	—	—	.50	—			
Light	−.48	—	—	.63	—	.44		

164

correlations were performed to more clearly identify relationships between particular environmental periodicities and rhythmicities of state. These analyses suggested that the rhythmicities of infant state and environmental events were related.

In the corridor unit, State 1 and handling were negatively associated ($r_{23} = -.58, p < .05$). State 1 was also negatively associated with speech in room ($r_{23} = -.54, p < .05$). Correlation coefficients decreased markedly when the common association of the two environmental events was removed ($r_{\text{handling} \cdot \text{SIR}} = .17$ and $r_{\text{SIR} \cdot \text{handling}} = -.30$, respectively), but showed high values when the other environmental rhythmicities were partialled out (partial correlations ranged from $-.49$ to $-.60, p < .01$—see Table 8.4).

Table 8.4. Partial correlations between periodic state and environmental events with other environmental effects held constant.[a]

	State 1	State 3	State 4	State 5
Corridor Unit				
Handling and State correlations				
Speech in Room constant	—	.69	—	—
Nonspeech in Room constant	−.53	.68	—	—
Speech Out of Room constant	−.57	.73	—	—
Illumination constant	−.58	.74	—	—
Speech in Room and State correlations				
Nonspeech in Room constant	−.49	—	—	—
Speech Out of Room constant	−.60	.57	—	—
Illumination constant	−.55	.46	—	—
Nonspeech in Room and State correlations				
Handling constant	−.47	(.35)	—	—
Speech in Room constant	−.47	(.37)	—	—
Speech Out of Room constant	−.51	—	—	—
Speech Out of Room and State correlations				
Handling constant	—	−.49	—	—
Speech in Room constant	(−.35)	−.58	—	—
Nonspeech in Room constant	—	(−.35)	—	—
Illumination constant	—	−.48	—	—
Open Unit				
Handling and State correlation				
Illumination constant	(−.38)	.42	—	—
Illumination and State correlation				
Handling constant	—	—	.53	—

[a] Only significant or marginally significant (in parentheses) correlations are presented.

State 1 was also associated with nonspeech in room ($r_{23} = -.53$, $p < .05$), and this association was independent of their joint association with any other event; that is, they remained significantly negatively correlated when each of the other environmental events was held constant (partial correlations ranged from $-.47$ to $-.51$, $p < .05$; Table 8.4). In the open unit, State 1 and handling were also negatively associated ($r_{23} = -.51$, $p < .05$). In this unit, however, partialling out of the effect of the other periodic environmental event (illumination) left a marginally significant negative association ($r_{\text{handling} \cdot \text{illumination}} = -.38$, $p < .10$), suggesting that in this unit State 1 was related primarily to handling.

The periodicity of State 3 was more clearly and uniquely related to the periodicity of handling than was that of State 1. Thus, in the corridor unit, the positive association between State 3 and handling ($r_{23} = .71$, $p < .05$) remained high when the effects of each of the other environmental events were partialled out (r values ranged from .68 to .74, $p < .05$; Table 8.4). Furthermore, when the effect of handling was removed, the only correlation that remained significant was a negative association with speech out of room ($r_{\text{SOR} \cdot \text{handling}} = -.49$, $p < .05$). Although the simple correlation between State 3 and handling was not significant in the open unit, it was sizeable ($r_{23} = .34$). When the effect of the periodicity of illumination was held constant, this association became more robust and significant ($r_{\text{handling} \cdot \text{illumination}} = .42$, $p < .05$). In the corridor unit, State 3 was also associated with each of the other measured environmental rhythms (r values ranged from .41 to .44, $p < .05$; see Table 8.3), except for illumination ($r_{23} = .02$). When the effect of partialling out various environmental rhythms was examined, a complex picture emerged. State 3 was negatively associated with speech out of room in all comparisons and positively associated with speech in room and nonspeech in room on some comparisons (see Table 8.4). In the open unit, State 3 was not associated with the other environmental periodicity (illumination) by simple or partial correlations.

It should be recalled that infants in the open unit (and not in the corridor unit) showed reliable periodicity of State 4. State 4 was significantly correlated with both handling ($r_{23} = .50$, $p < .05$), and illumination ($r = .63$, $p < .05$). However, holding illumination constant reduced the association with handling to nonsignificance ($r_{\text{handling} \cdot \text{illumination}} = .33$, NS). Holding handling constant left a strong and significant association with illumination ($r_{\text{handling} \cdot \text{illumination}} = .53$, $p < .05$). Thus, the State 4 periodicity seemed to be related primarily to illumination effects.

Unlike the other states, which showed reliable periodicities, State 5 was not clearly related to any of the measured environmental events in either unit.

Intensive Care Infants

For the open unit, where the rooms were larger and generally less crowded than in the corridor unit, comparable observations were made for infants under more intensive care. Data for these infants were compared with the data for the medically more stable infants housed in the same NICU. The infants under intensive care were handled as frequently as those in the intermediate care room (20.7% versus 21.4%). However, there was no diurnal rhythmicity in handling ($W = .41$, NS) and handling was related more to medical procedures and less to feeding and social interactions. Infants under intensive care were exposed to a higher mean illumination level (17.1 versus 14.3 footcandles; $t_{23} = 3.95, p < .01$). Illumination was periodic ($W = .57, p < .02$), and more homogeneous across the day, than for intermediate care infants. The mean sound level, which was higher than that in the intermediate care room (72.2 versus 67.9 dB; $t_{22} = 20.08$, $p < .001$), was also periodic from day to day ($W = .62, p < .01$). This contrasted with the intermediate care room in which no such reliable daily alteration in sound level was found. One reason for this difference was the visitation practices in the unit. Parents and family were encouraged to visit their infant at any time of the day or night; consequently, family visits and concomitant speech and noise occurred at variable times daily. However, such visits were more common when infants were in the intermediate care room. With regard to infant state, infants in the intensive care room were more often in State 1 (72.3% of the time versus 64.1%; $t_{22} = 2.91$, $p < .01$) and less often in State 4 (11.1% versus 4.5%; $t_{22} = 4.56$, $p < .01$) than were infants in the intermediate care room. They were in States 2, 3, and 5 for a percentage of observations (12.2%, 4.7%, and 6.6%, respectively), comparable to that in the intermediate care room. Unlike the infants in the intermediate care room, fluctuations in state were reliably circadian only with respect to state 3 ($W = .58, p < .02$). This state rhythm was associated only with illumination ($r_{23} = -.45$) and, because the sound and illumination periodicities were not correlated ($r_{23} = .10$), this association was the same when the effect of sound was held constant. Thus, infants housed in the intensive care room had lower levels of state rhythmicities than did infants in intermediate care.

Discussion

Infants in NICUs are exposed to considerable amounts of environmental stimulation. This exposure consists of almost continuous auditory stimulation (both speech and equipment sounds), relatively high levels of illumination, and handling during 10% to 20% of the day. In view of these data, it is clear that the NICU environments are not understimulating for infants. Simple generalizations about the amount of stimulation typical of NICUs cannot be drawn. To some extent, differences are mediated by the structure of the NICU. In this study, infants in the corridor unit were exposed to considerably higher levels of illumination and considerably less handling than the infants in the open unit. Although dissimilarities in observational measures and procedures between studies make direct comparison impossible, evaluation of reports by a number of investigators (Barnard and Blackburn, 1981; Gaiter et al., 1981; Gottfried et al., 1981; Jones, 1982; Lawson et al., 1977; Linn et al., 1981) support our finding that NICU environments provide considerable stimulation to infants but that there is no typical NICU with regard to amount of environmental stimulation.

The stimulation observed in the corridor unit entailed prolonged exposure to disjunctive stimulation (Lawson et al., 1977). For example, in the corridor unit, sounds from outside of the nursery were clearly audible in the nursery during 90% of the day, and the sources of these sounds were not visible, even if the infant turned toward them. Thus, such sounds consistently occurred independent of stimulation in other modalities, providing no possibility for the infant to form an association between a particular sound and its visual and tactile referents. In fact, it has been shown that in older infants the association between auditory and visual aspects of objects is not learned when presented in such a disjunctive manner (Lawson, 1980). Such a dissociation of stimulus inputs limits the infant's opportunity to integrate the multimodal aspects of the environment. In addition, if infant orienting responses fail to have consequences for the infant, this failure could produce habituation and nonresponsiveness to the environment. When prematurely born infants reared in the corridor unit reached term dates they uniformly failed to show responses to lateral auditory stimulation comparable to those of normal term newborns (Kurtzberg et al., 1979). In the open unit more sound sources were potentially visible, and a relatively high level of handling in the presence of speech and equipment sounds made it more likely that they occurred in conjunction with other types of stimulation. Preliminary data suggest that at 37 to 40 weeks gestational age infants cared for in the open unit showed better orientation to sound than did infants cared for in the corridor unit.

There were also marked differences in state distribution, with infants in the open unit being in States 2 and 4 more of the time observed. Infants in the corridor unit spent more time in States 3 and 5. The amount of time infants spent in these states may have consequences for their subsequent cognitive development. States 2 (Eyes Closed, Activity) and 4 (Eyes

Open, Activity) are states in which infants expend relatively large amounts of energy; thus, for premature infants high levels of either might be incompatible with optimal growth.

The data indicate that no one environmental event serves as a principal determiner of all aspects of infant state. The presence in the environment of one clear circadian rhythm will not suffice to produce general state organization in infants. Furthermore, environmental periodicities did not affect infant states equally in both units. Although illumination varied in a diurnally predictable manner in both units, State 4 was related to illumination only in the open unit. This may be attributable to greater variation in the amplitude of illumination in the open unit relative to that in the corridor unit.

In summary, there were significant differences between the units in the amount of stimulation to which infants were exposed and in the amount of time that infants spent in various behavioral states. Although most measured events and several states showed a reliable circadian rhythm in both units, the rhythmicities were, in general, not synchronous between units. The data clearly suggest that both the amount of time infants in NICUs spend in various states and the regular distribution of this time from day to day are influenced by the nature of the environmental events that occur in the units. Time spent in various states and the diurnal rhythmicity of such states may well affect cognitive and social development. It is therefore essential to examine both the state-environment relationships and relationships between different aspects of state-environment organization with subsequent infant functioning. Nonmedical aspects of the care of preterm and ill infants must take into account the manifold effects that are likely to accompany any environmental manipulation. The potential benefits for infants to be derived from effective environmental modifications may make such exploration well worth the effort.

Acknowledgments

We thank Cecelia Daum, who was integrally involved in the study of the NICU at Bronx Municipal Hospital Center, and Meredith Platt, who was involved in the study of the NICU of the Hospital of Albert Einstein College of Medicine. We also thank all of our observers for their help in data collection and the staff of both NICUs for their assistance.

References

Barnard, K. E., and Blackburn, S. 1981. Features of the premature infant's animate and inanimate environment in relation to infant activity. Paper presented at the meeting of the Society for Research in Child Development, April, Boston.

Davis, F. C. 1981. Ontogeny of circadian rhythms. In: J. Aschoff (ed.), Handbook of Behavioral Neurobiology, Vol. 4. Plenum Press, New York.

Dreyfus-Brisac, C. 1974. Organization of sleep in prematures: Implications for caretaking. In: M. Lewis and L. A. Rosenblum (eds.), The Effect of the Infant on Its Caregiver. John Wiley, New York.

Gaiter, J. L., Avery, G. B., Temple, C. J., Johnson, A. A. S., and White, N. B. 1981. Stimulation characteristics of nursery environments for critically ill preterm infants and infant behavior. In: L. Stern (ed.), Intensive Care for the Newborn, Vol. III. Masson Publishing, New York.

Gottfried, A. W., Wallace-Lande, P., Sherman-Brown, S., King, J., Coen, C., and Hodgman, J. 1981. Physical and social environment of newborn infants in special care units. Science 214:673–675.

Hellbrügge, T. 1960. The development of circadian rhythms in infants. Cold Springs Harbor Symp. Quant. Biol. 25:311–323.

Jones, C. L. 1982. Environmental analysis of neonatal intensive care. J. Nerv. Ment. Dis. 170:130–142.

Kurtzberg, D., Vaughan, H. G., Daum, C., Grellong, B. A., Albin, S., and Rotkin, L. 1979. Neurobehavioral performance of low-birthweight infants at 40 weeks gestational age: Comparison with normal fullterm infants. Dev. Med. Child Neurol. 21:590–607.

Lawson, K. R. 1980. Spatial and temporal congruity and auditory visual integration in infants. Devel. Psychol. 16:185–192.

Lawson, K. R., Daum, C., and Turkewitz, G. 1977. Environmental characteristics of a neonatal intensive-care unit. Child. Dev. 48:1633–1639.

Linn, P. C., Horowitz, F. D., Buddin, B. J., Leake, J. C., and Fox, H. A. 1981. A description of a neonatal intensive care unit. Paper presented at the meeting of the Society for Research in Child Development, April, Boston.

Parmelee, A. H. 1974. Ontogeny of sleep patterns and associated periodicities in infants. In: F. Falkner and N. Kretchmer (eds.), Modern Problems in Pediatrics, Vol. 13, Karger, Basel.

Parmelee, A. H., and Stern, E. 1972. Development of states in infants. In: D. Clemante, D. P. Purpura, and F. E. Mayer (eds.), Sleep and the Maturing Nervous System. Academic Press, New York.

Thomas, A., Chess, S., and Birch, H. G. 1968. Temperament and Behavior Disorders in Children. New York University Press, New York.

9

Thermal Aspects of Neonatal Care

Robert J. Moffat and Alvin Hackel

The birth of a human infant, as with other members of the mammalian species, is an amazing event. The newborn is confronted with a new environment that requires remarkable flexibility in order to respond to a new set of physiologic requirements. In particular, the newborn's thermal environment changes dramatically. From the warm surroundings of the amniotic chamber, newborns emerge into a cold world in which they are expected to provide their own thermal protection. Internal energy sources, the control of regional circulation, and anatomical protection provided by the skin are the primary mechanisms of temperature management with which infants can respond to their external environment. Unfortunately, this response is inadequate in all but the warmest climes. Clinical experience has emphasized the importance of providing an external environment that can assist the infant to sustain the required thermal state.

This chapter discusses temperature regulation of the newborn infant, presents thermal models, and discusses current techniques for thermal management in the clinical setting. This three-pronged presentation is necessary because current information is based on empirical methods without an adequate theoretical base. A theoretical framework may create a broader understanding of the subject of thermal regulation in the newborn.

The Effects of Hypothermia

The sicker the neonate and/or the more premature the infant, the harder it is to establish a neutral thermal environment. Newborn infants attempt to increase their body temperature by several mechanisms. In nonshivering thermogenesis blood flow is increased through specific areas of the body that contain deposits of "brown fat." The cells in these areas of the body are dense with mitochondria, and increased heat is generated at the expense of an increased oxygen consumption. Oxygen consumption is increased up to fourfold as the body's core temperature decreases from 37°C to 34°C. The newborn also attempts to conserve body heat through peripheral vasoconstriction, mediated by the autonomic nervous system. The neonate's surface-to-mass ratio is higher than that of an older child, and the skin is underdeveloped. The epidermis is thin, the dermis is thin and highly vascularized, and the subcutaneous layer is also underdeveloped. By centralizing blood flow, the infant can prevent loss of heat through the colder, external portions of his body. In the vasoconstricted regions, tissue perfusion decreases, resulting in a negative impact on tissue metabolism. There is an increase in lactic acid production.

These physiologic efforts are not effective to maintain a normal body temperature in sick and/or premature neonates—the infant remains cold. The main effect is a negative one—the utilization of valuable energy stores. This comes at a time when the infant can least afford the expenditure, particularly if he is ill already. Thus hypothermia is a severe type of physiologic trauma in the newborn infant. It can mean the difference between life and death in a sick infant. Several studies have reported that the mortality rate of transported neonates who arrive with rectal temperatures of $< 35.5°C$ is significantly greater than that of neonates whose rectal temperatures are $> 35.5°C$.

As hypothermia occurs, the impact is first noted in the lungs. At birth, the circulation goes through a transitional period, changing from a fetal to an adult pattern. As the lungs expand, pulmonary vascular resistance falls and right-to-left vascular shunts through the patent foramen ovale and the patent ductus arteriosus close. A number of physiologic factors can affect the pulmonary vascular resistance in a negative manner, preventing the anticipated drop in the pulmonary vascular resistance. The most important of these factors are hypoxia, acidosis, hypo- and hypervolemia, and hypothermia. The increase in pulmonary vascular resistance that occurs with hypothermia impedes the flow of blood through the lungs and can cause or increase hypoxia. As a consequence, there is a decrease in the amount of oxygen delivered to the body's tissues at a time when the demand for oxygen has increased.

Central nervous system function is decreased with hypothermia, and the body's fluid balance is altered. The functioning of the enzyme and hormonal systems of the body is significantly altered. In essence, many of the body's organ systems begin to shut down under hypothermia. The only one that "gears up" is the sympathetic (autonomic) nervous system, which, through the release of catecholamines, alters the distribution of systemic vascular resistance through peripheral vasoconstriction. Thus, there is pooling of the body's blood in the central portion of the body in an attempt to conserve heat. However, the catecholamine reserves are rapidly used up and, even if the infant is later warmed by external means, "the price has been paid." The energy stores are not rapidly replenished, and as much as 48 to 72 hours may be required for the catecholamines to return to normal levels.

The critical issue, then, is how to ensure a satisfactory body temperature with minimal demand on the infant's meager resources. For an understanding of the issues involved, the authors turn to engineering models of the infant's thermal responses.

Introduction to Thermal Modeling

A baby's body temperature depends on a dynamic balance between metabolic heat generation and heat loss. The physician must play an active role in this process by specifying an appropriate environment. In routine cases, a warm room and a light blanket are adequate, but premature infants and critically ill infants have special needs that require careful thermal management.

There is only one source of thermal energy within the infant: metabolic heat release. Babies lose energy to their surroundings by heat transfer or exchange and by mass transfer. They exchange heat with their surroundings by three mechanisms: conduction, radiation, and convection. They lose energy to their surroundings by mass transfer in three ways: transepidermal evaporation, respiratory evaporation, and ingestion of mass. For each of the exchange mechanisms, the rate of energy transfer can be expressed in terms of a *driving potential* (which causes the transfer) and a *coefficient* (which determines the rate of energy transfer). The latter are the engineering rate equations of energy transfer.

For infants the energy loss problem involves sophisticated aspects of thermodynamics, but the starting point is simple. The "First Law" of thermodynamics, which expresses the essential truth of conservation, is:

For any system, at any instant of time, the rate of energy inflow, minus the rate of energy outflow, equals the rate at which energy is being stored within the system.[1]

If the total energy losses from an infant and the total energy gains (metabolic, radiant warmer, or whatever) are accurately measured and the rate of increase of average body temperature accounted for, the data will always satisfy this law. In other words, to achieve an energy balance, the energy that can enter or leave the infant by each possible mechanism and the amount stored within the infant must be known.

Figure 9.1 is a schematic representation of the thermal problem in the neonate. The interior of the small circle represents the mass of the infant's body; the dotted area around the perimeter of the circle represents the skin. Metabolic heat generation is shown as a "source"(s) of thermal energy distributed within the tissue mass, and the six parallel paths by which energy is lost are shown by arrows.

The terms T_a, R_H, V, and IR refer to "appropriately averaged" values, a necessary simplification for modeling. Different authors use different ways of averaging, but the intent is always the same—to represent the conditions as they affect energy losses. The skin is shown as a separate entity to emphasize its importance in regulating water loss and, consequently, total energy loss. Each of the transports is shown as a double arrow, to show that energy can be transferred in either direction, depending on the conditions involved.

The heat losses along the conduction (q_{cond}), radiation (q_{rad}), and convection (q_{conv}) paths depend on the temperatures involved and the total "resistance" to heat transfer along that path. For a given temperature difference from one end of the path to the other, the heat transfer will go down as the resistance goes up. Energy transfer associated with evaporative water loss (e_{evap}) depends on the amount of water evaporated and its latent heat of vaporization. The amount of water evaporated depends on the moisture content of the air in the same sense that heat loss depends on the air temperature. Respiratory water loss (e_{trans}) depends on the "effectiveness" of the lung as a water-vapor exchanger and on the infant's respiratory parameters.

Metabolic processes in the infant's tissues generate heat, which is conducted through the tissues and carried by the blood to the skin and lungs, where it is dissipated to the surroundings. Because of this internal heat generation, the body temperature (rectal or esophageal) will always be higher than the skin temperature under *steady state* conditions (i.e.,

---

[1] A. L. London, unpublished lectures in thermodynamics, Stanford University, Stanford, California, 1960–1980.

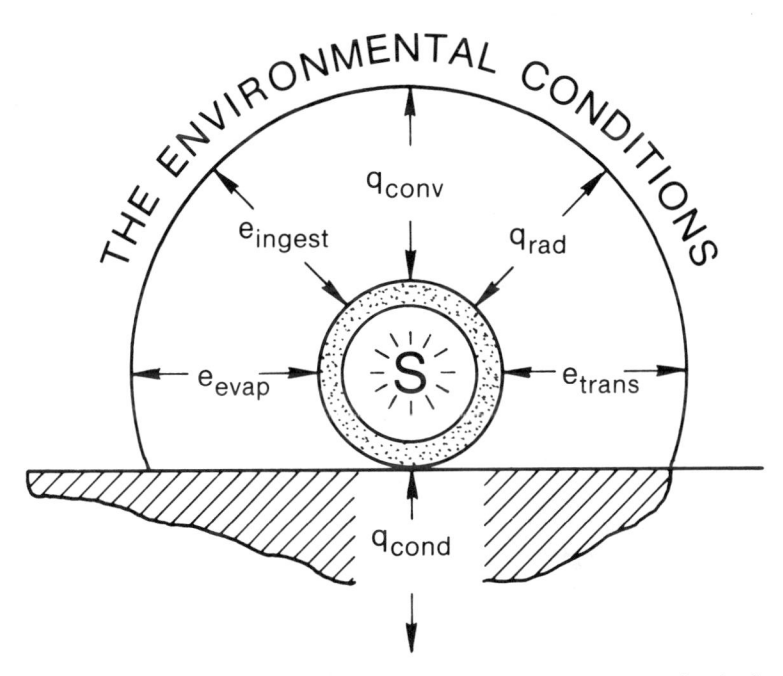

Figure 9.1. Schematic of the energy transport mechanisms operating in the neonate. T_a = ambient temperature; R_H = relative humidity; V = air velocity; IR = irradiation.

when the temperature of the infant is constant with time). If there were no transepidermal water loss, the skin temperature would be expected to always be above the air temperature. The fact is, however, that a premature infant's skin is frequently cooler than the surrounding air because of evaporative cooling.

Postnatal Heat Transfer Aspects

The infant is born warm and wet into a cold and possibly drafty place. At the moment of birth, the infant's core temperature is likely to be 37.5–38.5°C, between 0.5° and 1.0° warmer than the mother. Initially, the cooling rate is very high because of the high rate of evaporation of water from the infant's wet skin combined with a high rate of heat loss to the cold room (Hammarlund et al., 1980). The baby's skin temperature may drop

3°C within the first 10 seconds after birth (Tähti et al., 1972). Within a few minutes, however, the infant is dried and placed in a special environment—either a bassinet, a well baby incubator, or an intensive care incubator. At this time the infant should achieve a steady thermal state that will be favorable to his development. Whether this happens or not depends on the infant's metabolic rate and the temperature and humidity of the environment.

The metabolic rate depends on the infant's body weight and individual characteristics, but it is not very responsive to body temperature, especially in premature infants. As a consequence, the infant's energy inflow is relatively constant, whereas his losses depend on body temperature and environmental conditions. It is known that, if the rate of heat loss is greater than the metabolic heat generation rate, the infant's temperature will drop. As the body temperature drops, heat losses by conduction, convection, and radiation become smaller. The body temperature will continue to drop until the losses equal the metabolic generation.

Adequate thermal care of infants involves providing an environment within which the infant's body temperature remains stable at an acceptable level with minimal demand on the infant's reserves of stored energy. In other words, the environmental temperature, humidity, and air velocity must be selected so that the net energy lost to the surroundings, at the desired body temperature, equals the neutral thermal metabolic heat release. With a healthy term infant, an environmental temperature of 32°C with relative humidity of 50% provides a body temperature of 36.5–37.0°C (skin temperature of 35.2°C) for most infants nursed naked (Ryser and Jequier, 1972).

No such general rule applies for sick or premature babies. Premature infants lose much more heat and water than term infants. More attention must be paid to humidity control, and the air must frequently be kept significantly hotter than the desired body temperature in order to counterbalance the evaporative energy loss. An infant's skin is permeable to water, more so for prematures than for term babies and more so within the first postnatal week than later. Water is constantly evaporating from the skin. In addition, the infant breathes in air at ambient temperatures and humidity and breathes out heated and humidified air. Both of these energy loss mechanisms relate to the moisture content of the surroundings, not the temperature. The skin of a premature infant of 25 or 26 weeks gestational age may be 3° or 4° cooler than the air, and an ambient temperature as high as 40°C may be needed in order to maintain a body temperature of 36.5°C if the relative humidity is held at 50% (Hammarlund and Sedin, 1979).

Radiant warmers are frequently used to supplement the baby's metabolic heat release as an alternative to keeping the infant in a high temperature, high humidity environment. Once again, the water loss problem complicates the issue. The radiant warmer regulates its output so as to keep the temperature of its control sensor constant. That sensor is usually attached to the infant's abdomen with tape that is not as permeable as the infant's skin to water vapor. Through evaporation, the infant's skin loses considerable energy to the surrounding air, but the sensor is not cooled by evaporation. Hence, the radiant warmer runs hotter than the skin of the infant, causing it to shut off too soon (Belgaumkar and Scott, 1975).

The idea of a thermal "steady state" is easily expressed, but the state itself is difficult to measure. Steady state can be detected only by repeatedly measuring rectal, esophageal, and skin temperatures at periodic intervals over time. The reason is that the energy rates involved in infants are so low that changes in body temperature are very slow. Even if all of an infant's metabolic energy were being used to increase his body temperature (i.e., no losses by any means), the temperature would rise only 2.5°C per hour. Thus, if an infant's temperature drops even by as much as 0.5°C per hour, the infant is losing about 20% more heat than he is producing, and the body temperature will continue to drop until the infant has reduced his losses by 20%. There have been some reports of infants' rectal temperatures dropping below their skin temperatures under steady state conditions. This can only be the case if the infant is being heated from the outside; it cannot be the case for a steady thermal state. If rectal temperature seems to be below skin temperature under steady state conditions, this is most likely a measurement error.

Heat Transfer by Conduction

Heat loss by conduction from an infant to a dry mattress is seldom a significant part of the infant's overall heat loss (usually less than 5% of the total). When an infant is first placed on a mattress or any surface, however, there is significant heat loss by conduction across the area of contact. As heat continues to flow into the mattress, the contacted area becomes warmer and the rate of loss diminishes. After several minutes, a steady state condition is reached and the heat loss rate thereafter remains constant.

Two equations describe these processes (Holman 1981, p. 116):

$$\dot{q} = \frac{kA_c}{\sqrt{\pi \alpha \tau}} (T_o - T_i) \tag{1}$$

$$\dot{q} = \frac{kA_c S}{L}(T_o - T_i) \qquad (2)$$

where

$\dot{q}$ = Rate of transfer (W)
α = Thermal diffusivity (m^2/s)
k = Thermal conductivity (W/m - °C)
A_c = Contact area (m^2)
π = 3.14159
τ = Time after contact (seconds)
S = Conduction shape factor
L = Thickness of mattress (m)
T_o = Temperature of contact area (°C)
T_i = Initial mattress temperature (°C)

Equation 1 describes the instantaneous rate of heat loss as a function of time during the first few minutes after contact between the infant and the mattress. Equation 2 calculates the steady rate of heat loss after several minutes have elapsed. Typical values for these parameters are: $k = 0.05$ W/m-°C=C, $A_c = 17\%$ of body surface area, $\alpha = \pm 1.6 \times 10^{-7}$ m^2/s, and $S = 2.0$.

Transient heat loss may average 3 watts during the first minute of contact and settle out at 0.5 watts after 5 minutes. A new transient condition occurs each time the infant's position is changed on the mattress, and the heat loss rate is proportional to the new area brought into contact. Damp or wet mattresses act more like "marble slabs" than like mattresses, inducing high heat losses; mattresses and mattress pads must be kept dry. The transient conduction loss can be minimized by using lightweight mattresses of low thermal capacity, by preheating the mattress to body temperature, and by minimizing the number of times the infant is repositioned.

Water Mattresses Water mattresses induce large heat losses if the water is even a small fraction of a degree colder than the infant. Any person who has ever tried to sleep on a cold waterbed will recognize this problem. Very careful control of the water temperature is needed, and water mattresses should always be covered with several thicknesses of cloth or an insulating pad.

Radiation

Under ordinary nursing conditions, radiation heat transfer accounts for 35–65% of the heat loss of a naked term infant, and 20–40% of that of an infant under 30 weeks gestational age. This does not mean that prematures radiate less heat, but that their total losses (particularly because of evaporative loss) are higher. Radiant heat transfer depends on the temperature level of the objects involved and is independent of the air velocity.

Every object both emits and absorbs radiant energy all of the time. If the rates of emission and absorption are equal, there is no net heat transfer by radiation, even though there may be an appreciable energy transfer. The emission of radiant energy is governed by the Stefan-Boltzmann Law (Equation 3) and absorption is described by Equation 4 (Holman, 1981, p. 309):

$$\dot{e}_e = \varepsilon A(\sigma T^4) \qquad (3)$$

$$\dot{e}_a = \alpha A G \qquad (4)$$

where

$\dot{e}$ — Rate of energy emission (c_e) or absorption (c_a) (W)
α = Absorptivity
ε = Emissivity
σ = Stefan-Boltzmann Law constant (5.669×10^{-8} W/m²-K⁴)
G = Irradiation (W/m²)
A = Active area (m²)
T = Temperature (K)

The emissivity of human skin is a function of the wavelength of the radiation and varies from about 0.8 for visible light to nearly 1.0 for infrared. Only the infrared value need be considered for the heat transfer problems considered here. The emissivity and the absorptivity of human skin, for radiation in the infrared, are both approximately unity (Hardy, 1939).

The irradiation of a surface is defined as the total radiant energy striking it, from all sources, in watts per square meter. Some of this energy comes from the room, and some may come from a radiant warmer. The irradiation received by an infant from a surrounding room at 24°C is 441 W/m². About 65% of a naked infant's body surface area is exposed to the room radiation; the rest of the body is in contact with the mattress or very close to it. The radiation emitted from the infant's skin would be about 514 W/m², at a skin temperature of 35.5°C. Thus, there would be a net loss of energy by radiation of about 73 W/m² (about 15 W total for an average term infant) from the exposed area.

Radiant warmers can be used to deliver a net positive radiant heat transfer to an infant and to compensate for convective losses to the air. There is evidence that radiant warmers induce higher water loss rates than incubators, all other factors being equal. However, radiant warmers offer unequalled freedom of access to the patient and, for that reason, are the unit of choice in many cases in which the infant requires intensive care. When a radiant warmer is used, the irradiation reaching the infant is the sum of the irradiation from the radiant warmer and from the room.

Overhead radiant warmers are capable of delivering up to 300 W/m^2 at the infant's location, in addition to the irradiation from the room (Wheldon and Rutter, 1982). However, radiation from the warmer does not strike the entire exposed surface of the infant, whereas irradiation from the room does. This is because the warmer generates a somewhat collimated beam of radiation, aimed mainly at the infant's location. According to Baumgart et al. (1980), only about 32% of the infant's skin surface is bathed in radiation from such a collimated source. This is important in trying to calculate an energy balance, but it is not very important in practice because radiant heat losses from an infant are rarely calculated. The usual approach is to place a skin-temperature sensor on the infant and adjust the radiant warmer so that the infant's temperature remains constant.

Implications Even in a warm room, infants can lose heat by radiation to cold walls or windows that are not necessarily right next to the infant. Exterior windows should be double glazed or draped so that the interior surfaces are at room temperature; if these surfaces feel cool, they *are* cold.

Control Radiant heat transfer can be reduced by using aluminum foil as a reflector. Bright aluminum foil reflects more than 95% of the radiation incident upon it. When used to surround an infant, it reflects the infant's own radiation back to the infant, reducing the radiant loss to the surroundings.

Heat Transfer by Convection

Convective heat loss accounts for 25% to 50% of the heat loss from term infants and 15% to 30% of the loss from prematures. Once again, this does not mean that premature infants are less susceptible to convective loss than term infants; rather, that their total losses are higher because of their evaporation loss. Convective loss is proportional to the difference between the skin temperature and the air temperature; it increases as the air velocity increases, but not linearly.

Convection is the process whereby a solid exchanges heat with a liquid or gas. Infant convection losses usually occur through heat exchange to the surrounding air. If the fluid is at rest except for buoyant effects attributable to the heat transfer, the process is called *free* (or *natural*) *convection*. If the fluid is in motion as a result of a fan or blower, the process is called *forced convection*. There is an intermediate range, where the buoyant motions and the forced motions are both important. This region is called *mixed convection*.

In every case, the following equation (Equation 5) is used to calculate the heat transfer:

$$\dot{q} = hA(T_s - T_g) \tag{5}$$

where

$\dot{q}$ = Convective rate (W)
h = Heat transfer coefficient (W/m^2-°C)
A = Area (m^2)
T_s = Surface temperature (°C)
T_g = Gas temperature (°C)

The area used in Equation 5 is the "wetted" area, i.e., the area in contact with the fluid. The surface temperature must be described by a suitable average over the area in question, and the fluid temperature is measured far from the surface. Up to about 7 cm/sec, the air velocity has no effect on the heat transfer coefficient in the problems discussed. The situation is dominated by the free convection tendency. Even up to 15 cm/sec, the average heat transfer coefficient is not significantly different from what it would be in still air, and a value of 5.0 W/m^2-°C seems appropriate.

Clinical Implications As long as the air velocity is less than 20 cm/sec, there is little to be gained by trying to reduce it. Air circulation rates can be based on other criteria.

Evaporative Water Loss

All babies lose a significant amount of energy through evaporative water loss and, for prematures, evaporative energy loss may be the dominant mode. Evaporative loss can be as much as 90% of the total for very early premature infants born as early as the 26th week. For 32-week infants of about 1.5 kg birth weight in incubators, the evaporative energy loss (transepidermal plus respiratory) was found by Bell et al. (1980) to account for more than 60% of the total energy loss. Wheldon and Rutter (1982) reported somewhat lower values (around 35%). It has been suggested that the fraction is significantly higher under a radiant warmer.

Evaporative water loss occurs by two paths: through the skin (*transepidermal*) and in the lungs (*respiratory*). Respiratory water loss and energy loss are usually small compared to the totals and depend on the amount of air breathed and its initial humidity and temperature. If the air were breathed in at 100% relative humidity at body temperature, there would be no respiratory loss, either of water or of energy.

The transepidermal water loss depends on the body surface area and its permeability to water vapor. The surface area-to-mass ratio is high for premature infants, and the skin is much more permeable than the skin of a term infant. As a consequence of these two factors, transepidermal water loss is a very important problem for premature infants.

Transepidermal water loss can be calculated using the following equation:

$$\dot{m} = A \frac{m_{H_2O,o} - m_{H_2O,a}}{R_{tot}} \qquad (6)$$

where

$\dot{m}$ = Mass transfer rate (g/sec)
R_{tot} = Total resistance to water loss (m²-sec/g)
A = Area (m²)
$m_{H_2O,o}$ = Mass fraction of water in saturated air at skin temperature (g_{H_2O}/g_{mix})
$m_{H_2O,a}$ = Mass fraction of water in the ambient air (g_{H_2O}/g_{mix})

The total resistance to transepidermal water loss is the sum of two terms: the *epidermal resistance* and the *boundary layer resistance*. In term infants, about 98% of the total resistance is epidermal; at 26 weeks, the figure drops to about 75%. The epidermal resistance is a function of the gestational age at birth and the postnatal age, whereas the boundary layer resistance is a function of the air velocity.

For infants whose gestational age is 30 weeks or less, the problem of transepidermal water loss is most acute during the first postnatal week when the epidermal resistance is low. The rate of transepidermal water loss for a 25-week-old premature may be 15 times that for a term infant (in g/m²-hr), according to studies by Hammarlund et al. (1979). Under these conditions, the evaporative energy loss may account for 90% of the infant's metabolic output. These large effects are attributable to the latent heat of vaporization of water—the thermal energy required to change the state of water from liquid to vapor. When 1 gram of water is evaporated from the body, 2414.34 Joules of thermal energy are absorbed.

Implications Transepidermal water loss is an important factor in premature infants whose gestational age is 30 weeks or less, especially during the first postnatal week. After that, the skin matures and assumes more nearly "term" characteristics for the prevention of water loss.

The convective mass transfer coefficient plays little role in regulating water loss, except for the case of some of the most premature infants. For gestational ages of greater than 30 weeks, the transepidermal water loss can be expected to be independent of air velocity (within ± 5%). For the very early premature infant (25 weeks or less), air velocity is important because the resistance of the skin to water loss is very low.

Control The important variable at all gestational ages is the amount of water vapor in the surrounding air. If the ambient air could be held at body temperature and at 100% relative humidity, there would be no water loss, either by transepidermal or respiratory modes. Whether or not this is a desirable state for the infant is a matter for the attending physician to decide. However, the evaporative water loss and its associated energy loss can be controlled by this means.

Energy Loss Associated with Ingestion of Food, Fluids, or Medication

One often-ignored aspect of thermal regulation is the effect of food or medication ingestion by infants. Any food, fluid, or medication administered to an infant will equilibrate to the infant's temperature within a few minutes, and the thermal energy required for this process must come from the infant. The thermal load depends on the mass of material, its specific heat, and its initial temperature. The specific heat of water, for example, is 4.19 Joules/g-°C. A representative value for metabolic rate is 2.4 J/sec-kg.

A general equation describing this situation is:

$$q = mc(T_b - T_i) \qquad (7)$$

where

q = Total thermal energy required (J)
m = Mass of material (g)
c = Specific heat (J/g-°C)
T_b = Body temperature (°C)
T_i = Initial temperature of material at entry (°C)

Administration of 10 cc of water per kg of body weight at an initial temperature of 20°C creates the same heat load for the infant as would exposure to a 20°C environment for 5 minutes.

What matters in these instances is the temperature of the material as it enters the infant's body. It is not enough simply to warm a bottle of I.V. fluid. The bottle will cool before it is empty and the fluid will cool in the delivery line before it reaches the infant. Lines must be kept short and bottles kept warm.

Control All foods, fluids, and medications should be administered at body temperature at the point where they enter the body.

Equipment and Techniques for Managing Energy Loss

The infant should be kept in a neutral thermal environment by controlling the ambient temperature, humidity, and air flow. The techniques that should be used vary with the age of the infant, the degree of illness, and the theater in which clinical care is provided. If the infant is term and not ill, the creation of a neutral thermal environment presents minimal problems. A room heated to at least 26°C plus a blanket are usually all that is required. If the infant is premature and/or ill, the situation is quite different. This infant is less able to maintain his body temperature and, at the same time, can ill afford to utilize energy in the effort to keep warm. In addition, such infants often require intensive care, which means they cannot be swathed in protective blankets or garments. Continuous or frequent interventions requiring direct contact mandate the exposure of the infant.

For infants born after 30 weeks gestational age or more, control of the ambient temperature is the principal concern. For infants of less than 30 weeks gestational age, humidity control is as important as temperature control, and in very young infants (25 to 27 weeks) humidity control is mandatory. Sick babies and premature infants may require ambient temperatures up to 40°C, with relative humidity approaching 100%, to achieve a 37°C body temperature. It is not practical to maintain whole rooms at these conditions; hence, incubators and radiant warmers are used. These create local microclimates within which the infant's metabolic heat release can maintain a satisfactory body temperature, thus allowing normal activities in the rest of the room.

Nursery Incubators

Equipment for the care of a sick baby must provide four things: visibility, accessibility, temperature control, and humidity control. Incubators and radiant warmers are most frequently used for warming babies, but neither provides adequate humidity control for the intensive care of very premature infants. Although the incubator seems to offer the opportunity for humidity control, often it is not used for fear of bacterial growth. Radiant warmers have no capability for humidity control because the infant is directly exposed to the room air.

Most nursery incubators are transparent enclosures that control the infant's temperature through a servocontrol system. Most provide means for humidifying the air, although the available humidity control is not as sophisticated as the temperature control. In some incubators the infant can be reached through ports in the side of the unit, in others through the top cover, and in still others through rotation of a semicylindrical hood, which then allows access from the side.

Most incubators provide only limited access, at least without completely sacrificing thermal control. The extent to which thermal control is compromised by access to the infant differs from unit to unit and should be a factor in choosing which unit to use for a specific infant. The choice depends on the level of care the infant needs. A closed incubator can be used for infants requiring little and/or infrequent handling; it is the easiest artificial microenvironment to control. The classic example is the isolette incubator. In it, temperature, humidity, and air flow can be controlled.

Most units maintain the infant's temperature by regulating the air temperature through electric heaters, although some units use radiant heating inside the incubator and deliver the heat directly to the infant. Most units use servocontrol systems, which sense the infant's skin temperature. Two types of control system are used: *on/off* and *proportional*. With on/off control, the heater is either on or off, and control is achieved by controlling the fractional "on" time. Proportional control alters the level of power delivered to the heater, maintaining some power at (almost) all times. LeBlanc (1982) suggested that on/off control of environmental temperature leads to a higher metabolic rate (other factors remaining constant), but no controlled studies have clearly confirmed this report.

Radiant Warmers

In the 1960s, new therapeutic techniques were introduced for the care of premature infants with respiratory distress syndrome, including assisted ventilation, parenteral fluid and drug administration, and invasive arterial monitoring. Such techniques mandated an "open incubator" environment in which intensive care could be provided in a neutral thermal environment. Bassinets with overhead servocontrolled, radiant heat energy devices were developed and are now standard equipment in neonatal intensive care units (NICUs). These new devices have dramatically improved the ability of medical and nursing personnel to care for sick infants. Radiant warmers use arrays of infrared heat lamps that maintain the infant's skin temperature at a preselected level by radiation. The infant is nursed naked on a work table; hence, access is excellent. Radiant warmers are frequently used when the infant requires intensive care because of the free access they allow.

The infant is exposed to room air, usually maintained at about 26°C and 50% relative humidity, and loses considerable energy to the air. This is made up by the irradiation from the warmer. At the same time, however, humidification cannot be provided with these open bassinets. As a result, it is more difficult to manage the fluids and electrolytes in these infants. There is considerable evidence that insensible water loss is higher under a radiant warmer than in an incubator, all other factors being equal (Baumgart et al., 1981b; Bell et al., 1980; Jones et al., 1976; Wheldon and Rutter, 1982; Williams and Oh, 1974; Wu and Hodgman, 1974), and care must be taken to monitor fluid balance.

Fanaroff et al. (1972) reported high water loss from small infants (less than 1250 g) nursed under radiant warmers and also reported that this problem could be alleviated by covering the infant with a plastic shield. This was confirmed by Yeh et al. (1979), but subsequent research (Baumgart et al., 1980, 1981a; Marks et al., 1977) showed that a blanket of plastic bubble material is superior to a rigid hood in reducing water loss. This is probably because the plastic bubble blanket traps a smaller amount of air near the infant, thus reducing the demand on the infant for moisture to humidify the trapped air. The bubble material is better than single sheet material because of its superior heat-insulating properties. If a single sheet were used, moisture would probably condense on the sheet, which would then require more evaporation from the infant to maintain the humidity in the trapped air.

LeBlanc (1982) reported that, although incubators and radiant warmers can both maintain a desired body temperature, infants in incubators showed lower oxygen consumption by 5% to 10%.

Open-type radiant heat incubators are often used in delivery rooms and NICUs. Their success has prompted the use of mobile warming lamps for protection during other diagnostic and therapeutic procedures, e.g., cardiac catheterization, computed tomography (CT), and surgery. The effect of radiant heat units is sometimes supplemented by increasing the ambient temperature, heating the inhaled anesthesia gases, and warming the surgical rinsing solutions and intravenous fluids. The goal is always the same—to achieve and maintain a neutral thermal environment for the infant while providing the degree of access required by the attending staff.

Transport Incubators

With the popularization of regional care for critically ill newborn infants, emergency interhospital transport systems were developed to provide safe and effective transfer of critically ill patients between community hospitals and regional critical care facilities. Providing intensive care in a moving environment presents some major challenges for the transport team. Modern transport teams may bring all or most of the therapeutic modalities of the critical care unit to the patient's bedside in the referring community hospital and continue this same level of care during the transport.

The major technical problem involving intensive care during a transport is the maintenance of a neutral thermal environment while allowing easy access for the delivery of the required care. Medical transport teams may encounter cold weather during winter transfer of infants between hospitals and must also be prepared to cope with emergencies inside the transport vehicle, such as loss of electrical power. A transport incubator must be capable of providing an adequate internal environment in the worst foreseeable combination of conditions; the safety of the infant cannot be left to chance. The greater the tolerable environmental temperature range of the incubator and the more independent the system is, the larger the margin of safety.

There are several types of transport incubators available. The basic choice is between the radiant heat "open" type (see Figure 9.2) and the forced-air "closed" type. The open-type unit is recommended if intensive care is required during the transport. In 1972, Indyk discussed the deficiencies of available transport incubators, the most important being the inability to provide intensive care in a "closed isolette" without causing a drop in incubator temperature that persisted for a significant period of time. The closed isolette incubators do not afford easy access. Any entry causes a rapid and not easily recoverable temperature drop, which compromises the infant's body temperature. In 1973, Chance et al. noted the difficulty of providing adequate patient care when using less than optimal equipment. Studies published in 1975 indicated a 65% mortality rate in a group of 54 infants whose posttransport body temperatures were less than 35.5°C, as contrasted to a 25% mortality rate in 405 infants with posttransport body temperatures greater than 35.5°C (Hackel, 1975).

The transport incubator is an important component of a mobile intensive care system, and the development of such a system represents a significant challenge. The equipment must: provide the capabilities for life support and continuous monitoring of the patient to be transported; be self-contained; be lightweight; be portable; be easy to use; and allow uninterrupted intensive care throughout a transport, including the moments of entering and leaving the vehicle. A neonatal transport incubator system must include: 1) the ability to provide a neutral thermal environment under adverse environmental conditions; 2) easy access to

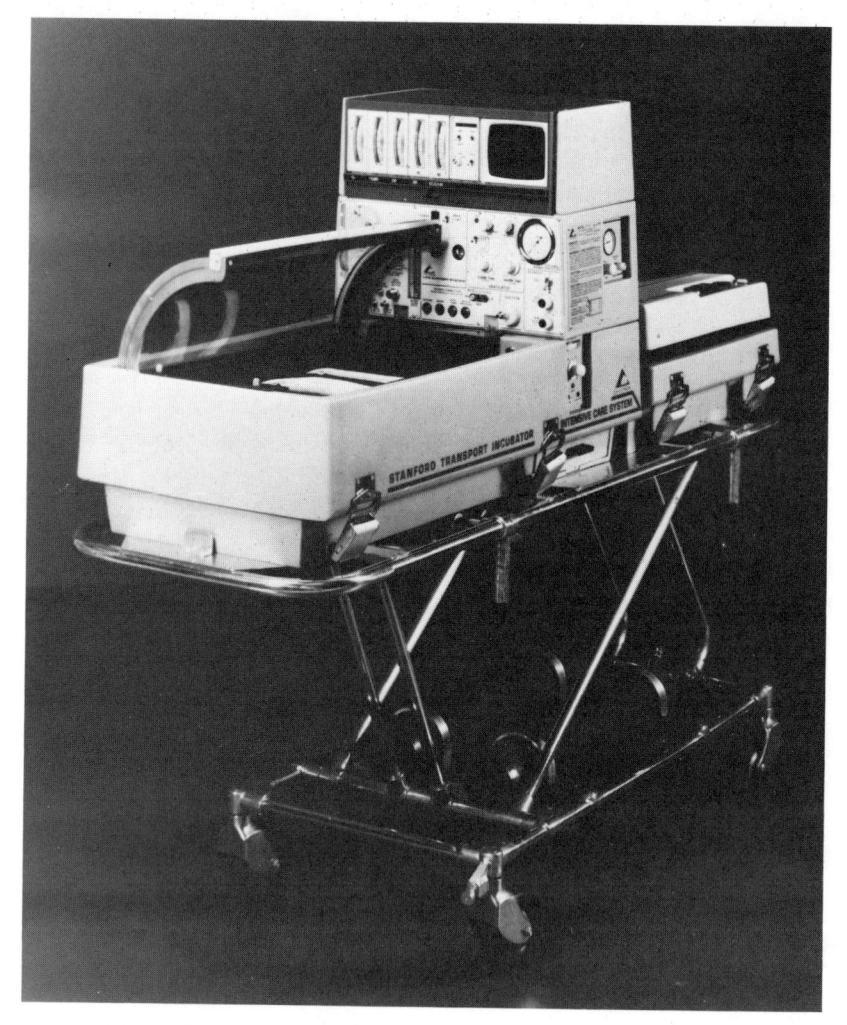

Figure 9.2. Radiant heat "open" type of transport incubator.

the infant for intensive care, including assisted ventilation; 3) monitoring of heart rate, blood pressure, inspired and transcutaneous oxygen, and core and/or skin temperatures; 4) a fail-safe humidified oxygen/air delivery system capable of delivering concentrations of oxygen between 21% and 100%; 5) adequate lighting under all conditions; 6) portable, self-contained, and lightweight rechargeable power for all electrical systems of the transport unit; and 7) a means of safely securing the incubator during transport to prevent injury in the event of sudden changes in speed or altitude.

Several new transport incubators have been developed in the past 10 years in an attempt to meet these requirements. The unit that most closely meets these requirements is the Healthdyne Transport Incubator. The prototype of this unit has been in use for 10 years. The commercially available unit has been in use for 7 years and has been used for more than 3000 transports at the Stanford University Hospital.

The transport incubator system consists of the incubator, the energy pack, and the life-support and monitoring modules represented in Figure 9.2. The transport incubator permits intensive care in a semi-open environment under severe external thermal conditions, with easy accessibility to the patient. Fully integrated life-support and monitoring modules have been added and combined with the transport incubator to form a transport-incubator system that is self-sufficient and capable of sustained operation for 2 hours or longer, depending on the external environment.

Thermal protection is provided by radiant heat, with a peak wavelength of 8.7μ, from a transparent, electrically heated membrane sandwiched between two layers of polycarbonate in a semicylindrical hood that covers the infant's bed. This hood rotates around the patient for storage under the bed. The usual mode of operation calls for the hood to be partly open, allowing access all along one side as well as through one end of the incubator. This position is designated as Procedure Mode I. Except under extreme environmental temperature conditions, the hood can be kept open in this position. An end cover is supplied for use when required. The radiant heat membrane is servocontrolled by a skin temperature probe placed on the infant's abdomen. A patient observation lamp is attached to the incubator. The combined weight of the incubator and life-support and monitoring modules is 50 pounds.

There are two alternative battery systems. One unit consists of 12 10-V, 9-amp/hr, sealed lead acid batteries and delivers 300 W of power at 120 V. The weight of this unit is formidable (130 pounds), but it will sustain a neutral thermal environment for 2 hours against a very low temperature ($-30°C$). A lighter 4.5 amp/hr battery pack or gel-cell battery units are also available for more moderate climates. Cold room tests were performed to ascertain the lowest external temperatures at which the incubator can maintain the desired neutral thermal environment in Procedure Mode I and in other more energy-conservative modes. These tests were conducted at the NASA Ames Research Laboratory at Stanford University and at the Dalmo Victor Corporation. Results of the three tests were entirely consistent with each other and are noted in Table 9.1.

The life-support module contains a time-cycled, constant-flow, pressure-limited ventilator and an oxygen/air delivery system. There is also provision for regulating continuous infusion of parenteral fluids and

Table 9.1. Permissible external temperatures for neutral thermal environment.

Procedure mode	Lowest permissible temperature
I. Hood open, end open	$-1°C$
II. Hood open, end closed	$-6°C$
III. Hood closed, end open	$-6°C$
IV. Hood closed, end closed	$-14°C$
V. Sealed, emergency closure	$<-30°C$

Reprinted by permission from Hackel, A., and Moffat, R. J. 1978. Provision of neutral thermal environment (NTE) during transport. Pediatric Research 12:525.

for airway suctioning. The monitor module contains FiO1 (inspiratory oxygen concentration), temperature, blood pressure, respiratory rate, and heart rate channels, as well as a two-channel display screen. The life-support and monitoring modules can be detached from the incubator and used separately. The equipment can be used in the hospital for transport and during special procedures outside the intensive-care nursery.

Other Methods for Control of Heat Loss and Water Loss

Incubators and radiant warmers are the most commonly used pieces of equipment, but other methods have been studied.

Topical Agents for Control of Water Loss Rutter and Hull (1981) reduced transepidermal water loss by 40–60% by topical application of a paraffin mixture (80% soft, 20% hard) over all of the skin except around the mouth and eyes. The benefit lasted 6 to 8 hours. The subject infants were 26 to 30 weeks gestational age and were in the age group most susceptible to transepidermal water loss. The paraffin did not irritate the skin. In later studies, the same team showed that an equal benefit could be achieved using a plastic bubble blanket (Brice et al., 1981).

Caps and Clothes Strothers (1981) reported reducing the heat loss from an infant by as much as 25% by insulating the head only, using a gamgee tissue-lined cap. The infants studied were term; hence, most of their heat loss was radiant and convective. Thus the benefit of such insulation is not surprising because the head accounts for about 21% of the body surface area.

Special clothing (caps and bunting) is available that combines a semipermeable inner liner with an effective thermal insulation (Minnesota Mining and Manufacturing Co., 1983). This material maintains a high humidity layer of air near the skin without allowing condensation and should have wide application. At the time of this report, there have not been any independent evaluations of its effectiveness, but it seems well designed and likely to be successful. Because it limits access, the full bunting seems suited only for use with well babies.

Problems That Arise in Special Theaters

Delivery and surgical areas impose special thermal burdens on the infant; thus, special equipment and procedures may be needed in order to provide a neutral thermal environment. In general, thermal problems arise whenever the environmental conditions are dictated by considerations other than the thermal response of the infant. Such situations arise when specialized equipment that requires certain environmental conditions in order to function properly (x-ray or CT equipment, for example) is used.

Delivery Rooms

In the delivery room, the infant's skin temperature may drop 3°C within 10 seconds, as shown by cinethermographic studies of infants during birth (Tähti et al., 1972). This combination of conditions imposes a severe thermal burden on the infant: "Wet infants exposed to room air may lose nearly five times more heat than those who were dried and warmed" (Tähti et al., 1972).

Dahm and James (1972) pointed out that initial cold stress may play an important role in stimulating breathing, so that providing complete thermal protection for the newborn may not be desirable. A little cold stress goes a long way, however, and the infant should be protected against excessive heat loss as quickly as possible. Dahm and James recorded rectal temperatures during the first 30 minutes after birth for groups of term (38–40-week-old) infants. The body temperature of infants exposed wet to the delivery room environment dropped 2°C or more within 30 minutes. Those who were dried and blanketed lost less than 1°C, and those dried and radiantly warmed lost as little as 0.5°C during the same period.

It is desirable to have a radiant warmer or other means of warming ready for depressed infants because drying and blanketing may not be enough. Plastic bubble wrap would also be useful, particularly for infants of less than 30 weeks gestational age, when transepidermal water loss is a major concern.

Sheldon (1974) recommended keeping sterile bowel bags available for use as thermal protectors. These would be used in case an infant was born with a skin defect, such as gastroschisis, which would expose moist tissue to the air. Water loss from such tissue is very rapid, more than 50 times the rate from the infant's skin, and it takes with it so much energy that the infant's body temperature could drop several degrees in a few minutes. The bowel bag should be used with blankets or a radiant warmer because it does not, by itself, prevent convective heat loss—only water loss.

Surgical Theaters

Surgical theaters are usually cool and highly ventilated. Free access to the patient is required, and thermal protective equipment can be tolerated only if it does not interfere with the surgeons' activities. Surgical procedures frequently expose significant amounts of moist body tissue to room air with the attendant water and energy losses. An infant patient is likely to be under considerable stress to begin with as a consequence of the condition requiring surgery, the thermal stress of transport to the surgery, and the anesthesia used during the procedures. All of these factors make surgery an especially challenging problem for thermal protection.

Transport incubators with full thermal protection are recommended even for "short" journeys within a hospital. Thermal equilibrium of the infant should be maintained throughout the transport.

Several reported methods of warming the infant surgical patient are: overhead radiant warmers (Russell et al., 1972; Shim and Halford, 1974); plastic bags (Rowe and Taylor, 1981); plastic surgical gowns (Hobbs et al., 1976); air-fluidized beds (Russell et al., 1972); and air-heated contact mattresses (Lewis et al., 1973). Even electrically heated rectal probes have been used (Roe et al., 1966).

Commercially available radiant warmers can be modified and supported from the ceiling tracks used for the surgical lights, leaving ample clearance between the surgeon and the heater (Poulos et al., 1974; Shim and Halford, 1974). The radiant field can be adjusted to cover the patient without unduly warming the surgeon. This approach does not reduce the infant's water loss.

Rowe and Taylor (1981) pointed out that cloth covers do not reduce water loss from infants and that a cloth mattress under a patient who is covered by a plastic drape absorbs enough water vapor to negate the protection of the plastic. To be effective, the plastic must completely surround the patient and should limit air flow as well. Hobbs et al. (1976) described a surgical gown made of transparent polyethylene that significantly reduces transepidermal water loss without impeding visibility or access.

Plastic bags and surgical gowns should be used in conjunction with a heat source, such as a radiant warmer, electrically heated surgical blanket, or chemical mattress. Without external heating, there may be condensation of moisture on the inside of the plastic; thus, water is lost from the infant just as effectively as though it had been carried away by the room air.

Russell et al. (1972) described an air-fluidized bed in which the patient is supported by siliconized glass microspheres perfused by heated and humidified air. The patient is bathed in a flow of conditioned air, and both heat loss and water loss can be controlled. If the air flow is reduced after the patient is placed on the bed, it defluidizes and "solidifies" around the patient, providing positive support. Contact mattresses that are heated electrically or chemically are also available. An air-heated contact mattress was described by Lewis et al. (1973).

X-Ray and Computer Tomography Areas

Rooms used primarily for x-ray or CT are kept cool because of equipment requirements. Bulky thermal protection equipment cannot be used because of interference with the primary function of the room; yet, the infant patient requires thermal assistance under these conditions. Marks et al. (1980) reported success using a combination of a chemically heated mattress with a plastic bubble blanket for in-hospital transport and CT scan procedures.

Hobbs et al. (1976) reported good results using transparent polyethylene surgical gowns during diagnostic x-ray procedures lasting up to 50 minutes. There was no interference with the x-ray imaging and no significant interference with access or with the placement of catheters. The x-ray rooms were cold (22°C), yet none of the infants lost more than 0.2°C in body temperature over the 50-minute period. No exogenous heat sources were used. The subjects ranged in weight from 1.45 to 3.4 kg.

Phototherapy

Three studies showed increased water loss associated with phototherapy, apparently beyond that which accompanies purely thermal irradiation. Oh and Karecki (1972) reported increased water loss by each individual mechanism (urine, stool, and evaporative water loss) when infants received phototherapy. Their data showed only small increases in body temperature (on the order of 0.2°C) but significant increases in respiratory rate.

Bell et al. (1979) found that phototherapy increased water loss beyond the value found using only a radiant warmer, even though, in all cases, the rectal temperature was maintained between 37.8°C and 37.1°C during the tests. It is not known whether the extra water loss was via the respiratory or the transepidermal path, and no recommendations were made regarding how to reduce the water loss.

Conclusion

Under normal environmental conditions, healthy term babies can regulate their own body temperatures, but premature and/or sick babies cannot. An infant of less than 30 weeks gestational age not only cannot regulate his body temperature but also loses considerable water through respiration and evaporation, further increasing heat loss. When a premature infant requires intensive care, the water loss problem is great. Radiant warmers, introduced in many intensive care nurseries over the past decade, offer unrestricted access but increase water loss. Thus, the attempt to solve the heat problem has increased the water loss problem.

The attending physician must understand how to assess infants' thermal problems and accompanying moisture loss, and how to provide the best possible environment. This chapter draws on thermal principles and clinical experience to present the best available knowledge on thermal management of infants. Eventually, research and practice will provide more refined and integrated models for more precisely predicting the thermal needs of infants.

References

Baumgart, S., Engle, W. D., Fox, W. W., and Polin, R. A. 1981a. Effect of heat shielding on convective and evaporative heat losses and on radiant heat transfer in the premature infant. J. Pediatr. 99:948–956.

Baumgart, S., Engle, W. D., Fox, W. W., and Polin, R. A. 1981b. Radiant warmer power and body size as determinants of insensible water loss in the critically ill neonate. Pediatr. Res. 14:1495–1499.

Baumgart, S., Fox, W. W., and Polin, R. A. 1980. Physiological implications of two different heat shields for infants under radiant warmers. J. Pediatr. 100:787–790.

Belgaumkar, T. K., and Scott, K. E. 1975. Effects of low humidity on small premature infants in servo-control incubators. Biol. Neonate 26:337–347.

Bell, E. F., Neidich, G. A., Cashore, W. J., and Oh, W. 1979. Combined effect of radiant warmer and phototherapy on insensible water loss in low-birth-weight infants. J. Pediatr. 94:810–813.

Bell, E. F., Weinstein, M. R., and Oh, W. 1980. Heat balance in premature infants: Comparative effects of convectively heated incubator and radiant warmer, with and without plastic heat shield. J. Pediatr. 96:460–465.

Brice, E. H., Rutter, N., and Hull, D. 1981. Reduction of skin water loss in the newborn. II. Clinical trials of two methods in very low birthweight babies. Arch. Dis. Child. 56:673–675.

Chance, G. W., O'Brien, M. J., and Swyer, P. R. 1973. Transportation of sick neonates 1972: An unsatisfactory aspect of medical care. Can. Med. Assoc. J. 109:847.

Dahm, L. S., and James, L. S. 1972. Newborn temperature and calculated heat loss in the delivery room. Pediatrics 49:504–513.

Fanaroff, A. A., Wald, M., Gruber, H. S., and Klaus, M. H. 1972. Insensible water loss in low birthweight infants. Pediatrics 50:236–245.

Hackel, A. 1975. A medical transport system for the neonate. Anesthesiology 43:258–268.

Hackel, A., and Moffat, R. J. 1978. Provision of neutral thermal environment (NTE) during transport. Pediatr. Res. 12:525.

Hammarlund, K., Nilsson, G. E., Öberg, P. A., and Sedin, G. 1979. Transepidermal water loss in newborn infants. II. Relation to activity and body temperature. Acta Paediatr. Scand. 68:371–376.

Hammarlund, K., Nilsson, G. E., Öberg, P. A., and Sedin, G. 1980. Transepidermal water loss in newborn infants. V. Evaporation from the skin and heat exchange during the first hours of life. Acta Paediatr. Scand. 69:385–392.

Hammarlund, K., and Sedin, G. 1979. Transepidermal water loss in newborn infants. III. Relation to gestational age. Acta Paediatr. Scand. 68:795–801.

Hardy, J. F. 1939. The radiating power of human skin in the infrared. Am. J. Physiol. 127:454.

Hobbs, J. F., Eidelman, A. I., MacKuanying, N., Weinberg, G., and Schneider, K. M. 1976. A new transparent insulating gown for the surgical neonate. J. Pediatr. Res. 11:453–460.

Holman, J. P. 1981. Heat Transfer, 4th ed. McGraw-Hill, New York.

Jones, R. W. A., Rochefort, M. J., and Baum, J. O. 1976. Increased insensible water loss in newborn infants nursed under radiant warmers. Br. Med. J. 2:1347–1350.

LeBlanc, M. H. 1982. Relative efficacy of an incubator and an open warmer in producing thermoneutrality for the small premature infant. Pediatrics 69:439–445.

Lewis, R. B., Shaw, A., and Etchells, A. H. 1973. Contact mattress to prevent heat loss in neonatal and paediatric surgery. Br. J. Anaesth. 45:919.

Marks, K. H., Friedman, Z., and Maisels, M. J. 1977. A simple device for reducing insensible water loss in low birthweight infants. Pediatrics 60:233–226.

Marks, K. H., Maisels, M. J., and Lee, C. A. 1980. Temperature control during computerized tomography and in-hospital transport of low-birth-weight infants. Am. J. Dis. Child. 134:1176–1177.

Minnesota Mining and Manufacturing Co. 1983. Product Bulletin. Minnesota Mining and Manufacturing Co.

Oh, W., and Karecki, H. 1972. Phototherapy and insensible water loss in the newborn infant. Am. J. Dis. Child. 124:230–232.

Poulos, P., d'Alessandro, E., Barbara, A., Falla, A., and Groff, D. B. 1974. Operating room infant warmer—modifications of a commercially available unit. J. Pediatr. Surg. 9:521–523.

Roe, C. F., Santulli, T. V., and Blair, C. S. 1966. Heat loss in infants during general anesthesia and operations. J. Pediatr. Surg. 1:266–274.

Rowe, M. I., and Taylor, M. 1981. Transepidermal water loss in the infant surgical patient. J. Pediatr. Surg. 16:878–881.

Russell, H. E., Jr., Othersen, H. B., Jr., and Hargest, T. S. 1972. Thermal regulation of pediatric patients in the operating room by means of an air fluidized bed. Am. Surg. 38:111–114.

Rutter, N., and Hull, D. 1981. Reduction of skin water loss in the newborn. I. Effect of applying topical agents. Arch. Dis. Child. 56:669–672.

Ryser, G., and Jequier, E. 1972. Study by direct calorimetry of thermal balance on the first day of life. Eur. J. Clin. Invest. 2:176–187.

Sheldon, R. E. 1974. The bowel bag: A sterile, transportable method for warming infants with skin defects. Pediatrics 53:267–269.

Shim, W. K. T., and Halford, P. 1974. Method for maintaining the neonate's intraoperative care temperature. Surgery 75:416–420.

Strothers, J. K. 1981. Heat insulation and heat loss in the newborn. Arch. Dis. Child. 56:530–534.

Tähti, E., Line, J., Osterlund, K., and Rylander, E. 1972. Changes in skin temperature of the neonate at birth. Acta Paediatr. Scand. 61:159–164.

Wheldon, A. E., and Rutter, N. 1982. The heat balance of small babies nursed in incubators and under radiant warmers. Early Human Dev. 6:131–143.

Williams, P. R., and Oh, W. 1974. Effects of radiant warmer on insensible water loss in newborn infants. Am. J. Dis. Child. 128:511–514.

Wu, P. Y. K., and Hodgman, J. E. 1974. Insensible water loss in pre-term infants: Changes with postnatal development and non-ionizing radiant energy. Pediatrics 54:704–712.

Yeh, T. F., Amma, P., Lilien, L. D., Baccaro, M. M., Matwynshyn, J., Pyati, S., and Pildes, R. S. 1979. Reduction of insensible water loss in premature infants under the radiant warmer. J. Pediatr. 94:651–653.

Recommended Readings

Adamson, K., and Towell, M. D. 1965. Thermal homeostasis in the fetus and newborn. Anesthesiology 26:531.

Bain, J. A., and Spoerel, W. C. 1972. A streamlined anaesthetic system. Can. Anaesth. Soc. J. 19:426.

Chang, J. A. T. 1979. Neonatal surgical emergencies. III. Congenital diaphragmatic hernia. Peri/Neonatology 3:22.

Cunio, R. L., Maibach, H. I., Khan, H., and Bloom, F. 1977. Skin barrier properties in the newborn. Transepidermal water loss and carbon dioxide emission rates. Biol. Neonate 32:177–182.

Dierdorf, S. F., and Krishna, G. 1981. Anesthetic management of neonatal surgical emergencies. Anesth. Analg. 60:204–215.

Dilworth, N. M. 1973. The importance of changes in body temperature in pediatric surgery and anesthesia. Anesthesiol. Intensive Care 1:485.

Graves, S. 1981. Fluid and electrolyte therapy in children. ASA Refresher Course #114, ASA Meeting, New Orleans, October 17.

Hammarlund, K., Nilsson, G. E., Öberg, P. O., and Sedin, G. 1977. Transepidermal water loss in newborn infants. I. Relation to ambient humidity and site of measurement and estimation of total transepidermal water loss. Acta Paediatr. Scand. 66:553–562.

Hammarlund, K., and Sedin, G. 1980. Transepidermal water loss in newborn infants. IV. Small for gestational age infants. Acta Paediatr. Scand. 69:377–383.

Hayckco, G. B., Schwartz, G. J., and Wisotsky, D. H. 1978. Geometric method for measuring body surface area: A height-weight formula validated in infants, children, and adults. J. Pediatr. 93:62.

Hendren, W. H. 1973. Pediatric surgery. N. Engl. J. Med. 289:456–461, 507–515, 562–568.

Inselman, L. S., and Mellins, R. B. 1981. Growth and development of the lung. J. Pediatr. 89:1.

Jonsen, A. R., et al. 1975. Critical issues in newborn intensive care: A conference report and policy proposal. Pediatrics 55:756.

Kays, W. M., and Crawford, M. E. 1980. Convective Heat and Mass Transfer, 2nd ed. McGraw-Hill, New York.

Kitterman, J. A., et al. 1969. Aortic blood pressure in normal newborn infants during the first 12 hours of life. Pediatrics 44:959.

Marks, K. H., Lee, C. A., Bolan, C. D., and Maisels, M. J. 1981. Oxygen consumption and temperature control of premature infants in a double-wall incubator. Pediatrics 68:93–98.

Orsmark, K., Wilson, D., and Maibach, H. 1980. In vivo transepidermal water loss and epidermal occlusive hydration in newborn infants: Anatomical region variation. Acta Derm. Veneriol. 60:403–407.

Rackow, H. 1970. Intraoperative fluid therapy in infants. Anesthesiology 32:298.

Rackow, H., and Salanitre, E. 1969. Modern concepts in pediatric anesthesiology. Anesthesiology 30:208.

Raphaely, R. D., and Downes, J. J. 1973. Congenital diaphragmatic hernia: Prediction of survival. J. Pediatr. Surg. 8:815.

Rudolph, A. M. 1974. Congenital Diseases of the Heart. Year Book Medical Publishers, Chicago.

Rudolph, A. M., and Yuan, S. 1966. Response of the pulmonary vasculature to hypoxia and H+ ion concentration changes. J. Clin. Invest. 45:399.

Rutter, N., and Hull, D. 1979. Water loss from the skin of term and pre-term babies. Arch. Dis. Child. 54:858–868.

Siebers, D., Moffat, R. J., and Kays, W. M. 1982. Mixed convection from a large vertical plate in a horizontal wind. HMT-30, Thermosciences Division, Department of Mechanical Engineering, Stanford University, Stanford, CA.

Sinclair, J. E. (ed.). 1978. Temperature Regulation and Energy Metabolism in the Newborn. Grune & Stratton, New York.

Smith, R. M. 1976. Pediatric anesthesia in perspective. Anesth. Analg. 57:34.

Smith, R. M. 1980. Anesthesia for Infants and Children, 4th ed. Mosby, St. Louis.

Stern, L., Lees, M. H., and Luduc, J. 1965. Environmental temperature, oxygen consumption, and catecholamine excretion in newborn infants. Pediatrics 36:367.

Sulyok, E., Jequier, E., and Prod'hom, L. S. 1973. Respiratory contribution to the thermal balance of the newborn infant under various ambient conditions. Pediatrics. 51:641–650.

Sulyok, E., Jequier, E., and Ryser, G. 1972. Effect of relative humidity on thermal balance of the newborn infant. Biol. Neonate 21:210–218.

Yeh, T. F., Vidysagar, D., and Pildes, R. S. 1975. Critical care problems of the newborn: Insensible water loss in small premature infants. Crit. Care Med. 3:238–241.

10

Consequences of Newborn Intensive Care

Joyce L. Peabody and Kathleen Lewis

> ... for every action there is an equal and opposite reaction...
> *Sir Issac Newton*
> Third Law of Motion

In the past 10 years, the survival rate of low birth weight infants has dramatically increased throughout the United States and abroad (Hack et al., 1979; Hirata et al., 1983; Reynolds and Taghizadeh, 1974). In 1972, at Children's Hospital of San Francisco, there was an overall survival rate of 48% for infants whose birth weights were under 1500 grams; this included no survival for infants less than 750 grams. By 1981, the overall survival rate had risen to 81%, with 53% of infants 500 to 750 grams surviving (Hirata et al., 1983). The impressive improvement in survival rates among these infants has been attributed to the development of sophisticated and effective centers to provide intensive care for sick newborns. The past 10 years have been characterized by marked progress in biomedical electronics and the application of this technology to the care of the fetus and newborn infant, the regionalization of facilities for perinatal care, and the development of techniques for mechanical ventilation of newborn infants. In addition, these years have brought new techniques for cardiorespiratory monitoring, expansion of neonatal pharmacology, widespread utilization of phototherapy for management of hyperbilirubinemia, and methods for delivery of high-caloric solutions parentally when oral alimentation is not possible.

Unfortunately, many studies of neonatal morbidity report essentially no change in morbidity over this 10-year period (Field, 1980; Fitzhardinge et al., 1976; Knobloch et al., 1982; Krishnamoorthy et al., 1980; Nelson et al., 1980). Of even greater concern is the increasing number of reports of complications directly related to procedures and interventions that characterize newborn intensive care in the 1980s (Brown and Glass, 1979; Moore, 1976; Rao and Elhassani, 1980). History has frequently shown a lag time of a generation or more before the deleterious effects of medical intervention become obvious. Such lessons include retrolental fibroplasia (Ashton et al., 1953; James and Lanman, 1976), thalidomide (Taussig, 1962), x-ray (Payne, 1899; Spear, 1973), and diethylstilbestrol (Herbst et al., 1978). Consider the environmental characteristics of the intensive care nursery (ICN) and their numerous potentially adverse effects on the newborn host. This chapter reviews what is known and what is unknown regarding the consequences of such newborn intensive care on the developing infant.

Physical Factors

Light

For many years it has been recognized that there are numerous effects of light on humans and other mammalian species. These include effects on various biologic rhythms, endocrine glands, gonadal function, and vitamin D synthesis (Aschoff, 1965; Halberg, 1975; Mills, 1966; Norman et al., 1962; Wurtman and Cardinali, 1976; Wurtman et al., 1964; Zacharias and Wurtman, 1969). Because of these effects there has always been a concern that exposure to light in an ICN might have deleterious effects on infants. Whereas there is currently little strong evidence regarding permanent sequelae (Behrman et al., 1974), long-term effects may still be possible.

All babies in ICNs are exposed to high levels of fluorescent lighting 24 hours each day. The Academy of Pediatrics guidelines recommend a minimum 100-footcandle intensity at the level of the infant at all times for adequate visualization in the ICN (American Academy of Pediatrics, 1977). It is known that there is no diurnal rhythmicity in the light exposure that infants receive in the ICN, and it has been speculated that this interferes with the development of their natural diurnal biologic rhythms. Although there is no proof that this prolonged, continuous, cool-white fluorescent lighting has adverse effects on newborn infants, there is strong evidence in animals, children, and adults that lighting conditions can have negative biochemical and physical effects. In many species, visible radiant energy has been shown to lead to various tissue injuries (Spikes and Glad,

1964). Intensive exposure to light in the visible spectrum was shown to kill or cause mutations in bacteria (Webb and Lorenz, 1970; Webb and Malina, 1970). Radiation in the visible light spectrum decreases the functional life span of mammalian spermatozoa (Norman et al., 1962). Recently, an increased risk of melanoma was reported in people with prolonged exposure to fluorescent light (Beral et al., 1982). Additional questions that remain unanswered include: Do photosensitization and photo-allergic reactions occur in infants cared for in an ICN who also receive certain drugs in the prenatal and neonatal period? Is there synergism between the vibratory phenomena of light and sound on infants in special care units? Do long-term endocrine changes occur in infants exposed to such continuous monotonous light?

In addition to the continuous exposure to ambient fluorescent lighting, many infants are exposed to such light for the treatment of hyperbilirubinemia. In the United States, it has been estimated that 90,000 infants annually are treated with phototherapy (Maisels, 1976). Various types of fluorescent light have been used, including broad spectrum, daylight, cool light, and blue or monochromatic (special blue) light. Blue light obscures the appearance of cyanosis and has been reported to cause nausea and other feelings of discomfort in the personnel working in the units. In addition, like sunlight, it may exacerbate herpes infections in caretakers.

Several investigations in recent years have delineated the biologic adverse effects of phototherapy, and many significant findings can be cited. Numerous changes in the skin have been reported in infants receiving phototherapy. Continuous exposure may cause an increase in peripheral blood flow and has caused erythema in adults. In addition, some of the photoenergy is absorbed by Plexiglas and may result in a rise in the incubator temperature and in infant hyperthermia (Wu and Berdhal, 1974) in single-wall incubators.

Some authors have described a change in the characteristics of stools of infants receiving phototherapy (Bakken, 1977; Lund and Peterson, 1974; Wu and Moosa, 1978). Many investigators have reported a more rapid transit time of materials such as electrolytes and nitrogen through the gut in infants receiving phototherapy (Bakken, 1977; Brown et al., 1970; Lund and Peterson, 1974; Wu and Moosa, 1978). Bakken (1977) demonstrated an impairment in lactase activity in light-treated jaundiced infants.

Insensible water losses are significantly increased during phototherapy in part because of the increase in skin blood flow and excessive stool water losses (Bell et al., 1979). This effect is particularly marked in infants who are under radiant warmers. In term infants, insensible water loss may increase by 40% (Oh and Karecki, 1972). In low birth weight infants, the increase may be as high as 80–190% in nonservocontrolled incubators (Wu and Hodgman, 1974).

Phototherapy has also been shown to have some acute hematologic effects. Maurer et al. (1976) reported an increased rate of platelet turnover resulting in lower mean platelet count. Kopelman et al. (1978) reported increased hemolysis in infants with glucose-6-phosphate dehydrogenase (G-6-PD) deficiency who are treated with phototherapy. However, in two controlled studies, no differences in hemoglobin or hematocrit levels were observed in G-6-PD–deficient infants who were treated with phototherapy compared to those who were not (Meloni et al., 1974; Tan, 1977).

In a series of studies, Speck and co-workers demonstrated that phototherapy is capable of damaging the DNA of cells growing in culture (Speck and Rosenkranz, 1975, 1976; Speck et al., 1975). Because it is likely that light penetrates the thin scrotal skin and perhaps even reaches the ovaries through the thin abdominal wall, it has been suggested that shielding gonads with diapers may be indicated when infants are treated with phototherapy (Speck, 1979). Many investigators have reported with confidence that no adverse effects have been seen in human infants during the 20 years that phototherapy has been in clinical use; however, long-term effects, such as DNA damage, will not be obvious until future generations.

Several other studies of animal species have demonstrated the potential toxic effect of light on the retina. Some of these studies are in question because midriatic drops were used or the animals that were selected had hypersensitivity of their retinas. Messner (1978) and co-workers studied the effects of clinical levels of phototherapy on the retina of newborn monkeys. They maintained the monkeys in standard nursery incubators and restrained them in a supine position facing the light. No midriatic drops were used, so that the monkeys could open and close their eyes as desired. One eye was suture-closed and covered with a patch to act as a control. The study showed that exposure of the eyes to phototherapy for as short as 12 hours and up to 7 days produced severe and progressive damage to the retina. To determine the rate of recovery, an additional series of monkeys were exposed to light for 3 to 10 days and returned to normal environments for 10 months before their eyes were examined. Substantial retinal healing was evident if the initial exposure lasted less than 3 days. However, there was some loss of rod and cone cells in all of the exposed retinas when compared to the controls. The loss is similar to the normal deterioration noted in aging photoreceptive cells. This description of the damage is important because visual acuity, electroretinography, and ophthalmic examinations may be normal in childhood even when an infant has suffered phototoxic retinal damage and considerable tissue damage. These observations indicate that it is prudent to continue to patch the eyes of infants receiving phototherapy. Once again, however, even in the patching of the eyes the cost-benefit ratio must be considered. Patching eyes has been reported to disturb parents and interfere with maternal-infant bonding. In addition, there have been reports of obstruction of the nares by eye patches, which leads to respiratory distress and hypoxemia (Harris and Smith, 1977; Konig and Mazzi, 1976). Finally, the eye patches have caused distortion of the face and, in some cases, excoriation of the periorbital area, corneal injury, or conjunctivitis (Rao and Elhassani, 1981).

In vitro studies as well as studies in humans and animals strongly suggest that the products of photodecomposition have no direct neurotoxic effects (Diamond and Schmid, 1968; Karon et al., 1970). However, physical growth may be affected. In one study of 120 infants receiving phototherapy from the second to sixth day of life, 44% of those receiving continuous phototherapy had regained their birth weight by the seventh day as compared to 57.6% of those receiving intermittent phototherapy and 80% of the control infants (Wu et al., 1974). The phototherapy group demonstrated catch-up growth during the next 2 weeks. These growth effects may have been caused by the increase in fluid and caloric losses reported in various studies of phototherapy. A two-year follow-up of these infants revealed no difference in weight, length, or head circumference (Teberg et al., 1977). In addition, there were no differences in developmental and neurologic performance in the phototherapy group when compared to the control infants.

Other adverse effects of phototherapy include hypocalcemia (Ramagnoli et al., 1979); changes in serum levels of gonadotropins (Dacou-Voutetakis et al., 1978); the "bronze baby syndrome" (when phototherapy is applied to infants with cholestasis) (Kopelman et al., 1972); a reduction in tryptophane, methionine, and histidine levels when amino acid solutions and multivitamin solutions are exposed to phototherapy (Bhatia et al., 1980); a shift to the right in the neonatal oxygen dissociation curve in vitro (Ostrea and Odell, 1974); and a depletion of riboflavin (Kostenbauder and Sanvordeker, 1973).

In summary, light and its possible adverse effects on infants are a major consideration as consequences of modern neonatal intensive care. It is unreasonable to expect that the absence of light in the uterus for the premature infant or the normal home lighting characteristics for the sick term infant can be reproduced in the nursery environment. Babies under intensive care are closely observed 24 hours a day, which requires a certain intensity of light within the nursery. In addition, the use of light to treat hyperbilirubinemia is considered to be less invasive and to cause less morbidity than the alternative of exchange transfusion. However, the advantages of light in the ICN should not lead to the belief that any level of light intensity is "safe." Keeping in mind the risk of light exposure, health care professionals should decrease the light intensity in areas in the nursery where infants are recovering and no longer need such close and intense observation. Phototherapy, although easy to apply, must be considered a drug that should be given in the lowest effective dose possible for the shortest effective time possible. Finally, follow-up studies must continue to try to identify any long-term effects of light exposure on nursery infants.

Noise

From the muffled but not soundless uterus, the newborn infant in an ICN is exposed to continuous variable noise. In utero, the fetus experiences the constant and regular auditory stimuli of the maternal heart rate and bowel sounds. External noises are transmitted but muffled by maternal tissues and amniotic fluid. In the ICN, noise levels are heightened, irregular, and often linked with other noxious stimuli. Noise levels have become a concern because of both their immediate effects on the premature or sick newborn's homeostasis and their long-term effects on hearing.

Noise levels in NICUs are significantly higher than those in a normal newborn nursery and are much higher and of a different quality than in the average home (Anagnostakis et al., 1980). Even higher noise levels are found inside incubators, particularly those that have ventilatory support systems. Sound measurements in two studies showed that infant incubators produce continuous noise levels between 50 and 86 decibels (dBs) on the A-weighted scale [dB(A)] (Blennow et al., 1974; Bell et al., 1979). In adults, noise levels above 80 dB(A), even for short duration, produce some degree of hearing loss in a small percentage of people (American Academy of Pediatrics, 1974). In addition, recent studies have suggested that young animals are more susceptible to noise damage than are adults (Falk et al., 1974). Finally, animal studies showed that noise-induced hearing loss can be potentiated by the use of ototoxic aminoglycoside antibiotics (Falk, 1972), a group of drugs commonly used in sick newborn infants.

In addition to the relatively high continuous noise levels in an incubator, there are peak noise levels during various procedures. Opening the door of an incubator may increase the decibel level tenfold (Anagnostakis et al., 1980). The highest levels measured in the intensive care unit itself occur when an infant is admitted to the unit (Anagostakis et al., 1980). Additionally, voices of caregivers peak during such times as emergencies and teaching rounds. Telephones, the dropping of equipment, and radios also contribute to sudden increases in noise levels.

The immediate and long-term effects of noise have been studied by several investigators. Noise levels of 65–75 dB(A) interfere with sleep in approximately 25% of adults. Studies in infants show that a level of 70–75 dB(A) for 3 minutes led to awakening in two-thirds of the children, and 75 db(A) for 12 minutes awakened all the infants (Gadeke et al., 1969). Increases in heart rate and peripheral vasoconstriction occurred with levels as low as 70 dB(A) (American Academy of Pediatrics, 1974). Lucey and co-workers showed that sudden loud noises cause agitation and crying, leading to a decrease in transcutaneous pO$_2$ (TcpO$_2$) followed by a rise in intracranial pressure (ICP) (Long et al., 1980a). The increased ICP was seen in some infants without any change in TcpO$_2$.

The long-term effects of this increased and unphysiologic noise exposure are less clear. The incidence of sensory hearing loss is higher among low birth weight infants (Schulman-Galambos and Galambos, 1979), but the contribution to this deficit made by noise exposure is controversial. Douek et al. (1976) showed that infants nursed in incubators for long periods of time have hearing losses. Abramovich et al. (1979), however, felt that the correlation was with illness and not with the incubators alone. Animal studies have shown that the very immature cochlea is more sensitive to "noise damage" than the mature cochlea (Falk et al., 1974). The additive effect of aminoglycosides and environmental noise is of additional concern, but no controlled studies have been done that show that noise levels contribute to hearing loss in infants with multiple problems. Addressing this concern, the American Academy of Pediatrics recommended that the manufacturers of incubators reduce the noise of motors to below 58 dB(A) and that physicians limit the use of aminoglycoside antibiotics and other potentially ototoxic drugs in newborns. It was further recommended that hospital personnel eliminate unnecessary noise, including radios, in the nursery. More carefully controlled studies are needed to evaluate the effect of this environmental factor on the outcome of preterm and sick infants.

Touch

As Dr. Hodgman outlined in the Introduction to this book, the history of perinatal care has vacillated between a minimal handling approach in the early premature infant nurseries in the 1930s and 1940s (Hess and Lundeen, 1941) and the aggressive medical intervention that characterized the first ICNs in the 1960s. In the 1980s, the direction has changed again, with mounting concern that infants are stimulated too much (Korones, 1976), that intensive care is too intense (Lucey, 1977), and that the quality of touching and stimulation is poor (Lawson et al., 1977). The reason for this vacillation is the concern that too much handling may cause trauma, sleep disturbances, and an increased infection rate in the premature infant and the recognition that, in order to survive, ICN infants need aggressive intervention and multiple diagnostic and therapeutic procedures. Because of this, in the last 15 years considerable attention has been directed toward the effects of various kinds of touch and stimulation on the physiologic state, neurologic maturation, and long-term outcome of infants who receive intensive care.

Of major concern is the difference in the sensory environment that a 28-week-old to 38-week-old fetus experiences in utero compared with that which the prematurely born infant experiences in the ICN. The fetus is bathed in a warm, water-filled environment with constant gentle oscillations. The prematurely born infant is delivered to a flat mattress, surrounded by a cool air-filled environment and has intermittent episodes of harsh, sometimes painful tactile stimulation. Immediately obvious physical consequences of this difference include: 1) position deformities, such as the flattened and narrow head of the premature infant (see Figure 10.1); 2) skin trauma from such things as electrocardiography leads, tape, restraints, and burns from transcutaneous blood gas monitoring; and 3) accidental trauma from other intensive care equipment. Skin infections are also frequent in this population and have been attributed to frequent handling and poor handwashing.

Of somewhat more subtle but equal importance is the observation that the developing infant cared for in an ICN is allowed little time for uninterrupted sleep (Korones, 1976; Lawson et al., 1977). The 28- to 32-week-old fetus sleeps approximately 80% of the time in utero. Much of this sleep is rapid eye movement (REM) sleep. Even the term newborn sleeps 17 to 19 hours a day in periods of 4 to 6 hours. Many physiologists speculate that these sleep periods are important for neuronal maturation (Oswald, 1969). However, the premature infant in an ICN was shown in one study to be disturbed at an average of 132 times each day. Furthermore, the frequency of disturbances was fairly constant throughout the day; 36% occurring from 7 AM to 3 PM, 31% from 3 PM to 11 PM, and 33% from 11 PM to 7 AM (Korones, 1976). The mean duration of an undisturbed rest period for 11 babies was only 4.6 to 9.2 minutes. It is difficult to determine the long-term effects of these constant interruptions of rest; however, it is clear that this is drastically different from conditions in utero and from the life of a normal newborn and therefore must be considered nonphysiologic. Furthermore, several investigators have reported hypoxemia (see Figure 10.2), hypertension, elevations in

Consequences of Newborn Intensive Care 207

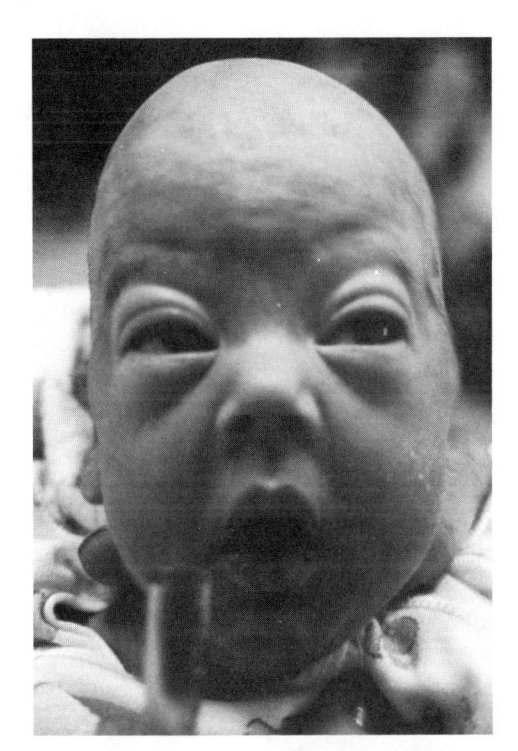

Figure 10.1. One-month-old infant who was born at 28 weeks gestation. Because of prolonged periods of time lying against the mattress, the head is flattened on both sides.

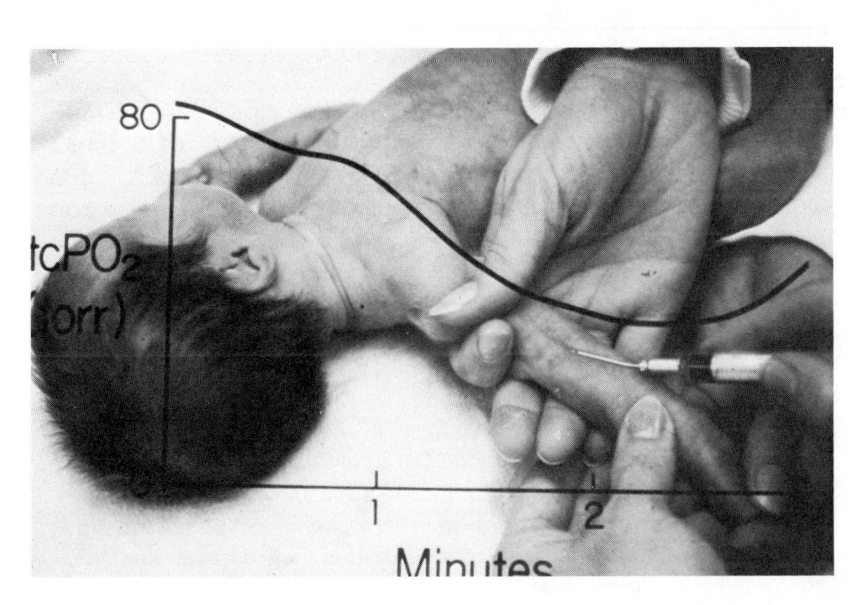

Figure 10.2. The effect of a venipuncture on transcutaneously measured pO_2. The pO_2 fell from the normoxemic range to hypoxemic values.

intracranial pressure, apnea, and feeding problems associated with such disturbances (Long et al., 1980b; Peabody et al., 1978b).

More recently, attention has shifted from the quantity of stimulation to the quality of stimulation. A clear distinction has been made between painful, harsh, tactile stimulation and the loving, gentle stimulation associated with mothering. Their effects on the infant may be quite different. Hasselmeyer (1964), in a study of 60 patients, showed that, by increasing the fondling of infants three times more than the control group for the first 14 days of life, crying activity decreased, bowel motility improved, periods of the quiet alert state increased, and there was general improvement in growth. Scarr-Salapatek and Williams (1973) reported that infants receiving extra play periods and increased visual stimuli achieved a higher developmental status at 1 year compared to a control group of premature infants. Several studies employed oscillating waterbeds to try to simulate the conditions of the amniotic fluid-filled uterus, showing repeatedly that this increases the regularity of breathing of premature infants and decreases periods of apnea (Korner, 1977). Furthermore, Long et al. (1980b) demonstrated that the frequency and severity of hypoxemic episodes caused by intensive care could be significantly reduced. In their study, caretakers were alerted to the effects of their procedures on oxygenation and were provided with continuous transcutaneous oxygen monitoring to assess how the infant responded to their care.

Temperature

Careful attention to temperature control has contributed to the improved survival of the premature or sick newborn (Schreiner et al., 1980; Silverman et al., 1958). However, even with careful attention to the thermal environment, temperature cannot be as carefully controlled in the intensive care unit as in utero. In utero, a "neutral thermal environment" is maintained by the maternal temperature plus the heat of metabolism of the infant. In most instances, there is no more than a 0.5°C variation in environmental temperature. This steady state condition cannot be reproduced in the ICU.

At delivery, the newborn is abruptly removed from a 38°C uterus and exposed to room temperatures as low as 22°C. Even with a radiant heat source present in the delivery room, the infant's temperature may fall as much as 3°C within the first 5 minutes of life through evaporative and convective heat losses. Such cold stress may play a physiologic role in the term infant, inducing an adrenergic and thyroid surge (Fisher and Oddie, 1964), but this occurs at the cost of markedly increased oxygen consumption. For the immature and sick newborn, who is already maximally stressed, acute hypothermia produces acidosis and exaggerates the effects of hypoxia (Gandy et al., 1964).

In an effort to create a neutral thermal environment and reduce the risk of cold stress, infants in an intensive care unit are routinely cared for in incubators or under radiant heaters. Incubators are convectively heated and do not control for changes in conductive, radiant, or evaporative heat loss. Servocontrol devices, which measure the skin surface temperature with a probe and adjust the incubator temperature to maintain temperature within set limits, are utilized to compensate for fluctuations in the thermal environment. However, there is an inherent lag time in the sensing mechanism, and environmental temperature changes as great as 10°C can occur between the "off" and "on" periods of the incubator heater. Furthermore, dislodged or displaced temperature sensors can result in overheating or overcooling an infant. Some of these large thermal fluctuations can be eliminated by introducing computerized control of the thermistors (Pearlstein, 1976). Radiant heat losses in an incubator may be decreased in the double-walled incubators now available, or by using a plastic heat shield inside the incubator (Fanaroff et al., 1972; Marks et al., 1981).

Evaporative losses also contribute significantly to heat exchange in the infant who weighs less than 1000 grams and is less than 28 weeks gestation (Hammerlund and Sedin, 1982). In an unhumidified incubator, the very tiny infant may require an ambient temperature of 40°C in order to maintain a normal body temperature. This is beyond the capacity of most available incubators, so an additional source of radiant heat, such as heating lamps, is often required. These contribute to more evaporative losses and may result in dehydration and hypernatremia (Wu and Hodgman, 1974).

Radiant warmers were initially developed for use in delivery rooms and adapted for use in intensive care areas. They provide ready access to the infant for procedures and easier visibility of the patient and his or her equipment. Similar to incubators, radiant warmers are regulated by skin servocontrol devices. However, it has not been conclusively established that they provide a neutral thermal environment. The only variable controlled is radiant heat loss. Very large evaporative losses occur under radiant warmers, particularly in the very low birth weight infant. Although the evaporative losses do not seem to increase oxygen consumption, they do result in large insensible water losses (Marks et al., 1980).

If the temperature probe should fall off and the sensor respond to the room or floor temperature, the infant may become overheated. If the skin sensor is covered by the infant's clothing or sandwiched between the mattress and the baby, the infant may become hypothermic. Because radiant warmers do not control for convective heat losses, wide swings in the infant's environmental temperature are common.

The final method used for warming infants is to place warm objects, such as water-filled gloves or heating pads, around the baby, increasing his or her temperature by conduction. Second- and third-degree burns have occurred when hot objects were placed on the very sensitive skin of the premature infant.

Radiation

Radiation exposure of newborn infants in ICNs is potentially hazardous and is at the center of ongoing research (Brent, 1980; Holbert et al., 1975). Radiation exposure takes several forms, including radiographic evaluation and the diagnostic use of ultrasound, which has recently become popular for the evaluation of heart disease and central nervous system (CNS) abnormalities (Allen et al., 1977; Babcock et al., 1980). Several questions are haunting, including the possible long-term effects of multiple and prolonged radiation exposures and the adverse effects on the immature developing infant. It is common for a premature infant with lung disease who is admitted to an ICN to receive 30 to 50 chest x-rays during his or her intensive care stay. If complications occur, this number may double or triple. Because even smaller and more immature infants are now surviving, it is impossible to say at this time what the impact of excessive radiation on these more immature infants will be.

The use of ultrasound radiation for the diagnosis of cardiac abnormalities and intracranial abnormalities has been an additional concern. Although there is extensive animal and adult literature regarding the safe dosages of ultrasound exposure and the average newborn exposure is well under this safety limit (AIUM Bioeffects Committee, 1978), this concern persists. The adverse effects on a developing newborn may be entirely different from the effects on other animal species or adult humans. It is mandatory that health care professionals be aware of the possible long-term effects of this radiation exposure so that infants are exposed to minimum amounts of radiation. Proper safety measures must be taken, especially shielding of the gonads and of other infants in the nursery when a portable x-ray is being taken. Active research and follow-up studies must continue to better define potential risk factors.

Electrical Hazards

One of the obvious environmental characteristics in any ICN is the number of electrical devices used for monitoring, diagnosis, and treatment of patients. The risk of electrical injury to the patient increases with each device employed. It has not been possible to determine the true incidence of mortality or morbidity that is attributable to exposure to electrical currents in newborn infants because infants receiving intensive care have a multitude of problems. Deaths and complications are often attributed to the obvious medical problems and not directly linked to small current, microshock injuries. Furthermore, injuries caused by electrical accidents demonstrate no specific tissue changes even at autopsy. It is mandatory that all ICN equipment be tested by trained engineers for safety and for use in an intensive care environment. Standards for safety must be meticulously followed, with more stringent standards used for patients with indwelling arterial lines and patients in surgery (Edwards, 1976). In addition, other precautions, such as the exclusive use of three-prong plugs and common grounding of all devices connected to a single patient, must be conscientiously followed. Finally, trained personnel must periodically check electrical devices within the unit for current leakage and the integrity of plugs, sockets, outlets, fuses, and grounds.

Miscellaneous Interventions

Respiratory Intubation and ventilation may be life-saving for infants with respiratory distress syndrome, meconium aspiration, severe pneumonia, diaphragmatic hernia, or extreme immaturity. However, the benefits gained by mechanical ventilation are not without some cost. Table 10.1 is a partial list of the complications reported for intubation and ventilation.

One of the most serious sequelae of mechanical ventilation is bronchopulmonary dysplasia (BPD). Both oxygen toxicity and barotrauma have been implicated in the lung damage that results in prolonged oxygen dependency, hypercarbia, cor pulmonale, and, occasionally, death. Infants who develop BPD have long-term as well as immediate problems. Abnormal pulmonary function may persist up to 5 years of age. A significant number of infants with BPD also have developmental delays (Mayes et al., 1983).

Intravascular Procedures

Catheters Umbilical artery and vein catheters are routinely used to aid in the management of the sick newborn, particularly those with respiratory problems. They provide easy access for blood sampling, pressure monitoring, and fluid infusion. Their use has made management of respiratory, cardiovascular, and metabolic disorders feasible in even the tiniest of infants. As with ventilatory support techniques, multiple complications have been reported with catheters. The magnitude of complications ranges from minor, with no clinical significance, to major,

Table 10.1. Complications in NICU infants from intubation and ventilation.

Endotracheal (ET) Tubes
  Subglottic stenosis (1–2%) (Drew, 1982)
  Erosion and ulceration of trachea (Joshi et al., 1972)
  Airway obstruction—blocked ET tubes (25%) (Elton and Berkowitz, 1981)
  Deformation of nares (Jung and Thomas, 1974)
  Cleft palate (Biskinis and Herz, 1978)
  Perforation of trachea and esophagus (Touloukian et al., 1977)
  Infection (4.3%) (Joshi et al., 1972)
  Unilateral lobar emphysema with suctioning (Miller, 1981)
Ventilators
  Pneumothorax (10–30%) (Borg et al., 1975; Ogata et al., 1976)
  Pneumomediastinum
  Pneumoperitoneum
  Chronic lung disease (5–30%) (Mayes et al., 1983)
Continuous positive airway pressure
  Endotracheal tube
    Pneumothorax
    Hyperoxia
    Hypercarbia
  Mask
    Apnea (from global pressure)
    Cerebellar hemorrhages (ventilation) (Pape et al., 1976)
    Flattened facies
  Nasal cannula
    Loss of oxygen and pressure when crying
    Excoriated nostrils

with death resulting (Rao and Elhassani, 1980). Table 10.2 lists some of the complications reported with umbilical vessel catheters (see also Figure 10.3).

Central venous catheters are used to provide nutrition to infants who are unable to obtain adequate nutrition enterally. Their use has enhanced the survival of infants who have required abdominal surgery for gastrointestinal anomalies or who have had necrotizing enterocolitis. Infection rates of 11% to 30% are reported with central venous lines. Right atrial thrombus formation and perforation have occurred (Mahoney et al., 1981).

Even peripheral venous cannulation is not without risks. Placing an intravenous fluid line in a small baby can cause hypoxemia and bradycardia. Infiltration of the infusing solution has caused complications ranging from local edema to total necrosis of the hand (Yosowitz et al.,

Table 10.2. Complications in NICU infants from umbilical vessel catheters.

Arterial
  Umbilical artery catheters
    Vasospasm
    Ischemia
    Thrombosis
    Embolus
    Hemorrhage
    Infection
    Hemiplegia
      (Krishnamoorthy et al., 1976)
    Perforation (Miller et al., 1979)

  Peripheral artery catheters
    Vasospasm
    Emboli with ischemia (Cartwright and Schreiner, 1980)
    Central nervous system emboli with hemiplegia (Simmons et al., 1978)
    Infection

Venous
  Umbilical vein catheters
    Portal vein thrombosis
      (Oski et al., 1963)
    Hepatic necrosis
      (Oski et al., 1963)
    Pulmonary emboli
      (Scott, 1965)
    Hepatic abscess
      (Brans et al., 1974)
    Cardiac arrhythmias
      (Johns et al., 1972)
    Perforation of atrium
      (Egan and Eitzman, 1971)
  Peripheral vein catheters
    Tissue sloughs
    Venous occlusion
    Local infection
    Necrosis 2° to infiltration
      (Yosowitz et al., 1975)

1975). Injection of sclerosing substances into small veins may also result in skin necrosis (Figure 10.4).

An additional recognized risk associated with all methods of fluid delivery in the neonate is the presence of plasticizers in the intravenous equipment. Di-2-ethylhexylphthalate (DHEP) has been found in significant levels in the tissues of neonates with indwelling umbilical artery catheters. One study suggested that the blood and tissue level of DHEP may be causally related to the development of necrotizing enterocolitis (Hillman, 1975). The immediate toxic effects of DHEP in animals is the abolishment of the vascular response to physiologic stimuli. DHEP is toxic to rapidly growing cells in tissue culture (DeHaan, 1971). The long-term potential of this exposure in the developing neonate is not known.

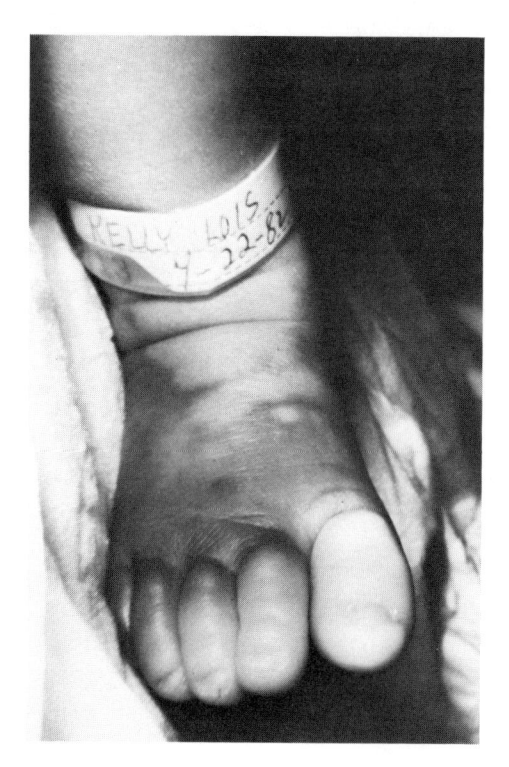

Figure 10.3. Toes of a premature infant with an umbilical artery catheter. The toes and the dorsum of the foot are blanched, reflecting vasospasm.

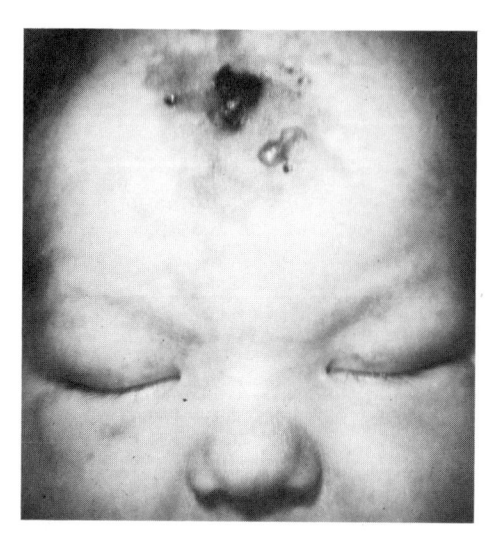

Figure 10.4. Area of tissue injury on the forehead of a premature infant. Hypertonic solutions had been infused through an indwelling peripheral vein catheter, causing sclerosis and some permanent scarring.

Chemical Factors

In utero, the placenta performs a number of impressive and important regulatory functions. It provides nutrients, removes waste products of metabolism, acts as a barrier to many toxins, and, along with the maternal liver, detoxifies many substances. Furthermore, the uterus provides a sterile environment for the developing fetus. Although NICUs attempt to recreate a controlled chemical microenvironment for the sick and immature infant, each measure employed potentially adds to the burden of environmental exposures. The list of known consequences from these exposures grows with each year of experience with intensive care. Although many of the adverse effects are acutely recognized, some may not become apparent for years.

Gases

The fetus is entirely dependent on its mother for the supply of oxygen and the elimination of carbon dioxide. The intervillous space in the placenta has been compared to the newborn alveolus and the placenta to the lung. Despite this analogy, there are some very major differences in the characteristics of the gaseous composition of the fetal environment and the environment of ICNs. In the fetus, the passage of oxygen and carbon dioxide between the mother and the fetus is controlled merely by diffusion. With a healthy mother, a constant supply of oxygen and removal of carbon dioxide to the fetus takes place throughout gestation without any respiratory work required of the fetus. At the time of labor and delivery and during the neonatal period in ICNs, this constancy is disrupted. It has been well documented that the process of labor and delivery stresses the gas exchange by the placenta and that all fetuses are born somewhat asphyxiated relative to their blood gas status prior to labor and delivery. Once a fetus has assumed extrauterine life, he or she must take responsibility for his or her own gas exchange.

Many problems in the newborn period hamper this adaptation. In fact, the most common reason for admission to an ICN is one of these respiratory disorders and the need for medical intervention to regulate the arterial blood partial pressures of oxygen and carbon dioxide. However, despite the recent advancements in respiratory equipment and the availability of competent medical personnel, the constancy of oxygen and carbon dioxide experienced in utero is rarely, if ever, reproduced in the ICN. Many recent investigations (Hansen and Tooley, 1979; Peabody et al., 1978a; 1979) utilized continuous monitoring of transcutaneous oxygen and carbon dioxide to document the intense and frequent fluctuations in these gases (see Figure 10.5). Nonphysiologic levels of

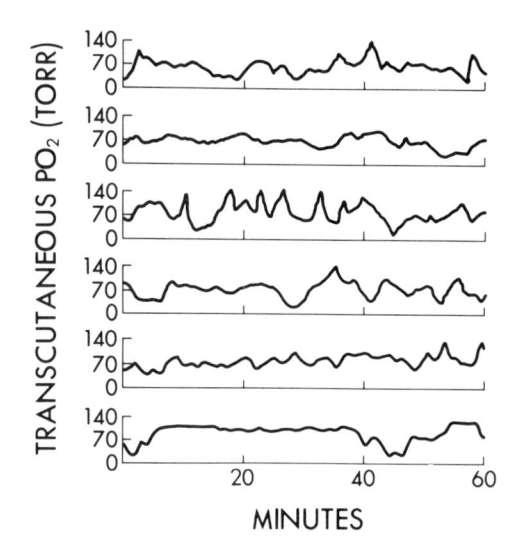

Figure 10.5. One-hour recording of transcutaneous pO_2 from six sick premature infants receiving intensive care. Frequent episodes of hypoxemia and hyperoxemia are present (adapted from Peabody, 1979).

these gases have been associated with a number of morbidities, including retrolental fibroplasia (Aranda et al., 1971), pulmonary fibrosis (Philip, 1975), and brain injury (Volpe, 1976). In addition, current medical knowledge lacks a precise definition of a "safe" level of oxygen and carbon dioxide for a sick infant, particularly if he or she is premature. Additional research is needed to improve the capability of medical technology to reproduce the role of the placenta in gas regulation.

Gaseous pollutants are an additional potential hazard to infants. Carbon monoxide has been shown to be present in excess in incubators (Behrman et al., 1971). ICNs that are located near freeways have also been found to have excessive levels of this gas. Mercury vapor poisoning has been reported from a broken mercury expansion switch in the heating unit on an incubator (McLaughlin et al., 1980) and from contamination of infant incubators (Waffarn and Hodgman, 1979).

Disinfectants

At the time of rupture of amniotic membranes and delivery, the infant loses the protection of the sterile amniotic cavity. It is widely recognized that infection is a major cause of neonatal morbidity and mortality. Several factors contribute to this incidence. Nosocomially acquired infections account for a distressingly high percentage; crowded nursery spaces, frequent handling and procedures, and poor handwashing have also been implicated (Goldman et al., 1978). Widespread use of broad spectrum antibiotics has resulted in a high rate of colonization with relatively resistant strains of bacteria in infants (Sprunt et al., 1978). Blood transfusions, required to maintain blood volume, probably contribute to the high rate of cytomegalovirus infection found in premature infants (Yeager et al., 1981). In addition, transfusions with blood products may cause risk of hepatitis and possibly acquired autoimmune diseases (Purcell, 1978).

Environmental decontaminants employed to reduce the risk of infection represent a special hazard to the newborn. Efforts to ensure a sterile environment have, in some instances, substituted chemical contamination for bacterial contamination. The story of hexachlorophene is now well known. Originally, hexachlorophene was introduced to the nursery as a handwashing agent. It was so effective at decreasing the rate of staphylococcal colonization on the hands of nursery personnel that it was soon used as a bathing solution for infants. Eighteen years after its introduction as a bacteriostatic agent, toxicity studies in animals began to question its safety (Lockhart, 1972). Both animal and human histopathologic studies showed that topical application of 3% hexachlorophene for more than 3 days resulted in vacuolar encephalopathy of the brainstem reticular system. Epidemiologic studies of treated infants found that the most immature infants were at the highest risk (Sherman et al., 1974).

Phenolic compounds are commonly used as cleansing agents in hospitals. Use of phenolic detergent to clean a nursery area has been implicated as a cause of an outbreak of severe neonatal hyperbilirubinemia. The chemical is postulated to interfere with normal bilirubin metabolism (Wysowski et al., 1978).

Isopropyl alcohol (80% solution) is routinely used as a skin disinfectant prior to venipuncture or invasive procedures. Its effectiveness as a disinfectant is questionable but, even more significantly, it can cause third-degree burns in the very immature infant (Rao and Elhassani, 1980).

Disinfectants that contain iodine (like betadine) may be absorbed through very immature skin. Significant increases in serum iodine levels have been found in premature infants after topical application of these agents (Pyati et al., 1977). The effect of this increase on thyroid activity is not yet fully known, but with the renewed interest in the relationship between thyroxin and respiratory distress syndrome, it may ultimately be found to be adverse.

Parenteral Solutions

Fluids and Nutrition Still another adaptation required of the newborn is the establishment of adequate oral nutrition. Many sick infants cannot tolerate enteral feedings or cannot achieve adequate calories for growth by this route. In these instances, parenteral alimentation is necessary.

The reported complications of total parenteral nutrition (TPN) solutions are as numerous as the ingredients within the solution (Brans, 1977). Hypoglycemia, hyperglycemia, metabolic acidosis (Hend et al., 1972), abnormal plasma aminograms (Das, 1975), fatty acid deficiency (Holman et al., 1982), and trace element deficiencies (James and MacMalion, 1976) have all been reported with TPN.

Even routine intravenous fluid administration is potentially harmful to infants. The adverse effect of benzyl alcohol, used to preserve these solutions, is now well documented (Gershanik et al., 1981; Kimura et al., 1971). Sixteen deaths in newborns weighing less than 2500 grams have been reported when normal saline with 0.9% benzyl alcohol was used to clear intravascular catheters. The toxicity may be related to reduced detoxification capacity in the immature liver or to the relatively larger dose per body weight given to these small infants (Meyer, 1982).

Intravenous fluids do not present the only risk to the preterm baby. The perfect oral nutrition has yet to be devised. Mother's milk may not provide the rapidly growing premature infant with enough protein, minerals, or calories. Proprietary formulas, which have been compounded to provide a more concentrated source of nutrients, are often poorly tolerated and may not be well absorbed.

Drugs

Finally, a major consideration in the chemical exposure of infants cared for in ICNs are the chemicals used for therapeutic intervention. Every drug used to treat problems of the newborn is associated with some risk. Adverse drug effects may be caused by excessive drug administration, excessive serum levels attributable to poor metabolism by the patient, synergism with other drugs or therapies, an inappropriate route of administration of the drug, an idiosyncratic reaction by the patient, or a known but undesirable effect of the drug. Unfortunately, excessive drug administration has accounted for a significant degree of neonatal morbidity in recent years. Mathematical errors in calculating drug dosages are easily made, particularly during an emergency situation. Poisonings have included theophylline toxicity, causing seizures, tachycardia, and gastrointestinal disorders (Soyka, 1977). Digitalis toxicity has been reported as causing arrhythmias and, in rare instances, sudden death (Krasula et al., 1974). Synergism between drugs is frequent. For example, the ototoxicity of aminoglycosides, used as antibiotics in newborns, may be synergistic with Lasix when used as a diuretic. Most drugs used in the ICN have known undesirable effects, and the need for their use must always be weighed against the risk of these adverse effects. Examples are the platelet dysfunction and renal insufficiency associated with indomethacin, used for the treatment of patent ductus arteriosus (Friedman, 1978). Hypotension associated with morphine and tolazoline and hypochloremia associated with Lasix are further examples. Unfortunately, drugs given through inappropriate routes also contribute to neonatal morbidity (see Figure 10.6).

Summary

Despite the dramatic improvement in neonatal survival since the 1970s, morbidity in infants managed in ICNs remains high. Every characteristic of these highly technical nurseries has the potential to harm as well as to help. Some of the adverse effects of intensive care have been recognized and reviewed in this chapter. Other hazards remain hypothetical and will require further study to delineate. Continuing awareness of the potential harmful effects of intensive care and ongoing research are very much needed in the decade to come.

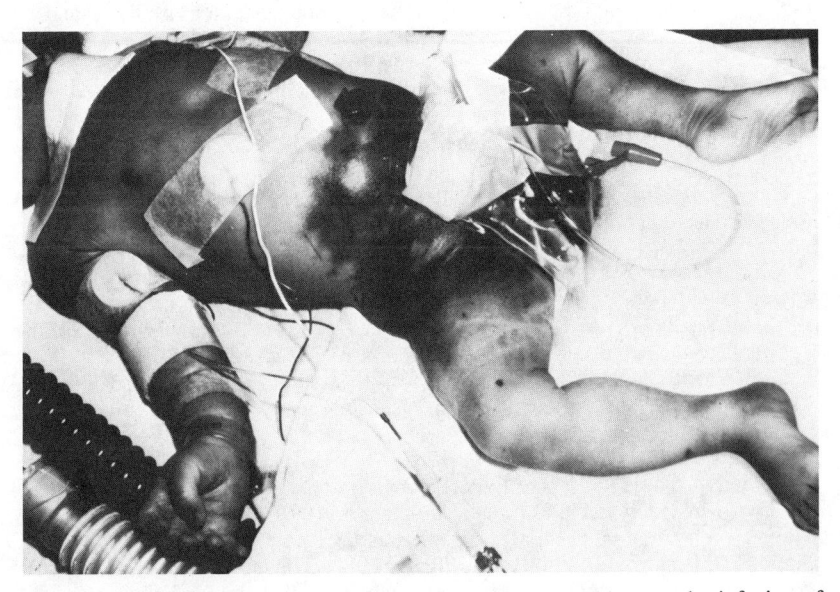

Figure 10.6. Marked tissue ischemia and necrosis secondary to the infusion of calcium into an umbilical artery catheter.

Acknowledgment

The authors wish to express their sincere appreciation to Ms. Myrna Pantangco for her patience and expert assistance in the preparation of this chapter.

References

Abramovich, S., Gregory, S., Slemick, M., et al. 1979. Hearing loss in very low birth weight infants treated with neonatal intensive care. Arch. Dis. Child. 54:421.

AIUM Bioeffects Committee. 1978. Statement on Mammalian In Vivo Ultrasonic Biological Effects. Revised Oct. AIUM, Oklahoma City.

Allen, H. D., Goldberg, S. J., Sahn, D. S., et al. 1977. Suprasternal notch echocardiography: Assessment of its clinical utility in pediatric cardiology. Circulation 55:605.

American Academy of Pediatrics. 1974. Noise pollution: Neonatal aspects. Pediatrics 54:476.

American Academy of Pediatrics. 1977. Standards and Recommendations for Hospital Care of Newborn Infants, p. 27. American Academy of Pediatrics, Springfield, IL.

Anagnostakis, D., Petmezakis, J., Messaritakis, J., et al. 1980. Noise pollution in neonatal units: A potential health hazard. Acta Pediatr. Scand. 69:771.

Aranda, J. V., Saheb, N., Stern, L., et al. 1971. Arterial O_2 tension and retinal vasoconstriction in newborn infants. Am. J. Dis. Child. 122:189.

Aschoff, J. 1965. Circadian rhythms in man: A self-sustained oscillator and an inherent frequency underlies human 24 hour periodicity. Science 148:1427.

Ashton, N., Ward, B., and Serpel, G. 1953. Role of oxygen in the genesis of retrolental fibroplasia: Preliminary report. Br. J. Ophthalmol. 37:513.

Babcock, D. S., Han, B. D., and LeQuesne, G. W. 1980. B-mode gray scale ultrasound of the head in the newborn and young infant. Am. J. Roentgenol. 134:457.

Bakken, A. F. 1977. Temporary intestinal lactase deficiency in light-treated jaundiced infants. Acta Pediatr. Scand. 66:91.

Behrman, R. E., Fisher, D. E., and Paton, J. 1971. Air pollution in nurseries: Correlations with a decrease in oxygen carrying capacity of hemoglobin. J. Pediatr. 78:1050.

Behrman, R., Brown, A. K., Currie, M. R., et al. 1974. Preliminary report of the committee on phototherapy in the newborn. J. Pediatr. 84:135, 145.

Bell, E. F., Neidich, G. A., Cashore, W. J., et al. 1979. Combined effect of radiant warmer and phototherapy on insensible water loss in low birth weight infants. J. Pediatr. 94:810.

Beral, V., Evans, S., Shaw, H., et al. 1982. Malignant melanoma and exposure to fluorescent lighting at work. Lancet 2:290.

Bess, F., Finlayson Peck, B., and Chapman, J. 1979. Further observations on noise levels in infant incubators. Pediatrics 63:100.

Bhatia, J., Mims, L. C., and Roesel, R. A. 1980. The effect of phototherapy on amino acid solutions containing multivitamins. J. Pediatr. 96:284.

Biskinis, E., and Herz, M. 1978. Acquired palatal groove after prolonged orotracheal intubation. J. Pediatr. 92:512.

Blennow, G., Svenningsen, N. W., and Almquist, B. 1974. Noise levels in infant incubators (adverse effects?). Pediatrics 53:29.
Borg, T. J., Pagtakhan, R. D., Reed, M. H., et al. 1975. Bronchopulmonary dysplasia and lung rupture in hyaline membrane disease: Influence of continuous distending pressure. Pediatrics 55:51.
Brans, Y. W. 1977. Parenteral nutrition of the very low birth weight neonate: A critical view. Clin. Perinatol. 4:367.
Brans, Y. W., Ceballos, R., and Cassady, G. 1974. Umbilical catheters and hepatic abscesses. Pediatrics 53:164.
Brent, R. L. 1980. X-ray, microwave, and ultrasound: The real and unreal hazards. Pediatr. Ann. 9:469.
Brown, A., and Glass, L. 1979. Environmental hazards in the newborn nursery. Pediatr. Ann. 8:698.
Brown, R. J. K., Valman, H. B., and Daganah, E. G. 1970. Diarrhea and light therapy in neonates. Lancet 1:498.
Cartwright, G. W., and Schreiner, R. L. 1980. Major complication secondary to radial artery catheterization in the neonate. Pediatrics 65:139.
Dacou-Voutetakis, C., Anagnostakis, D., and Matsaniotic, N. 1978. Effect of prolonged illumination (phototherapy) on concentrations of luteinizing hormone in human infants. Science 199:1229.
Das, J. B. 1975. Studies of amino acid metabolism in infants. In: R. W. Winters and E. G. Hasselmeyer (eds.), Intravenous Nutrition in High Risk Infants. John Wiley, New York.
DeHaan, R. L. 1971. Toxicity of tissue culture media exposed to polyvinyl chloride plastic. Nature 231:85.
Diamond, I., and Schmid, R. 1968. Neonatal hyperbilirubinemia and kernicterus: Experimental support for treatment by exposure to visible light. Arch. Neurol. 18:699.
Douek, E., Bannister, L. H., Dodson, H. C., et al. 1976. Effects of incubator noise on the cochlea of the newborn. Lancet 2:1110.
Drew, J. H. 1982. Immediate intubation at birth of the very-low-birth-weight infant: Effect on survival. Am. J. Dis. Child. 136:207.
Edwards, M. K. 1976. Specialized grounding needs. Clin. Perinatol. 3:367.
Egan, E. A., and Eitzman, D. V. 1971. Umbilical vessel catheterization. Am. J. Dis. Child. 121:213.
Elton, D. R., and Berkowitz, G. P. 1981. Endotracheal tube obstruction in neonates. Perinatol. Neonatol. 5:75.
Falk, S. A. 1972. Combined effect of noise and ototoxic drugs. Environ. Health Perspect. 2:5.
Falk, S. A., Cook, R. O., Haseman, J. K., et al. 1974. Noise induced inner ear damage in newborn and adult guinea pigs. Laryngoscope 84:444.
Fanaroff, A. A., Wald, M., Gruber, H. S., et al. 1972. Insensible water loss in low birth weight infants. Pediatrics 50:236.
Field, T. 1980. Infants born at risk. In: S. Friedman and M. Sigman (eds.), Preterm Birth and Psychological Development. Academic Press, New York.
Fisher, D. A., and Oddie, T. M. 1964. Neonatal thyroid hyperactivity. Am. J. Dis. Child. 107:574.
Fitzhardinge, P. M., Pape, P., Arstikaitis, M., et al. 1976. Mechanical ventilation of infants of less than 1,500 gm birth weight: Health, growth, and neurologic sequelae. J. Pediatr. 88:531.
Friedman, Z. 1978. Indomethacin disposition in indomethacin induced platelet dysfunction in premature infants. J. Clin. Pharmacol. 18:272.

Gadeke, R., Doring, B., Keller, F., et al. 1969. The noise level in a children's hospital and the wake-up threshold in infants. Acta Pediatr. Scand. 58:164.

Gandy, G., Adamson, K., Jr., and Cunningham, N. 1964. Thermal environment and acid-base homeostasis in human infants during the first hours of life. J. Clin. Invest. 43:751.

Gershanik, J. J., Boecler, G., Sola, A., et al. 1981. The gasping syndrome: Benzyl alcohol poisoning? Clin. Res. 29:895.

Goldman, D. A., LeClair, J., and Macone, A. 1978. Bacterial colonization of neonates admitted to an intensive care environment. J. Pediatr. 93:288.

Hack, M., Fanaroff, A. A., and Merkatz, I. R. 1979 Current concepts: The low birthweight infant—Evaluation of a changing outlook. N. Engl. J. Med. 301:1162.

Halberg, F. 1975. Chronobiology. Annu. Rev. Physiol. 31:675.

Hammarlund, K., and Sedin, G. 1982. Transepidermal water loss in newborn infants (IV). Heat change with the environment in relation to gestational age. Acta Pediatr. Scand. 71:191.

Hansen, T., and Tooley, W. H. 1979. Skin surface carbon dioxide tension in sick infants. Pediatrics 64:942.

Harris, F., and Smith, C. S. 1977. More on apnea resulting from obstruction of nares by an eye shield. J. Pediatr. 90:995.

Hasselmeyer, E. G. 1964. The premature neonate's response to handling. Am. Nurs. Assoc. 11:15.

Heird, W. C., Driscoll, J. W., Jr., Schullenger, J. W., et al. 1972. Intravenous alimenation in pediatric patients. J. Pediatr. 80:351.

Herbst, A. L., Scully, R. E., Robberty, S. J., et al. 1978. Complications of prenatal therapy with diethystilbestrol. Pediatrics 62:1151.

Hess, J. H., and Lundeen, E. C. 1941. The Premature Infant: Its Medical and Nursing Care. Lippincott, Philadelphia.

Hillman, L. S., Goodwin, S. L., and Sherman, W. R. 1975. Identification and measurement of plasticizer in neonatal tissues after umbilical catheters and blood products. N. Engl. J. Med. 292:381.

Hirata, T., Epcar, J. T., Walsh, A., et al. 1983. Survival and outcome of infants 501–750 gm: A six year experience. J. Pediatr. 102:741.

Holbert, C. L., Frey, G. D., Levkoff, A. H., et al. 1975. Radiographic technic, safety, and interpretation in the newborn nursery. J. Pediatr. 87:968.

Holman, R. T., Johnson, S. B., and Hatch, T. F. 1982. A case of human linolenic acid deficiency involving neurological abnormalities. Am. J. Clin. Nutr. 35:617.

James, B. E., and MacMalion, R. A. 1976. Balance studies of nine elements during complete intravenous feeding of small premature infants. Aust. Paediatr. J. 12:154.

James, L. S., and Lanman, J. T. 1976. History of oxygen therapy and retrolental fibroplasia. Pediatr. Suppl. 57:591.

Johns, A. W., Kitchen, W. H., and Leslie, D. W. 1972. Complications of umbilical vessel catheters. Med. J. Aust. 2:810.

Joshi, V. V., Mandavia, S. G., Stern, L., et al. 1972. Acute lesions induced by endotracheal intubation. Am. J. Dis. Child. 124:636.

Jung, A. L., and Thomas, G. K. 1974. Stricture of the nasal vestibule: A complication of nasotracheal intubation in newborn infants. J. Pediatr. 85:412.

Karon, M., Imach, D., and Schwartz, A. 1970. Effective phototherapy in congenital nonobstructive, nonhemolytic jaundice. N. Engl. J. Med. 282:377.

Kimura, E. T., Darby, T. D., Krause, R. A., et al. 1971. Parenteral toxicity studies with benzyl alcohol. Toxicol. Appl. Pharmacol. 18:60.

Knobloch, H., Malone, A., Ellison, P. H., et al. 1982. Considerations in evaluating changes in outcome for infants weighing less than 1,501 grams. Pediatrics 69:285.

Konig, H., and Mazzi, E. 1976. Apnea resulting from obstruction of nares by an eye shield. J. Pediatr. 89:652.

Kopelman, A. E., Brown, R. S., and Odell, G. B. 1972. The "bronze" baby syndrome: A complication of phototherapy. J. Pediatr. 81:466.

Kopelman, A. E., Ey, J. L., and Lee, H. 1978. Phototherapy in newborn infants with glucose-6-phosphate dehydrogenase deficiency. J. Pediatr. 93:497.

Korner, A. 1977. A polygraphic study of the sleep and respiratory patterns of apneic premature infants on and off an oscillating water bed. In: J. F. Lucey, D. C. Shannon, and L. Soyka (eds.), Apnea of Prematurity. Report of Seventy-First Ross Conference. Ross Laboratories, Columbus, OH.

Korones, S. B. 1976. Disturbance and infants' rest. In: T. Moore (ed.), Iatrogenic Problems in Neonatal Intensive Care. Report of the 69th Ross Conference on Pediatric Research. Ross Laboratories, Columbus, OH.

Kostenbauder, H. B., and Sanvordeker, D. R. 1973. Riboflavin enhancement of bilirubin photocatabolism in vivo. Experientia 29:282.

Krasula, R., Yanagi, R., Hastreiter, A. R., et al. 1974. Digoxin intoxication in infants and children: Correlation with serum levels. J. Pediatr. 84:265.

Krishnamoorthy, K., Fernandez, R., Todres, I. D., et al. 1976. Paraplegia associated with umbilical artery catheterization in the newborn. Pediatrics 58:443.

Krishnamoorthy, K. S., Shannon, D. C., DeLong, G. R., et al. 1980. Neurologic sequelae in the survivors of neonatal intraventricular hemorrhage. Pediatrics 64:233.

Lawson, K., Daum, C., and Turkewitz, G. 1977. Environmental characteristics of a neonatal intensive care unit. Child. Dev. 48:1633.

Lockhart, J. 1972. How toxic is hexachlorophene? Pediatrics 50:229.

Long, J. G., Lucey, J. F., and Philip. A. G. S. 1980a. Noise and hypoxemia in the intensive care nursery. Pediatrics 64:143.

Long, J. G., Philip, A. G. S., and Lucey, J. F. 1980b. Excessive handling as a cause of hypoxemia. Pediatrics 65:143.

Lucey, J. F. 1977. Is intensive care too intensive? Pediatrics (Neonatol. Suppl.) 59:1069.

Lund, H. T., and Petersen, I. 1974. Beta glucuronidase in duodenal bile of jaundiced newborn infants treated with phototherapy. J. Pediatr. 85:268.

Mahoney, L., Snider, R., and Silverman, N. 1981. Echocardiographic diagnosis of intracardiac thrombi complicating total parenteral nutrition. J. Pediatr. 98:469.

Maisels, M. J. 1976. Phototherapy. In: T. Moore (ed.), Iatrogenic Problems in Neonatal Intensive Care: Report of the 69th Ross Conference on Pediatric Research, p. 54. Ross Laboratories, Columbus, OH.

Marks, K. H., Gunther, R. C., Rossi, J. A., et al. 1980. Oxygen consumption and insensible water loss in premature infants under radiant warmer heaters. Pediatrics 66:228.

Marks, K. H., Lee, C. A., and Bolan, C. D., Jr. 1981. Oxygen consumption and temperature control of premature infants in a double-walled incubator. Pediatrics 68:93.

Maurer, H. M., Fratkin, M., McWilliams, N. B., et al. 1976. Effects of

phototherapy on platelet counts in low birthweight infants and on platelet production and lifespan in rabbits. Pediatrics 57:506.
Mayes, L., Perkett, E., and Stahlman, M. 1983. Severe bronchopulmonary dysplasia: A retrospective review. Acta Pediatr. Scand. 72:222.
McLaughlin, J. F., Telzrow, R. W., and Mae Scott, C. 1980. Neonatal mercury vapor exposure in an infant incubator. Pediatrics 66:988.
Meloni, T., Costa, S., Dore, A., et al. 1974. Phototherapy for neonatal hyperbilirubinemia in mature infants with erythrocyte G-6-PD deficiency. J. Pediatr. 85:560.
Messner, K. H. 1978. Light toxicity to newborn retina. Pediatr. Res. 12:530.
Meyer, H. M. 1982. Food and Drug Administration, Dept. of Health and Human Services, May 28 (letter).
Miller, D., Kirkpatrick, B. V., Kodroff, M., et al. 1979. Pelvic exsanguination following umbilical artery catheterization in neonates. J. Pediatr. Surg. 14:264.
Miller, K. 1981. Acquired lobar emphysema in bronchopulmonary dysplasia. Radiology 138:589.
Mills, J. N. 1966. Human circadian rhythms. Physiol. Rev. 14:128.
Moore, T. (ed.). 1976. Iatrogenic Problems in Neonatal Intensive Care. Report of the 69th Ross Conference on Pediatric Research. Ross Laboratories, Columbus, OH.
Nelson, R., Resnick, M., Nelson, L., et al. 1980. Differential outcomes: Mortality and morbidity for extremely premature infants (abstract). Pediatr. Res. 14:437.
Norman, C., Goldberg, E., and Porterfield, D. 1962. The effect of visible radiation on the functional life span of mammalian and ovian spermatozoa. Exp. Cell. Res. 28:69.
Ogata, E., Gregory, G., Kitterman, J., et al. 1976. Pneumothorax in the respiratory distress syndrome: Incidence and effect on vital signs, blood gases and pH. Pediatrics 58:177.
Oh, W., and Karecki, H. 1972. Phototherapy and insensible water loss in the newborn infant. Am. J. Dis. Child. 124:230.
Oski, F. A., Allen, D. M., and Diamond, L. K. 1963. Portal hypertension—A complication of umbilical vein catheterization. Pediatrics 31:297.
Ostrea, E. M., and Odell, G. B. 1974. Photosensitized shift in the O_2 dissociation curve of fetal blood. Acta Pediatr. Scand. 63:341.
Oswald, I. 1969. Human brain protein, drugs and dreams. Nature 233:893.
Pape, K. E., Armstrong, D. L., and Fitzhardinge, P. M. 1976. Central nervous system pathology associated with mask ventilation in the very low birthweight infant: A new etiology for intracerebellar hemorrhage. Pediatrics 58:473.
Payne, E. 1899. Notes on the effects of x-rays. Arch. Roentgen. 3:67.
Peabody, J. L., Gregory, G. A., Willis, M. M., et al. 1978a. Transcutaneous oxygen tension in sick infants. Am. Rev. Resp. Dis. 118:83.
Peabody, J. L., Willis, M. M., Gregory, G. A., et al. 1978b. Clinical limitations and advantages of transcutaneous oxygen electrodes. Acta Anaesth. Scand. Suppl. 68:76.
Peabody, J. L., Gregory, G. A., Willis, M. M., et al. 1979. Failure of conventional monitoring to detect apnea resulting in hypoxemia. In: A. Huch, R. Huch, and J. F. Lucey (eds,), Continuous Transcutaneous Blood Gas Monitoring: Original Article Series—Birth Defects, p. 275. National Foundation March of Dimes. Liss, New York.
Pearlstein, P. H. 1976. Thermal control. In: T. Moore (ed.), Iatrogenic Problems

in Neonatal Intensive Care: Report of the 69th Ross Conference on Pediatric Research. Ross Laboratories, Columbus, OH.
Philip, A. G. S. 1975. Oxygen plus pressure plus time: The etiology of bronchopulmonary dysplasia. Pediatrics 55:44.
Purcell, R. H. 1978. The viral hepatitides. Hosp. Prac. 13:51.
Pyati, S., Ramamurthy, R., Krauss, M., et al. 1977. Absorption of iodine in the neonate following topical use of povidone iodine. J. Pediatr. 91:825.
Ramagnoli, G., Polidori, G., Catalbi, L., et al. 1979. Phototherapy-induced hypocalcemia. J. Pediatr. 94:815.
Rao, H. K. M., and Elhassani, S. B. 1980. Iatrogenic complications of procedures performed on the newborn. Perinatol. Neonatol. 4:25.
Rao, H. K. M., and Elhassani, S. B. 1981. Iatrogenic complications of procedures performed on the newborn. Perinatol. Neonatol. 5:23.
Reynolds, E. O. E., and Taghizadeh, A. 1974. Improved prognosis of infants mechanically ventilated for hyaline membrane disease. Arch. Dis. Child. 49:505.
Scarr-Salapatek, S., and Williams, M. L. 1973. The effects of early stimulation on low-birth weight infants. Child. Dev. 44:94.
Schreiner, R. L., Kisling, T. A., Evans, G. M., et al. 1980. Improved survival of ventilated neonates with modern intensive care. Pediatrics 66:985.
Schulman-Galambos, C., and Galambos, R. 1979. Brain stem evoked response audiometry in newborn hearing screening. Arch. Otolaryngol. 105:86.
Scott, J. M. 1965. Iatrogenic lesions in babies following umbilical vein catheterization. Arch. Dis. Child. 40:426.
Sherman, R. M., Leech, R. W., and Alvoid, E. C. 1974. Neurotoxicity of hexachlorophene in the human (I): A clinicopathological study of 248 children. Pediatrics 54:689.
Silverman, W. A., Fertig, J. W., and Berger, A. P. 1958. The influence of the thermal environment upon the survival of newly born premature infants. Pediatrics 22:876.
Simmons, M. A., Levine, R. L., Lubchenko, L. O., et al. 1978. Warning: Serious sequelae of temporal artery catheterization. J. Pediatr. 92:284.
Soyka, L. 1977. Pharmacology of aminophylline in the neonatal period. In: Apnea of Prematurity, 71st Ross Conference, Ross Laboratories, Columbus, OH.
Spear, F. G. 1973. Early days of experimental radiology. Br. J. Radiol. 46:762.
Speck, W. T. 1979. Effect of phototherapy on fertilization and embryonic development. Pediatr. Res. 13:506.
Speck, W. T., Chen, C. C., and Rosenkranz, H. S. 1975. In vitro studies of effects of light and riboflavin on DNA and HeLa cells. Pediatr. Res. 9:115.
Speck, W. T., and Rosenkranz, H. S. 1975. The bilirubin-induced photodegradation of deoxyribonucleic acid. Pediatr. Res. 9:703.
Speck, W. T., and Rosenkranz, H. S. 1976. Intracellular deoxyribonucleic acid-modifying activity of phototherapy lights. Pediatr. Res. 10:553.
Sprunt, K., Leidy, G., and Redman, W. 1978. Abnormal colonization of neonates in an intensive care unit: Means of identifying neonates at risk of infection. Pediatr. Res. 12:998.
Tan, K. L. 1977. Phototherapy for neonatal jaundice in erythrocyte glucose-6-phosphate dehydrogenase deficient infants. Pediatrics 59:1,023.
Taussig, H. B. 1962. A study of the German outbreak of phocomelia: The thalidomide syndrome. JAMA 180:1106.
Teberg, A. J., Hodgman, J. E., and Wu, P. Y. K. 1977. Effect of phototherapy on

growth of low birthweight infants—Two year follow-up. J. Pediatr. 91:92.
Touloukian, R., Beardsley, G. P., Ablow, R. C., et al. 1977. Traumatic perforation of the pharynx in the newborn. Pediatrics 59:1019.
Volpe, J. J. 1976. Perinatal hypoxic–ischemic brain injury. Pediatr. Clin. North Am. 23:383.
Waffarn, F., and Hodgman, J. 1979. Mercury vapor contamination of infant incubators: A potential hazard. Pediatrics 64:640.
Webb, R. B., and Lorenz, J. R. 1970. O_2 dependence and repair of lethal effects of near ultraviolet and visible light. Photochem. Photobiol. 12:283.
Webb, R. B., and Malina, M. M. 1970. Mutagenic effects of near ultraviolet and visible radiant energy on cultures of E. coli. Photochem. Photobiol. 12:457.
Wu, P. Y. K., and Berdhal, M. 1974. Irradiance in incubators under phototherapy lamps. J. Pediatr. 84:754.
Wu, P. Y. K., and Hodgman, J. E. 1974. Insensible water loss in preterm infants: Changes with postnatal development and nonionizing radiant energy. Pediatrics 54:704.
Wu, P. Y. K., Lim, R. C., Hodgman, J. E., et al. 1974. Effect of phototherapy in preterm infants on growth in the neonatal period. J. Pediatr. 85:563.
Wu, P. Y. K., and Moosa, A. 1978. Effect of phototherapy on nitrogen and electrolyte levels and water balance in jaundiced preterm infants. Pediatrics 61:193.
Wurtman, R. J., Axelrod, J., and Fisher, J. E. 1964. Melatonin synthesis in the pineal gland: Effect of light. Science 143:1328.
Wurtman, R. J., and Cardinali, D. P. 1976. The effects of light on man. In: D. Bergsma and S. H. Blondheim (eds.), Bilirubin Metabolism in the Newborn, Vol. 2, p. 110. American Elsevier, New York.
Wysowski, D., Flynt, J. W., Goldfield, M., et al. 1978. Epidemic neonatal hyperbilirubinemia and use of a phenolic disinfectant detergent. Pediatrics 61:165.
Yeager, A., Grumet, C., Hafleigh, E., et al. 1981. Prevention of transfusion-acquired cytomegalovirus infections in newborn infants. J. Pediatr. 98:281.
Yosowitz, P., Ekland, D. A., Shaw, R. C., et al. 1975. Peripheral intravenous infiltration necrosis. Ann. Surg. 182:553.
Zacharias, L., and Wurtman, R. S. 1969. Blindness and menarche. Obstet. Gynecol. 33:603.

11

The Impact of the Environment on the NICU Caregiver
Perspectives of the Nurse, Pediatric House Officer, and Academic Neonatologist

Richard E. Marshall, John L. Roberts, and Joan H. Walsh

The environment of the neonatal intensive care unit (NICU) has a significant impact on the lives of those who work there (Marshall et al., 1982). This chapter focuses upon the impact of the NICU upon three different caregivers—the staff nurse, the pediatric house officer, and the attending academic neonatologist. No one perspective can capture the complex milieu and, like the patterns in a kaleidoscope, we each tell our story in a different manner. Each of us sees different stresses and proposes different coping strategies; however, certain common themes emerge. All discuss the specific stresses imposed by the complex patient load, the death of many patients, and the frequent necessity for making ethical decisions. Moreover, the fragility of sick premature patients requires special levels of competence in caregivers so that issues about one's ability to perform become important. Since caregivers must work as a team in the NICU. Thus, considerable attention is focused upon interpersonal relationships, especially upon the nurse-doctor relationship as well as nurse-nurse and doctor-doctor interactions. Finally, each of us provides a perspective on how to cope with the challenging tasks presented by working in the NICU environment.

A Nurse's Perspective, by Joan Walsh, R.N., B.S.N.

The neonatal intensive care unit has been described as a stressful environment. It is hectic and noisy, especially at shift changes. Technology has become essential in any NICU, and its ever-changing nature creates increasingly greater demands on the caregiver. The number of patients, the acuteness of their illnesses, and their familes often push the nursing staff to the limits of their coping capabilities. Complex issues emerge, only to confuse and frustrate the caregiver. These include controversies over nursing and medical management of patients, ethical dilemmas, and increasing involvement of the neonate in research projects. In short, the NICU is an abnormal environment not only for the infant and family, but for the caregiver as well.

Yet many nurses continue to choose the subspecialty of neonatal nursing. Student nurses request it as a part of their elective curriculum. New graduates, experienced R.N.s seeking a new field, and experienced ICU nurses changing from one unit to the next continue to flock into the NICU environment.

This raises a question or two about the impact of the NICU on the staff nurse. First, with all the opportunities in nursing in the 1980s, why would a staff nurse choose to work in an NICU? Second, with all the stressors described in the literature, how can a professional nurse derive any personal satisfaction or achieve professional growth in an NICU?

This section describes not only the hardships and coping strategies of staff nurses but, more important, the rewards and avenues for growth potential in an NICU.

An Attractive Sub-Specialty

From the outside looking in, the NICU appears to be an attractive area of nursing. This is evidenced by the constant influx of new staff members. The "orientees" are comprised of new graduates, R.N.s changing from one specialty to another, and NICU veterans changing from one unit to the next. Student nurses are also anxious to acquire some exposure to the NICU. Their experiences can be limited to observation only or they can be provided the challenge of hands-on experience through supervised delivery of patient care. Although these educational experiences are quite varied, at St. Louis Children's Hospital we witness a great student demand for clinical exposure to the NICU.

What is it, then, that draws so many nurses to this intriguing yet demanding work environment? For some, like myself, it can be an inherent attraction to newborns. Others have a strong desire to nurture these helpless creatures and provide comfort for them throughout their extensive hospital stay. Most NICU nurses desire the challenge of working with sick newborns as well. The highly specialized patient population affords the nurse many opportunities for exposure to, and management of, patients with unique and diverse disease entities. The NICU is generally associated with prematurity and the "premie" population. However, even though prematurity is the most frequent condition of their patients, NICU nurses are confronted with a variety of challenging neonatal illnesses. Those who work in university medical centers are often exposed to the most unusual and oftentimes sensationalized cases, e.g., conjoined twins, multiple congenital anomalies, and the "tiny" (less than 800 grams) babies. Although the nature of such cases can be very frustrating for family and staff, nurses tend to develop a strong sense of pride in their abilities to manage such a select group of patients and hope for opportunities to do so at some time in their careers. Success stories with patients can bring health care professionals closer together as a team, ultimately enhancing patient care.

Some nurses are attracted more to the intensive care setting than to the infants in an NICU. Most nurses who choose to work in the NICU prefer intensive care nursing or want to accept the challenge of adapting to a demanding yet exciting pace. Although the patient care is often more complex than on a general floor, the patient load is drastically reduced— the nurse-patient ratio, at 1:1–3, is much more manageable than a 1:5–10 patient assignment on a general floor. Other nurses tend to thrive on the hectic pace and the emergency nature of ICUs.

The NICU environment also affords the nurse many opportunities to acquire highly technical clinical skills and strive for professional growth. Those who develop their theoretical knowledge base and refine their clinical skills realize that the NICU can provide more avenues for professional growth than other sub-specialities of nursing. Although the extent of the nurse's role expansion will depend upon the size and nature of the NICU (private versus university setting), the highly specialized nature of an NICU lends itself to the development of expanded roles, such as nurse transport teams, nurse clinicians, primary nursing, nurse specialists, or the adaptation of the clinical ladder concept to an NICU.

Adaptation to the NICU

Reflecting back on personal experience in an NICU will take most nurses through an adaptive process that progresses through stages based on their level of expertise. Each stage is, at one time or another, accompanied by strong emotional responses, such as fear, pride, discouragement, disgust, apathy, and eventually acceptance. Nurses who commit themselves to working in an NICU for several years eventually experience these peaks, valleys, and plateaus—some sooner and some more noticeably than others.

Stage I: The Novice Many nurses find that becoming an integral part of the NICU is an overwhelmingly painful process. Orientation can certainly be equated with fear, especially for those who have never been exposed to an NICU. I recall a general uneasiness during those first few months: butterflies in my stomach, frequent headaches, inability to eat, and occasional nightmares. However, all of these symptoms were masked every morning at 0700 by a bright smile and friendly demeanor, in the hope of denying it all.

When hired into a staff position a nurse soon discovers that the NICU, which once looked so intriguing, can take on a new character. The workplace is unfamiliar and extremely technical. The physical structure can be overwhelming. In the beginning, even one's previous neonatal experience may offer very little consolation for the mounting fears. When I entered the NICU as a new staff member, the unit seemed larger and much noisier than I expected; the equipment seemed different; and, worst of all, none of the faces were familiar. Where were the support systems that I thought were there? Even the babies may take on a new character. What once looked like such cute, helpless creatures are actually fragile, often tiny complex technical challenges. Even the growing premature infant can present the new graduate with a multitude of problems. Fears and questions begin to surface. How does one successfully manage to prevent hypothermia when giving a bath or learn to gavage feed without fear of causing aspiration? Use of the most basic skills can contribute to a sense of insecurity in the new NICU nurse.

A nurse's lack of confidence can have a direct effect on ability to perform certain skills, which contributes significantly to the fears of the new neonatal staff nurse. As a result, the complexity of patient care in these early days and months is greatly magnified by fears. However, as confidence builds, fears begin to dissipate, and the required skills eventually become second nature.

Some of the methods utilized to overcome these initial fears include: 1) developing strong ties with other orientees who are experiencing the same frustrations, 2) having access to a well-rounded orientation staff who not only teach the necessary skills to an orientee, but also help to instill confidence, and 3) addressing stress in the didactic portion of the orientation program, which ultimately encourages the development of support systems.

For some nurses, the security of the orientation group is shattered as they become integrated into the general nursing staff in the unit. The peer group is split apart as nurses venture onto their assigned shifts. Here novices are confronted once again with unfamiliar and oftentimes threatening personalities. No longer can they fall back on their "orientator" but, instead have to establish new sources of guidance and support with a new peer group. Once these hurdles have been overcome, novices can begin to feel that they, too, are becoming an integral part of the NICU staff, and they can start to enjoy the work that has to be done.

Stage II: The First Year The first year is a period of rapid growth for most nurses. The first six months are generally an extension of the orientation program, with the most challenging patient care assignments reserved for the less experienced nurses. This enables the first-year nurses to develop their recently attained bedside skills and to broaden their knowledge base in neonatal nursing. It is helpful to have a "charge" nurse designated on all three shifts so that there continues to be an organized method of supervision of new staff nurses during this time, especially for less experienced R.N.s or new graduates. Permanent charge nurses can be excellent role models, encouraging new staff members to take on increasingly complex patient care assignments. Their direction, teaching, and praise can have a significant impact on the nurse's ability to adapt to a new shift and complex situations. Confidence will build quickly as the new NICU nurse becomes more adept at technical skills, especially those that are highly visible to others, such as starting intravenous fluid lines. These skills become mechanisms by which new nurses prove themselves to their peers, thus gaining their acceptance. Positive reinforcement and continued guidance is essential at this time if the first-year nurse is to feel comfortably integrated into the NICU staff.

If all goes well, secure confidence appears at about 6 months. The "new" nurse can start to assume additional responsibilities. Assuming charge nurse, team leader, or primary care nurse roles are milestones. Once these responsibilities are managed in addition to patient care, individuals are no longer "new" staff nurses. At this level of experience, these nurses will reach out to other staff members who are less experienced, very eager to lend a helping hand. More satisfying experiences start to emerge and stand out over the fearful ones. Complex patient care assignments are now regarded as challenging, with positive rewards. The nurse is confident that he or she can appropriately manage an admission, an extubation, and even a major resuscitation.

Stage III: The Second and Third Years As the NICU nurse settles into her second and third years of staff nursing, professional growth becomes a more important issue. The challenges in patient care have been confronted and, by some, mastered. Nurses with this level of expertise are generally considered to have "refined" patient care skills and often act as resource persons to new staff. They will investigate other avenues for growth potential within the unit or decide to find a new challenge outside of the NICU.

Some seek positions as charge nurses in addition to patient care. These nurses enjoy interacting with the entire health team and take great pride in their ability to manage larger numbers of patients. Years ago, when the St. Louis Children's Hospital NICU functioned under the team leader system, this was easily demonstrated. A "good" nurse could competently manage patient care for two to three patients as well as act as team leader for nurses caring for as many as 13 patients. These nurses were required to be present on rounds, to communicate pertinent problems to physicians, to transcribe and communicate new orders to the nurses on their team, and to present shift-to-shift reports, all in addition to providing patient care. In retrospect, those of us who have worked under these conditions often wonder how we did it. Although it is hard to find the answer, one thing is certain—taking on a multitude of responsibilities in addition to providing high-quality patient care gained us the respect of the entire health team, which was essential to our self-esteem. Busy periods were often the most challenging and rewarding, as long as patient care did not suffer. However, once that fine line distinguishing quality care from sub-standard care was crossed, frustration became paramount and burnout often ensued.

Some nurses decide that this is the time to venture into expanded nursing roles. Each institution differs in what it can and will offer a staff nurse in terms of an expanded role. Generally this includes opportunities for the transport team, nurse clinician roles, clinical nurse roles (at St. Louis Children's Hospital this includes the NICU nurses responsible for orienting new employees and for direct clinical supervision of staff nurses during each shift, as well as the nurses in charge of the transport team and outreach education), and nurse specialists. Opportunities for the expanded role of the nurse is one aspect of NICU nursing that is unique. Fewer pediatricians are seeking out neonatology, because of its highly specialized nature, which opens the door ever wider for nurses who wish to take on expanded roles.

Regardless of the choice a nurse makes for role expansion and professional growth, continued job satisfaction depends heavily on families, co-workers, and unit administrators recognizing a job well done. Otherwise, frustration can mount, leading to burnout and lack of motivation. Second- and third-year nurses are expected to function as patient advocates and sometimes must take risks on behalf of their patients. If their observations and recommendations go unnoticed, or their patients' medical and nursing needs are minimized by the health care team, nurses start to question their role as patient advocate and their reasons for staying in the field. Feelings of "no one can do it as well as I" will surface. These feelings can be directed at other nurses as well as physicians, but are generally directed at less experienced house staff. More experienced nurses learn not to exhaust themselves trying to fight with and persuade individuals about methods of management, but rather take such issues to the attending neonatologists or nurse managers. This is where recognition by administration can be of greatest value. If nurses' judgments, opinions, and beliefs are respected by unit managers, they know that they can deal with issues on this level. Consequently, frustrations will be minimized and actions rewarded.

Stage IV: Three Years and More   At this point in the staff nurse's career, personal fulfillment is no longer the most critical issue. Typically, these nurses have peaked in their level of clinical expertise, have advanced into expanded roles and have achieved previously established professional goals. In short, NICU nurses with more than 3 years of experience are accomplished clinicians. Superiors must recognize their achievements and address the issue of employee recognition and compensation if they hope to hold on to these senior staff members. If an NICU is well managed and supported by administration, staff satisfaction will continue to mount and turnover rates will begin to decrease.

Staff nurse needs at St. Louis Children's Hospital are highly regarded not only by patient care managers, but also by the Director of Nursing. Over the last 9 years, staffing strategies and policies have changed considerably and have had a major impact on turnover rates. Five years ago it was unusual to have more than a handful of staff nurses whose length of stay in the NICU was more than 3 years. In 1982, 23% of our staff nurses had been employed for more than 5 years (these numbers do not include the senior nurses in managerial roles), and half of these nurses are still full-time employees. Many changes have arisen through the combined efforts of the patient care manager, her staff, and the Director of Patient Care, with many positive outcomes (Marshall et al., 1982). These changes include: 1) instituting the 4-day, 10-hour shift schedule, including extended (3-day) weekends; 2) striving for maximum staffing by the patient care manager; 3) providing cyclical time schedules for the staff; 4) offering straight-day positions for senior staff members (for full-time personnel this is a 4-day, 10-hour workweek); and 5) creating opportunities for staff involvement in unit and hospital-wide committees with compensation for a greater-than-40-hour workweek.

These measures have boosted morale in several ways. The stresses incurred by the 5-day workweek have been eased tremendously by reducing the work week to 4 days. This is especially true for the nurses who work straight-night shifts. Cyclical staffing allows for greater flexibility in planning time off because the staff nurses always know their work cycles. Straight-day positions for staff nurses are quite rare and are a highly revered benefit of the senior staff nurse. Finally, the provision for involvement by staff nurses in activities removed from direct patient care fosters creativity, motivation, and a continued sense of professional growth. As a result of these measures, two unique staff re-entry patterns into the NICU have occurred along with a dwindling turnover rate: 1) clinical nurses are returning to staff nurse positions; and 2) some staff nurses who leave the unit return within 6 months.

Those nurses who advance into clinical positions seem to experience the same degree of burnout in these positions, but for different reasons. Each position offered in an NICU seems to have its own tolerance level, whether it involves new staff orientators, shift clinical advisors, patient care managers, or outreach education coordinators. As a result, over the last 5 years several nurses in clinical roles at St. Louis Children's Hospital have returned to staff nursing rather than leaving the field altogether.

Several nurses also returned to the NICU after terminating their positions for various reasons. Most returned within 6 months, having been more dissatisfied with positions outside the unit. It still remains unclear whether these re-entry patterns are unique to St. Louis Children's Hospital, but they do reflect the desirability of and contentment with the workplace.

Conclusion

Reflecting back on 9 year's experience in an NICU raises many issues. As discussed, the NICU is a stressful work environment, but it is also a highly desirable one. Balancing the two extremes is largely dependent upon two factors: 1) the individual's inherent ability to confront and cope with the pressures; and 2) the administrative support of the unit so that the staff have some degree of control over their environment. If these factors coexist, the impact of the NICU on the staff nurse will be positive. Ultimately, such coexistence will provide nurses who choose the NICU workplace with greater job satisfaction, less disillusionment, and exciting opportunities for professional growth.

A Pediatric House Officer's Perspective, by John L. Roberts, M.D.

The highly technical and critical nature of the NICU environment is very stressful for the inexperienced pediatric house officer. Much of the stress occurs because of an imbalance between the house officer's resources (knowledge, technical skills, interpersonal skills, and support systems) and the demanding service requirements of the NICU. Several reports have emphasized the stress experienced by the pediatric house officer during the internship year (Adler et al., 1980; Alpert et al., 1973; Levine et al., 1969; Roughman et al., 1975; Schowalter, 1970; Seigel and Donnelly, 1978; Smith and Harlan, 1977; Valko and Clayton, 1975; Werner et al., 1979). A few have explored the stresses experienced in the pediatric intensive care units (Marshall and Kasman, 1980; Rosini et al., 1974; Todres et al., 1974; Waller et al., 1979). In many respects, the stresses in the NICU, except for quantity, seem to be the same as those experienced throughout the internship. In the NICU, workdays are longer, patients are more critically ill, and relationships with allied health personnel and parents are more intense.

Stresses

Fatigue is thought to be a major stress for the house officer in the NICU. In most NICUs, house officers work 80 to 100 hours per week during a 4-week rotation. During this time, they average eight 30-hour shifts. By the end of the rotation, most house officers are fatigued. However, pediatric training programs that reduced the number of hours on duty found that fatigue is not the only stress experienced by pediatric house officers (Reynolds and Bict, 1971).

House staff training programs were devised because of two needs: practical training for the house officer and the hospital's need for patient care. Often in the NICU, the latter is dominant. The busy work schedule and acute nature of the care do not lend themselves to controlled and scheduled learning. Teaching sessions are frequently interrupted because of the need to transport an infant or because of a crisis in the nursery. Most house officers question the value of their experience in the NICU, feeling that it is not useful in their general pediatric careers. Because the NICU service is a major portion of most pediatric house officer training programs, commanding a full one-sixth of the training years in some, it is understandable why some house officers find it unduly stressful.

Another stress felt by the pediatric house officer in the NICU centers on the expectations made of him or her by others to react correctly to the rapidly changing, life-threatening situations that arise in the NICU. Parents expect house officers to cure their baby, nurses expect them to perform proficiently and to have logical answers to their patient-related questions. Hospital administrators and medical superiors expect them to be available when crises arise, to react in a professional manner, and to prevent problems when possible. In truth, there is a covert hope that the inexperienced house officer can function as a seasoned neonatologist. Initially, interns are intellectually, technically, and professionally unable to fulfill that role. Pediatric house officers may feel psychological pressures when the NICU experience does not meet their expectations for education, or if they feel that their performance does not meet the expectations of parents, nurses, or physician colleagues.

Certain categories of patients, such as patients with terminal (Todres et al., 1974) or chronic (Reynolds and Bict, 1971) illnesses and patients with private physicians (Marshall and Kasman, 1980) are more stressful than others to the house officer-in-training. In addition to these types of patients, patients in the NICU can have multiple serious problems. Cardiorespiratory, metabolic, neurologic, and hematologic abnormalities often occur simultaneously in babies weighing less than 2 pounds. It is difficult and sometimes impossible for the most experienced neonatologist to correctly identify and correct these abnormalities. For the young pediatrician still trying to learn about normal babies, sick premature infants represent an almost incomprehensible challenge.

"The responsibility of each physician is to prevent, to diagnose, to prognosticate, and to treat when, and if necessary" (Andrews, 1976, p. 84)—but above all, the physician's responsibility is to console. Not all babies in the NICU survive, nor is the outcome of the survivors always favorable. Hence, physicians are frequently in the position of consoling bereaved or grieving parents. This is tremendously stressful for junior house officers whose training has not adequately prepared them for such intense interpersonal relationships (Benfield et al., 1978). Indeed, they are often asked to help parents cope when they, themselves, are trying to cope. Often, a patient's death or handicap is viewed by the house officer as a personal failure. Intense parental reactions, such as denial, anger, console parents who blame them for the outcome of an infant is difficult, if not impossible (Kravath, 1977).

Finally, house officers experience a great deal of stress because of the necessary ethical decisions that must be made in the NICU every day. Deciding when to withhold or withdraw extraordinary therapy is generally done by the attending physician, with input from the neonatal health care team and the parents. Although junior house officers do not directly make the decisions, they are often involved in implementing them, and because house officers are in the NICU almost constantly throughout the day, they often witness the outcome. Inexperience may result in passivity in the management of a premature infant weighing less than 1 kilogram, but unwillingness to surrender a term infant with a terminal illness. Watching a beautiful term newborn die may be unbearable.

Support System

How house officers handle these stresses depends upon their knowledge about sick newborns, their proficiency at technical and interpersonal skills, and available support systems. Generally, much of the knowledge and the proficiency at technical skills needed to function as a competent intern are gained early in the course of training. Because of the lack of formal training in interpersonal skills, however, many house officers never master the "art" of talking to parents. This remains a source of stress, even later in practice.

Besides developing self-confidence and a feeling of competence, there are potentially many sources of support available to the house officer in the NICU. Perhaps the greatest support is the comradery with other house officers. The fact that some have "made it through before" may make the rotation endurable. The fact that other house officers are having difficulties with the rotation reassures the house officer that the problem does not lie within himself or herself. Furthermore, house officers can learn from each other in a less threatening way than from a superior who might have certain expectations.

NICU nurses can be a tremendous source of support for the fledgling house officer. Nurses who have many years of experience are often conditioned to seeing certain occurrences responded to in specific manners. They can help the inexperienced house officer to respond appropriately to a crisis. In addition, nurses assume many of the technical duties needed to run the unit, relieving the house officer of some of the necessary service-related tasks in the nursery.

Many NICUs employ social workers to help parents cope with

having a newborn in the NICU. Social workers are also a tremendous source of support for NICU physicians. They are able to provide feedback to supplement the physicians' communication with the parents. For junior house officers who have limited experience in physician-parent interactions, this feedback can reassure them that they are getting their point across to the parents. In addition, because social workers are often trained counselors, they may be able to identify the house officer who has difficulty with the NICU and offer emotional support.

Attending and other senior physicians in the NICU help the intern by imparting some of their knowledge about the subspecialty and by offering an extra pair of hands to get the work done. The attending physician further decreases the stress load on the house officer by making many of the ethical and difficult decisions and by ensuring that the NICU runs smoothly. Finally, by providing a comprehensive orientation to the NICU early in the rotation, the attending physician can allay many of the junior house officer's fears.

Besides the sources of support that originate from NICU personnel, each house officer has various other support systems. Family, hobbies, sports, and routines all impart to the house officer a certain baseline personal stability, allowing him or her to remain emotionally coherent despite the stresses. The extent to which these personal support systems enable a house officer to endure the NICU rotation is immeasurable.

Coping

Most house officers survive the NICU rotation, most do not seem to mind it, and some may even begin to enjoy it. The reaction of the house officer probably depends upon the balance achieved between stresses and support systems. The degree of imbalance manifests itself in the emergence of various coping behaviors; some will be more appropriate than others. Appropriate coping behaviors will be manifest as confidence, knowledge, and skill emerge during the rotation. Priorities will include important family responsibilities and recreation away from the unit.

The following behaviors indicate inappropriate coping and are displayed by many house officers some time during the rotation: depression (Wolraich and Reiter, 1979), withdrawal, aggressive or passive-aggressive attitudes toward other staff members, recurrent nightmares relating to aspects of the unit, derogatory attitudes toward patients, avoidance of responsibility, and deterioration of friendships or family life. These aberrations are frequently subtle but may progress to the extent that they affect patient care and the functioning of the NICU. If they occur sporadically, it may be that the house officers are not cognizant of or are not using available support systems. However, if inappropriate coping styles occur in every house officer, then the NICU rotation may indeed be too strenuous and unrewarding and may need to be improved.

Modification of the NICU Rotation

NICU rotations are part of every pediatric training program; obviously, then, it is possible for most pediatric house officers to adapt to the NICU environment. But is the NICU rotation optimal from the standpoint of patient care as well as house officer training? With NICUs getting larger and more technical, just what are the limits to which the average house officer can be expected to cope? Is NICU training necessary for every pediatrician? What should be the goals of the NICU experience for the house officer? What should be the house officer's responsibilities in the NICU? The answers to these questions await the design of an appropriate scientific model to objectively measure the effect of the NICU on the house officer. Only with such a model can modifications of the present system be logically addressed.

Some welcomed changes have already been proposed in various NICUs throughout the country:

1. The house officer's workload has been decreased, by hiring more house officers, assigning house officers fewer patients and nights on call (Wolraich and Reiter, 1979), or giving nurses more responsibilities.
2. Technical and educational objectives have been outlined for the house officer during the NICU rotation (Kravath, 1977) and he or she has been given an orientation before being given responsibilities (Todres et al., 1974).
3. Some centers have organized intern support groups (Seigel and Donnelly, 1978; Werner and Korsch, 1979) or scheduled weekly meetings of all NICU personnel to identify stresses (Rosini et al., 1974; Todres et al., 1974).

Another possible improvement is to include rotating the more experienced house officers through the NICU rather than the newly graduated interns. This would allow the intern to learn some technical skills and develop some confidence at a less demanding pace.

Regardless of modifications, the NICU, because of its size and intensive nature, will continue to be stressful for all who work there. Therefore, support systems should be identified and utilized by all NICU personnel.

An Academic Neonatologist's Perspective, by Richard E. Marshall, M.D.

My perspective is that of an academic neonatologist in charge of a program that includes three other staff colleagues on the faculty of a medical school. Some of the problems that I address may be unique to the leadership position, but I believe others are common to my colleagues.

Priorities

Perhaps the most difficult problem facing a productive academic neonatologist is how to organize one's time in an effective manner. There are unusually heavy clinical requirements in an NICU that make it particulary difficult to satisfy the demands that one be an effective teacher and published investigator, as well as an accomplished clinician. Obviously, there are difficulties in being superman/superwoman and performing incomparably at all times, but perhaps there are a few clues through the maze. First, the neonatologist must recognize that no one can do all things equally well all of the time. The fact is that, as professionals, each task at work—teaching, clinical care, and research—has to be performed at a competent level. When one teaches or acts as an attending physician, that activity must take precedence over other tasks and be done well. Second, such an ability to do different things well requires that there be enough neonatologists to do the work. There must be sufficient time for diverse activities to be pursued by everyone.

Research

The usually heavy clinical responsibilities of the NICU impose special problems for the neonatologist who wishes to conduct independent research. Young neonatologists are often told that research is not essential and that clinical service and teaching will be rewarded by promotion committees. Although that may be true for some universities, it may not remain true because priorities change with different administrative leadership. Certainly in times of economic hardship, funding for neonatal research is a major problem. External funding is scarce and neonatologists may be forced to conduct investigations that can be done with modest resources and diligent observations. There are unique opportunities for research on the impact of the NICU environment on both the patient and the caregivers that have just begun to be explored. Moreover, money for neonatal research may need to be derived from the clinical activities of the investigators. However, in many circumstances, the monies derived from neonatologists' clinical work are directed elsewhere for other programs within a department or a medical school. Arriving at a just distribution of clinical income is not an easy task.

Patients

NICUs have diverse patients with many kinds of illnesses, and yet there are two types of patients that I think cause particularly intense stresses for neonatologists—small prematures under 1000 grams and chronic lung patients. Small prematures are difficult to care for since there is virtually no margin for error, and everyone is aware of this. In addition, one not infrequently asks, when placing a 750-gram patient with severe hyaline membrane disease on a ventilator, what am I doing this for? However, the facts are comforting. NICUs are saving many more such patients, and statistics on follow-up demonstrate that some survivors do well neurologically.

Chronic lung patients, those with bronchopulmonary dysplasia, who require assisted ventilation or supplemental oxygen for weeks or months, represent a unique frustration for the NICU staff. In my opinion, many caregivers who gravitate into NICU work have high expectations of themselves and need rapid resolutions of their patients' illnesses in order to feel rewarded. In short, they want quick recoveries and have relatively low thresholds for frustration. Unfortunately, the very technology that can save lives produces chronic patients, and both nurses and doctors become disappointed and angry at one another. The nurses imply that, if the doctors were more adequate, there wouldn't be "chronic patients" and doctors wish the nurses would stop expecting miracles. I know of no easy answers to this situation, although some NICUs are finding it best for the infants and their families to send many of these patients home earlier than before. Meanwhile, all must strive for the highest standard of nursing and medical care so that "preventable" illness is minimized. Of course, patience, tolerance, and more patience and more tolerance are required from all parties involved.

Relationships

The NICU cannot function without a team approach. No one neonatologist can emit enough energy to make an NICU work without the support of many other physicians, nurses, social workers, and technicians, as well as enlightened hospital administrators. Thus, it becomes imperative to develop mutually supportive relationships with many others.

Relationships with House Staff
Within the neonatal unit itself, there must be cordial relationships with the house staff. The perspective of

how the house staff views the NICU experience is discussed elsewhere in this chapter by John L. Roberts. What I am concerned with here is how the neonatologist relates to the young physicians. The interns and residents are called upon to work long hours in the NICU and usually get only 1 to 2 hours of sleep when they are on call at night. They are required to perform intricate technical procedures on critically ill patients with minute veins and small lumbar spaces. Patients die unexpectedly and ethical problems arise at inopportune times. It is only natural that interns and residents are nervous during their NICU rotation.

Neonatologists must be as supportive as possible while maintaining the highest possible standards of care. Support can take many forms. Physical presence in the NICU is mandatory for significant periods of time if crises are to be avoided and burdens are to be shared. Role modeling for problems around dying patients and ethical discussions is obligatory. Teaching, both at the bedside and in the conference room whenever clinical conditions permit, is required. Also, it is crucial to be discreet and private about correcting mistakes that are inevitable, given the nature of the problems. Suggestions or criticisms should be given in private, whenever possible, to avoid an adversary relationship; such discretion can help more than giving vent to a screaming rage reaction.

Relationships within Neonatology Group Relationships within the neonatology group also require nurturing. In our program, each faculty neonatologist has an independent research program so that each has a distinct area of expertise and recognition. Because there is so much autonomy with this structure, it is relatively easy for each of us to spend most of our time doing what we enjoy and are good at. Yet, there are still areas of responsibility in which consensus becomes essential, especially in clinical matters. Two approaches have been helpful. One, we hold weekly business meetings with formal agendas where clinical issues are openly addressed. Two, we have a manual of clinical care written jointly that outlines common approaches.

Relationships with Other Hospital Personnel Relationships with other colleagues within the clinical faculty require careful attention. Neonatology was not a recognized subspecialty when some senior faculty members were in their house staff training. At times they, and others, view neonatology as a growth that knows no limits. This is not surprising when, in our hospital, the NICU employs about 25% of the nursing staff. There arises, then, at times, questions not only of appropriate personnel allocation, but also bed and space allocation for NICU graduates when there is an occupancy problem. In addition, at times there can be legitimate differences of opinion about patient care in grey areas of jurisdiction. Who, for example, should best write the respirator orders on postoperative surgical patients or decide if a patient requires cardiac catheterization? These problems of jurisdiction can be usually solved by discussing them with the involved parties, but may require adjudication by the chairmen of surgery and pediatrics. Conflict about space allocation may be solved by negotiating agreement on maximal NICU overflow beds in other parts of the hospital in such a way that other subspecialists are not overwhelmed by too many babies.

Another potential source of conflict within the clinical faculty revolves around the belief that NICU patients are not available to non-neonatologists for research. Since there is a wealth of clinical research material in an NICU such an insular attitude is unreasonable, yet consistency in patient care must be maintained. We have found that, when investigators discuss their research protocols early in their formulation, it is possible to integrate multiple studies with quality patient care.

Relationships with Nursing and Social Work Neonatologists can establish significant professional friendships with their colleagues in social work and nursing. Often social workers can identify problems before a physician is aware of them. They can let you know when your interactions with the nurses or house staff are destructive rather than supportive or when negative feelings are brewing in the unit. What might become a big problem may be nipped in the bud. Social workers can also help by providing insight into problem families. Perhaps the most valuable service that the social worker can provide is listening to the neonatologist as a true professional friend who has no medical or nursing responsibilities and thus may have a unique perspective.

Nurses can also become genuine professional friends, but there are many nurses and the interactions thus tend to become more complex. In our hospital the clinical nurse specialist works closely with the social worker as part of the support staff for families and staff. She provides the background of a nurse and facilitator and provides a rare blend of clinical experience and balanced discipline. Open communications must exist between the hospital nursing administration and neonatologists if the inevitable staffing problems are to be solved. The head nurses and other members of the management staff must be able to have candid discussions with their neonatology group. We meet as a group—neonatologists and management nurse—twice a month, and I meet with the head nurse privately once a month. These meetings, while sometimes not fulfilling all our expectations, have been generally productive. The neonatologists must work hard at developing and maintaining communication with the staff nurses so that they can obtain important medical information from those who spend the most time at the bedside making crucial observations. It is important to stay and talk with nurses when one is in the unit. Such contact enhances professional relations that are of mutual benefit and may serve as a key to nurturing professional friendships.

The morale of the nursing staff must be an essential concern of the neonatology group. The neonatologists can be supportive of the nursing staff in a variety of ways. For example, they can hold regular weekly meetings with an open agenda—we do this and have found it helpful, if a bit frustrating for all. Neonatologists can demonstrate their concern for patients by their physical presence in the unit and their availability when out of the unit. They can come to NICU activities, such as parties for NICU graduates and NICU staff picnics, and remember holidays with a gift to the nursing staff. They should elicit nurses' opinions during bedside rounds. They must act as a role model in their behavior to the nurses, making sure that their demeanor is always respectful and courteous, especially when they are asked questions that are provocative and even embarrassing. Finally, the neonatologists can try to work with the nursing leadership to stimulate them, and can, in turn, be responsive to constructive changes in the nursing organization that are designed to enhance staff nurse satisfaction.

Relationships with Administration No academic NICU can survive without generous support from the hospital. Adequate medical, nursing, and social work personnel as well as adequate ancillary technical personnel such as x-ray and laboratory technicians are necessary. Old equipment requires continuous maintenance and new equipment is frequently required. The only criteria for adequacy of personnel or equipment is whether or not excellent patient care can be maintained without making unrealistic demands on all who are called on to provide such care.

Neonatologists must be prepared to justify their requests and be available to help the administration understand their unique problems. Tours of the unit can help administrators and trustees grasp the ambience of the NICU. A well-respected NICU can generate significant income and reputation for the hospital in which it is located, and this may have to be pointed out. On the other hand, if the state or federal government is unable or unwilling to pay costs for nonpaying patients, the administrations of private hospitals may be forced to regulate the expenses of the NICU or face bankruptcy.

Team Approach

There are two areas in which the team approach of the NICU can make lonely responsibilities more tolerable: 1) death of patients, and 2) ethical decisions.

Death of Patients   Although physicians and social workers all have a difficult time in accepting a perinatal death, each group of caregivers grieves in ways related to their roles. The physicians bear the ultimate responsibility for the diagnosis and treatment of the patient. Many physicians believe that their function is to save lives and prevent death. They interpret a baby's death as a personal failure. Physicians then feel guilty and become angry at the impotent situation in which they find themselves. They may go to unusual lengths to avoid talking to the parents of a dying infant. It is almost as if by denying the reality of the death situation they can reaffirm their own control.

Caregivers need to be allowed to react to death and to permit feelings to be expressed. Expressing emotions does not make caregivers less professional; they may not grieve equally over every death. There is no reason why a doctor, nurse, or social worker should not cry on occasion and grieve with a family. An expression of grief may be therapeutic both to the caregiver and to the family. Such an attitude presupposes that the health care team members have somehow dealt with the issue of their own mortality. It is hard to help families cope with infant death when one is confusing the fact of the baby's death with one's own fear of death.

Some neonatal deaths are more painful than others for both the families and the health care team. It is prudent to anticipate which kinds of neonatal death are most traumatic so that appropriate efforts can be made in these sensitive areas. Additional support may be offered to the health care team by holding open meetings to discuss feelings surrounding a special case. The opportunity to share these painful experiences with other caregivers can be a valuable source of support for the individual team member. In some cases, encouraging staff members to attend funerals if they so desire can also be helpful. In our institution there are three types of neonatal death that cause the most anxiety: 1) whenever the family and physician decide, after thorough discussion, to withhold further support; 2) the death of a chronic patient who has been in the hospital for 2 months or more and to whom the family and health care team have become deeply attached; and 3) the death of a term baby who has no major external malformations. In our unit the death of a critically ill premature infant weighing under 1200 grams is easier to cope with than that of a 3.5-kilogram baby who dies from congenital heart disease.

The perinatal health care team needs to be organized so that it can be mutually supportive. Caregivers need an opportunity to discuss their feelings while the infant is dying as well as after the death. Most caregivers will not be able to continue to function at optimal levels until they have been able to vent some of their frustrations and anger. The attending physician must be available to help the interns and residents deal with their own feelings so that they, in turn, can help families. Experienced nurses must support their junior colleagues. Social service workers can be indispensable in providing support to all staff members and can provide immeasurable strength during times of crises. Members of each group must be willing to talk openly with each other. Regular, formal conferences in which the attending physicians, experienced nurses, and social workers can discuss these issues with their younger, less experienced colleagues are invaluable to all participants.

Ethical Dilemmas Physicians are taught that it is their responsibility to save lives. However, little systematic attention is focused in medical schools or hospital training programs on the quality of the life they are called upon to save. Whether he or she likes it or not, a neonatologist is forced by patients to deal with issues of life and death. With the increase in technical advances, many patients who used to die rapidly now survive for indeterminate periods. Neonatologists confront many different medical situations that try their consciences. The most demanding classes of patients for me are: 1) respirator-dependent infants under 1000 grams whose ultrasound scans show evidence of intracranial hemorrhage with massive hydrocephalus; and 2) infants with severe chronic lung disease (stages 3–4 bronchopulmonary dysplasia) who require supplemental oxygen of near 100% and the ventilator at 3 to 4 months of age.

What is the wisest course of action? How should the family's wishes be considered? What is best for the patient? What can or should be done? There are no universal solutions for dealing with the ethical problems posed by either group of infants. It further complicates matters that there is often an urgent need to make a decision.

Some approaches that we recently adopted may be helpful to others. First, attending physicians, fellows, and any other appropriate consultants meet as a group to make certain that there is unanimity as to the dismal medical prognosis. All consultants must agree that there is no opportunity for the patient to have a normal emotional or mental life. An overall plan to limit care is then formulated. After this, meetings are held with social workers and appropriate nurses to discuss the family situation. Many meetings may be required between the neonatologists, social workers, and nurses at this time to ensure that there is understanding and acceptance by all about the prognosis and plan.

A meeting is then held with the patient's family at which the neonatologist, the social workers, the nurses and, in some situations, the house staff and the chaplain may be present. The family is informed of the medical opinion and told that further respirator support does not seem to be medically indicated. This discussion can only be broached if the social workers, nurses, and neonatologist have determined that the family is prepared for it (insofar as anyone can be said to be prepared for such a decision). Under certain circumstances, medical/legal considerations dictate that the parents sign a witnessed note saying that they understand, agree, and consent to the decision proposed.

I must emphasize that these decisions are the most stressful and painful experiences that I, as a neonatologist, have yet endured. However, if one defines the role of a physician as a professional who must try to minimize suffering, such decisions are forced upon us. It is too soon to know the impact of parental participation in these decisions upon the future coherence of family life. Benfield et al. (1978) have published data suggesting that the immediate impact may not be deleterious, but further investigation is required.

Rewards

What are the rewards and satisfactions associated with a career in neonatology? I think there are many. It is a pleasure to be part of a new subspecialty that saves many high risk patients. I consider neonatology an achievement of major medical significance. As a former internist, the satisfaction of salvaging newborns can be more gratifying than working with older patients whose life expectancy is much briefer after they get well. A newborn can look forward to 70 plus years. Academic neonatology, with its diverse demands, provides challenges that permit multiple talents to be nourished. For many who have multiple interests, each of the tasks we must learn to master offers different rewards. The opportunities for personal growth, forged in the crucible of hope and despair of clinical practice, are significant and real. Our communities appreciate our efforts, and I, for one, look upon the future with optimism and faith. Faith comes, in part, with humility from the number of "unexpected outcomes" that could not be predicted. After all, how many careers in this age permit the full use of a person's abilities in a manner that is socially rewarding?

Summary

Each of us has written from our own perspective. We have all found that the unusual diversity of premature and critically ill newborns is both a major stress and source of satisfaction when we are rewarded in knowing that our skills have been instrumental in saving a baby. We have all found that support from other peers and superiors is essential in doing our daily jobs and ensuring the continued growth that is required for professional competence. Each, in his or her own way, has recognized that a team approach is essential for both the caregivers and the patients and families that they serve.

Yet it is not surprising that each of us dwells on those aspects of the NICU experience that are specific to our vantage point. The staff nurse focuses upon the essential details of working at the bedside. Both of the physicians mention how painful patients' deaths and ethical dilemmas are for them. The academic neonatologist finds it important to discuss research, funding, and the diverse responsibilities that are part of a faculty position in a university medical service.

One of the most striking differences is the tone that each perspective emits. To the house officer, the NICU is a place where he or she is faced with what are initially almost overwhelming problems. Because the house officer is not permanently committed to a neonatology career, he or she is not in a position to undergo the prolonged maturation discussed by the nurse and the neonatologist. Certainly, neonatology can be a rewarding career for nurse and neonatologist; it remains a challenge to make the experience as rich and meaningful for the house officer.

Acknowledgments

Joan Walsh wishes to express her gratitude to the following colleagues for their assistance and support: Helen Gibbs, R.N., B.S.N., Linda Cape, R.N., M.S.N.; and Beth Shinners, M.S.W.

References

Adler, R., Werner, E. R., and Korsch, B. 1980. Systematic study of four years of internship. Pediatrics 66:1000.

Alpert, J. J., Youngerman, J., Breslow, J., and Kosa, J. 1973. Learning experiences during the internship year: An exploratory study of pediatric graduate education. Pediatrics 51:119.

Andrews, B. F. 1976. Childrens' rights against abuse and neglect. J. Kentucky Med. Assoc. 74:84.

Benfield, D. G., Leib, S., and Vollman, J. 1978. Grief responses of parents to neonatal death and parent participation in deciding care. Pediatrics 62:171.

Kravath, R. E. 1977. Educational objectives for house staff in the pediatric intensive care unit. Crit. Care Med. 5:159.

Levine, M. D., Robertson, L. S., and Alpert, J. J. 1969. A descriptive study of a pediatric internship. Pediatrics 44:986.
Marshall, R. E., and Kasman, C. 1980. Burnout in the neonatal intensive care unit. Pediatrics 65:1161.
Marshall, R., Kasman, C., and Cape, L. (eds.). 1982. Coping with Caring for Sick Newborns. Saunders, Philadelphia.
Reynolds, R. E., and Bict, T. W. 1971. Attitudes of medical interns toward patients and health professionals. J. Health Soc. Behav. 12:1307.
Rosini, L. A., Howell, M. C., Todres, I. D., and Dorman, J. 1974. Group meetings in a pediatric intensive care unit. Pediatrics 53:371.
Roughman, K., Pizzo, P., Graham, E., Graham, D., Guyer, B., and Harris, P. 1975. The pediatric internship as a teaching technique: A comparison of learning experience in five hospitals. Pediatrics 56:239.
Schowalter, J. E. 1970. Death and the pediatric house officer. J. Pediatr. 76:706.
Seigel, B., and Donnelly, J. C. 1978. Enriching personal and professional development: The experience of a support group for interns. J. Med. Educ. 53:908.
Smith, S. M., and Harlan, W. R. 1977. A pediatric residence program revisited. South. Med. J. 70:784.
Todres, D. I., Howell, M. C., and Shannon, D. C. 1974. Physician reaction to training in a pediatric intensive care unit. Pediatrics 53:375.
Valko, R. J., and Clayton, P. J. 1975. Depression in the internship. Dis. Nerv. Sys. 36:26.
Waller, D. A., Todres, D. I., Cassem, N. H., and Anderten, A. 1979. Coping with poor prognosis in the pediatric intensive care unit. Am. J. Dis. Child. 133:1121.
Werner, E. R., Adler, R., Robison, R., and Korsch, B. 1979. Attitudes and interpersonal skills during pediatric internship. Pediatrics 63:491.
Werner, E. R., and Korsch, B. M. 1979. Professionalization during pediatric internship: Attitudes, adaptation, and interpersonal skills. In: E. C. Shapiro and L. M. Lowenstein (eds.), Becoming a Physician, pp. 113–138. Ballinger Publishing Co., Cambridge, MA.
Wolraich, M. L., and Reiter, S. 1979. Training physicians in communication skills. Dev. Med. Child Neurol. 21:773.

12

Environmental Neonatology
Implications for
Intervention

Allen W. Gottfried

The information presented in the preceding chapters demonstrates the importance and necessity of investigating the environment of newborn special care units. For the most part, the architecture and structure of these units as well as their functions were designed to maximize staff efficiency and, in turn, enhance the quality of care for sick newborns (Korones, Chapter 2 in this volume; also see Brans, 1983). There is no doubt that great strides have been made in the medical care and technology for premature newborns. The fact is that neonatal mortality and morbidity have both been substantially reduced.

However, the issue at hand is whether greater progress could be accomplished by well-designed environmental interventions beneficial to the newborn. Such interventions should be conducted during the neonatal period, not because of any notion of it being a critical period or of what premature newborns lack by not being in utero or of the stimulation term healthy newborns receive, but because of current environmental conditions that exist in most modern newborn special care facilities (intense, constant illumination, high noise levels, etc.). Intervention is defined as manipulations geared not only toward improving the status of premature newborns but also toward promoting the developmental requirements of

---

The preparation of this chapter was supported by a California State University, Fullerton, President's Grant.

fetuses during the neonatal period. It is not assumed that intervention during this period will completely eliminate or prevent sequelae associated with prematurity. Overcoming adverse consequences of prematurity or potential developmental problems in any at-risk population of children may involve extensive and/or continuous environmental interventions (see Brown et al., 1980; Zigler and Berman, 1983).

Although it is difficult to define what is meant by an abnormal or aberrant environment, data presented in this volume certainly suggest that the environment of special care units is far from what newborns would be experiencing if still in utero or what is typically observed in the environment of term healthy newborns (see, e.g., Linn et al., Chapter 5 in this volume). It has not been established that all environmental characteristics of special care units are harmless to newborns. It has been pointed out that certain environmental characteristics may have a detrimental effect on the medical and developmental status of premature newborns.

Neonatal environmental intervention programs aimed at improving the developmental status of premature infants emerged rapidly during the 1970s. Virtually all of the investigators of these programs readily adopted the position that hospitalized premature newborns are sensorily deprived. This sensory deficit hypothesis, which served as the basis of intervention strategies, was accepted in the absence of knowledge about the environment or ecology of newborns in special care units. Without exception, all of the experimental intervention programs for premature newborns conducted to date have provided additional stimulation of one sort or another. More stimulation was the guiding remedy. Furthermore, the stimulation schedules were without an empirical foundation.

Suggestions for Intervention

What is proposed here is not a prescription but instead suggested directions for environmental engineering and interventions. The suggested modifications involve substitutions, reductions, and alterations as well as increases in stimulation. The direction of change is variable-specific and based on our current environmental literature. The variables of concern include light, sound, vestibular-kinesthetic, and social stimulation. There are other important environmental characteristics in newborn special care units (e.g., temperature, radiation, electrical hazards, and gases). These latter variables have been addressed by other investigators (Kellman, 1980; Moffat and Hackel, Chapter 9 in this volume; Peabody and Lewis, Chapter 10 in this volume; Perlstein, 1983). Issues concerning methodology and assessment of intervention programs with premature newborns are not discussed here because they have been given attention elsewhere (see Cornell and Gottfried, 1976; Gottfried, 1981). It is important to emphasize that the impact of many environmental characteristics on premature newborns has yet to be established. These suggestions are based primarily on the author's appraisal of special care unit environments and, unfortunately, not on an extensive body of knowledge of environment-developmental relationships in premature newborns. Hence, positive outcomes and potential negative side effects must be continually monitored.

Lighting

With respect to lighting conditions, there are two major considerations for modification or intervention: 1) the use of cool-white fluorescent lighting; and 2) the need for 24-hour continuous lighting in the entire unit. Cool-white fluorescent lighting systems, which have replaced incandescent lights, produce greater illumination, generate no heat, and allow accurate examination of infants' skin tones. However, as noted by Gottfried (Chapter 3 in this volume) and Peabody and Lewis (Chapter 10 in this volume), prolonged continuous exposure to cool-white lights may have undesirable effects on premature newborns. Such lighting systems could be readily substituted either completely or partially by full-spectrum lights.[1] The latter approximates the spectrum of solar light and has been found in experiments (e.g., Wurtman and Weisel, 1969) to eliminate the negative consequences associated with cool-white fluorescent lights without any side effects. The use of full-spectrum light may entail some adjustments in the assessment of infant skin color.

Although continuous light is necessary for surveillance of some infants (Korones, Chapter 2 in this volume), many infants and particularly those in convalescent care units do not require constant observation. Continuous light is primarily a convenience for the staff (i.e., lights do not have to be turned on in order to see the infants) and is a result of the large-room concept that became popular in the 1960s. Because a number of infants do not need to be observed constantly and 24-hour lighting serves no developmental or medical function for many infants, lighting schedules should be instituted. Specifically, lighting conditions should be altered to simulate day/night cycles. This could be accomplished by using rheostats, particularly in cubical-type units (see Frayer, 1983) or an individual or localized type of lighting arrangement over each incubator. It would be

---

[1] My associate Patricia Wallace-Lande must share acknowledgment for this recommendation.

useful to determine whether day/night lighting schedules facilitate certain circadian rhythms in premature newborns. Such schedules could dovetail those instituted subsequently in the infant's home environment. Overhead lighting is not a major issue because, most of the time, most infants do not face directly upward. However, side-, directional- or track-lighting fixtures have advantages in terms of regulating lighting conditions. It is noteworthy that, in a survey by Sheridan (1983), 47% of newborn intensive care facilities attempted to simulate day/night lighting conditions. However, to the author's knowledge, there are no reports or collaborative investigations of these conditions on the development of premature infants.

Sound

Sound levels need to be normalized and reduced in newborn nurseries. There is no reason for staff and infants to be exposed to intense noise levels characteristic of modern newborn special care facilities. If nothing else, abating noise in special care units would make this environment a less tense place to work. Reduction of sound levels could be accomplished by a number of methods:

1. Washable sound proofing for ceilings and walls (i.e., acoustic tile) and possibly for floors could be installed. Although most units have vinyl floor covering and painted walls, a small number of facilities do have carpeted floors and wallpaper (Sheridan, 1983). Further consideration should be given to sound reduction materials on the perimeter of units.
2. The noise generated from telephones, monitors, and alarm systems could be replaced by light signal systems (see Korones, 1983).
3. Manufacturers of medical equipment and incubators should be encouraged to muffle noise levels in their products. Also, forceful closing of incubator ports should be eliminated. In some informal observations by the author and his associates, such closing of the ports was found to increase sound levels in excess of 100 dB (linear) in the incubator, with rapid increases in the infant's cardiac activity.
4. If feasible, noisy equipment should be moved to a room adjoining the unit. In a recent study by Long et al. (1980a), reduction of noise levels was conducted by removing the capillary tube centrifuge from the nursery and by silencing the systolic beep on cardiac monitors and bells on the telephones. The results showed a reduction in the incidence of hypoxemia and elevated intracranial pressure in premature infants.

In view of these findings and the potential hazards of being continuously exposed to high sound levels, intervention strategies should be aimed at reducing the noise present in the environment of special care units.

Vestibular-Kinesthetic Stimulation

Vestibular-kinesthetic stimulation may prove to be one of the most promising modes of intervention for premature infants. It has been the most widely used form of intervention during the neonatal period. Furthermore, a growing body of interesting studies of premature and term newborn and older infants in hospital- and home-based programs indicates positive effects on a range of outcome measures involving stimulation administered by machines, humans, and (more recently) waterbeds (see Gottfried, 1981; Korner, Commentary 1 in this volume). However, a number of questions need to be answered before determining the most effective intervention program employing these types of stimulation:

1. At what point in development should intervention be applied, and by what means? Both Speidel (1978) and Long et al. (1980b) reported that handling of sick prematures may be associated with hypoxemia. Thus, waterbeds may be helpful.
2. Should vestibular-kinesthetic stimulation be restricted to one method of intervention, or should it include various procedures (e.g., oscillating waterbeds, handling, rocking) at differing points in the course of hospitalization?
3. How much vestibular-kinesthetic stimulation should be applied, at what rate, and at what schedule?
4. In view of the vast individual differences in the amount of contact and handling infants receive in special care units, should vestibular-kinesthetic interventions be tailored to individual infants?
5. Should vestibular-kinesthetic programs take into account the behavioral state of the infant when stimulation is applied?

Because of the number of investigators whose data indicate benefits from vestibular-kinesthetic types of stimulation, more extensive research should focus on this form of intervention.

Social Stimulation

Social stimulation of premature newborns should be increased. The sources of such stimulation should include both staff and family. Such stimulation should serve the dual purpose of enriching the social-sensory experiences of infants and encouraging and establishing early parent/infant interactions. Newborn special care units are intimidating places. The experience of having a sick newborn, plus the hospital environment in which the newborn is cared for, often is emotionally overwhelming for parents. Data indicate that the preponderance of contacts between staff and infants are devoid of social interactions. The impact of this lack of social climate on families is not known. However, it seems reasonable to hypothesize that the low occurrence of social activities with infants by staff may inadvertently convey signals that discourage families from visiting their infants and/or may transmit information that families should be cautious or hesitant in engaging in social support activities with their sick infants. These modeling influences may be differentially effective on families that vary in socioeconomic or educational levels. Families of lower status may be more vulnerable to these influences.

Enhancement of social stimulation should include more of the following activities: 1) verbal stimulation; 2) tactile contact with the infant; 3) soothing responses to infants' distress during contacts; and 4) sensory integrated social experiences. If in fact such activities are difficult to incorporate into the staff's medical or nursing responsibilities, perhaps foster grandparent programs may be helpful to this end. Evidence indicates that parents should be given the opportunity to directly observe their infant and gain knowledge about his or her behavioral and interactional capabilities. Studies by Widmayer and Field (1980) and Worobey and Belsky (1982) demonstrated with preterm and term infants, respectively, that, when mothers participated in Brazelton neurobehavioral assessments of their newborns, the quality of subsequent parent-child interactions was enhanced. These findings are important because longitudinal investigations have shown that the social home environment is an important determinant in the subsequent developmental outcome of prematures (see Beckwith and Cohen, 1984; Siegel, 1984). Hence, intervention should encompass social stimulation as well as a socioeducational component.

Conclusions

The suggestions put forth here are not easy to carry out, may be expensive, and involve considerable administrative decisions. However, they provide a focus for intervention with premature newborns—a direction based on emerging knowledge from environmental studies of newborn special care units.

References

Beckwith, L., and Cohen, S. E. 1984. Home environment and cognitive competence in preterm children in the first 5 years. In: A. W. Gottfried (ed.), Home Environment and Early Cognitive Development: Longitudinal Research, pp. 235–71. Academic Press, New York.

Brans, Y. W. (ed.). 1983. Clinics in Perinatology, Vol. 10. Saunders, Philadelphia.

Brown, J. V., La Rossa, M. M., Aylward, G. P., Davis, D. J., Rutherford, P. K., and Bakeman, R. 1980. Nursery-based intervention with prematurely born babies and their mothers: Are there effects? J. Pediatr. 97:487–491.

Cornell, E. H., and Gottfried, A. W. 1976. Intervention with premature human infants. Child Dev. 47:32–39.

Frayer, W. W. 1983. Neonatal intensive care unit renovation. Clin. Perinatol. 10:153–165.

Gottfried, A. W. 1981. Environmental manipulations in the neonatal period and assessments of their effects. In: V. L. Smeriglio (ed.), Newborns and Parents, pp. 55–61. Lewis Erlbaum, Hillsdale, NJ.

Kellman, N. 1980. Risks in the design of the modern neonatal intensive care unit. Birth Fam. J. 7:243–248.

Korones, S. B. 1983. Evolution of nursery design and function: The Memphis story. Clin. Perinatol. 10:127–140.

Long, J. G., Lucey, J. F., and Philip, A. G. S. 1980a. Noise and hypoxemia in the intensive care nursery. Pediatrics 65:143–145.

Long, J. G., Philip, A. G. S., and Lucey, J. F. 1980b. Excessive handling as a cause of hypoxemia. Pediatrics 65:203–207.

Perlstein, P. H. 1983. Physical environment. In: A. Fanaroft and R. Martin (eds.), Behrman's Neonatal-Perinatal Medicine, pp. 259–277. Mosby, St. Louis.

Sheridan, J. F. 1983. The typical perinatal center: An overview of perinatal health services in the United States. Clin. Perinatol. 10:153–165.

Siegel, L. S. 1984. Home environmental influences on cognitive development in preterm and full-term children in the first 5 years. In: A. W. Gottfried (ed.), Home Environment and Early Cognitive Development: Longitudinal Research, pp. 197–233. Academic Press, New York.

Speidel, B. D. 1978. Adverse effects of routine procedures on preterm infants. Lancet 1:864–865.

Widmayer, S. M., and Field, T. M. 1980. Effects of Brazelton demonstrations on early interactions of preterm infants and their teenage mothers. Infant Behav. Dev. 3:79–89.

Worobey, J., and Belsky, J. 1982. Employing the Brazelton scale to influence mothering: An experimental comparison of three strategies. Dev. Psychol. 18:736–743.

Wurtman, R. J., and Weisel, J. 1969. Environmental lighting and neuroendocrine function: Relationship between spectrum of light source and gonadal growth. Endocrinology 85:1218–1221.

Zigler, E., and Berman, W. 1983. Discerning the future of early childhood intervention. Am. Psychol. 38:894–906.

13

Ethical Considerations in the Intensive Care Nursery

Gordon B. Avery

The Current Public Debate

The rapidly advancing technology of newborn intensive care has allowed smaller and sicker premature infants to survive and major birth defects to be corrected or ameliorated surgically. Yet, with this new power to heal has come a set of ethical questions that have been vigorously debated, first in medical centers and, more recently, in the media and courts. Should inevitable death be prolonged by technically possible but ultimately futile, life-support systems? In cases of near hopeless prognosis, is highly invasive care justified if survival is unlikely and only an extremely damaged survivor is possible? Is natural selection being reversed, leaving terribly handicapped children to be cared for by parents with meager personal resources? Are these policies justified in an era where cost-containment has caused the government to reduce Medicaid benefits, cut crippled children's funds, and curtail public resources available to distressed families with enormous medical bills? To what extent is neonatal intensive care itself cost effective?

A recent article reduced the bottom line to dollars and cents. Boyle et al. (1983) compared the cost of care per salvaged infant with an estimated economic value of that individual over his or her lifetime. The potential earning power of the survivor is adjusted for handicap in an appropriate proportion, and a cost per salvaged life-year is computed. There is a mathematical allowance for the possibility of a life worse than death. The authors allow a factor of -0.3 for infants totally without economic productivity but with such intense suffering that their parents feel that their care has produced a negative social value. The conclusion of the authors is that neonatal intensive care is cost effective in prematures of 1000 to 1500 grams birth weight but not in those 500 to 1000 grams at birth.

At the opposite end of the spectrum are the arguments of some "right-to-life" lobby groups. Their assertion is that life is sacred and meaningful under all circumstances, and they actively seek to prevent withholding life-saving and life-support techniques regardless of prognosis, the parents' wish, or the recommendations of the health care team.

Recently, there has been pressure for federal intervention to prevent arbitrary withholding of medical care from newborns. An example of this is the so-called Baby Doe rule, promulgated by the Secretary of Health and Human Services (March 22, 1983) as an administrative ruling (Federal Register, 1983). It applies a law guaranteeing handicapped individuals access to rehabilitative services to the special case of handicapped newborns. In order to protect the civil rights of these babies, it was declared a violation of federal law to withhold food or customary medical care to an infant on the basis of a handicapping condition. The institution was made responsible for the actions of its staff, and the penalty was withdrawal of all federal support. Because the Secretary suspected that violations of this ruling would not be reported in a timely manner, a toll-free hotline was set up so that anonymous informants could report suspected violations, and an immediate federal investigation would follow to determine if the institution was guilty of a violation. It was not clear what standards would be applied to define "customary medical care" or what type of investigation would be conducted to determine compliance. The rule was only in force 2 weeks before being struck down by Judge Gerhard Gesell as being promulgated without adequate consultation and consideration of its disruptive consequences, too vague, and a questionable application of the intent of the civil rights law on which it was based. During this interval, there were 400 calls on the hotline without any instance of a violation being uncovered (Culliton, 1983). The Department of Health and Human Services has since released a revision of the rule, clarifying the infants to whom it applies, and suggesting local institutional review boards to help formulate guidelines and review appropriate cases.

Curiously enough, the President's Commission for the Study of Ethical Problems in Medicine and Biomedical and Behavioral Research made its official report the day after the Baby Doe rule became effective (President's Commission Report, 1983). This commission, composed of experts in medicine, ethics, law, theology, and public affairs, spent 2 years studying a broad range of issues in medical ethics. The report covered some of the same concerns implicit in the Department of Health and Human Services rule, but reached rather different conclusions. The Commission acknowledged that there were complex decisions regarding what advanced medical care is appropriate for which babies in the face of grave prognosis and often multisystem disease. The family and medical team were judged to be most competent to make these decisions within the limits of law and usual medical practice. The Commission recognized that there were conditions that, although handicapping, do not in themselves constitute grounds for withholding even drastic medical intervention; a prominent example in this category is Down's syndrome. On the other hand, the Commission acknowledged that so many situations exist in the intensive care of newborns that any attempt at detailed codification of expected medical care would be doomed to produce arbitrary oversimplification. It suggested the creation of institutional review boards to oversee and guarantee the integrity of decisions in this area. Similar institutional review boards have worked well in representing the rights of human subjects in medical research.

Within intensive care nurseries (ICNs) around the country, health care teams and involved families continue to work out, on a case-by-case basis, the appropriate care for individual critically ill newborns. Considerations in making these decisions are discussed elsewhere (Avery, 1981), and are not recapitulated here.

The Potential for Violence in the ICN

Despite its benign purpose, an ICN can unwittingly be severely hurtful to infants and their parents. Other chapters in this book deal with details of the ICN environment and its impact on the sick newborn patient. A few of the necessarily painful aspects of newborn intensive care are mentioned here by way of example.

The ICN deprives the baby and family of the opportunity for privacy and the feeling of intactness as a family. The child is denied substantial intervals of undisturbed rest. Many of the human interactions first experienced by the infant involve painful stimuli. Gratifications normally experienced by a healthy newborn, such as holding, gentle handling, nursing, and being talked or sung to, are sharply curtailed. The lighting is continuous and too bright for the comfort of the baby, who is often supine and looking up at brilliant fluorescent lights while his or her caretakers look down with the light behind them. Medical devices, such as intravenous fluid lines or chest tubes, may mandate long periods of physical restraint. Instead of a single set of parents in constant attendance, caretakers rotate from among a large team, potentially depersonalizing the feeling and texture of handling. Parents are not kept abreast of many of the details concerning their baby's care and must come to the medical team to receive news about *their* child. Parents must simultaneously mourn the loss of their expected normal child, balance fear and hope with respect to the strange and tiny infant seemingly overwhelmed with medical devices, deal with prolonged uncertainty about survival and the possibility of grave brain damage, and transmit an attitude of cheerfulness and "appropriate" concern in the relatively public environment in which they must visit their baby.

In ethical terms, these treatment regimens represent assaults on the person and the dignity of the infant and are only justified if directed at a beneficial result, such as a reasonable chance for meaningful survival.

The Gentle ICN

In the meantime, while science improves outcome and prognosis and society and medical institutions clarify decision making regarding "heroic" intensive care of the newborn, we must respond to yet another ethical imperative—the requirement to care for newborns with gentleness and love. Precisely because they are small and helpless, newborn babies above all others call on our basic humanity for support and nurture. Many of the elements of care are the same in the gentle nursery as in any "high-tech" ICN, but the attitude behind each detail of care colors its impact on baby and family and may lastingly affect the outcome for both. This is especially true in the battlefield setting of newborn intensive care, where many survive but others die—where some continue chronically ill and not a few are discharged with lasting handicaps.

Gentle care requires that, no matter how complex the medical situation, how desperate the circumstances, or how harried the staff, the baby and his or her parents remain the center of awareness and concern of all. The baby deserves to be called by name, to be assigned the proper sex, and to be accorded human dignity. The possibility that even a premature infant is experiencing pain should be considered, and at times appropriate sedation should be given. Even small measures aimed at comfort must be seized as opportunities to make up for the inevitable discomforts of intensive care. Although bedside rounds may require attention to a series of problems, system by system, the whole baby should be remembered at the beginning and end of this exercise and perhaps touched or spoken to as an affirmation of his or her personhood.

Interventions should be clustered so that times are allowed for undisturbed rest. Parents should be allowed to take on small aspects of care in even the sickest baby. The terrifying physical aspect of the ICN, which looks more like a space station than a nursery, can be modified by pictures, mobiles, and even teddy bears, which are more likely to bring comfort than infection. Parents must be greeted warmly and made to feel welcome, with the realization that they are forced to be with their baby under bizarre circumstances in what rightfully should be their home. A dying baby should never be left alone. If the parents are unable to be there, the child should be held and perhaps spoken to as the parents would like to have done. Parents who can be with their dying baby should be given a sensitive mixture of companionship and privacy, and their wishes should be paramount once medical care has clearly failed. After-care ought to include an offer of help with funeral arrangements and a plan for follow-up visits for further support and reinterpretation of the baby's illness.

The moral obligation for gentle care brings with it the opportunity for healing staff as well as patients. The privilege of being with families in their time of crisis can allow an affirmation of life even in the presence of death. The joy of seeing a tiny premature go home can only be fully appreciated by those who have shared the vigil with the mother and father. Whatever the resolution of the scientific and societal issues around neonatal intensive care, the requirement that the ICN strive to be gentle, nurturing, and compassionate seems certain to remain.

References

Avery, G. B. 1981. The morality of drastic intervention. In: G. B. Avery (ed.), Neonatology, p. 13. Lippincott, Philadelphia.

Boyle, M. H., Torrance G. W., Sinclair J. C., and Horwood, S. P. 1983. Economic evaluation of neonatal intensive care of very-low-birth-weight infants. N. Engl. J. Med. 308:1330.

Culliton, B. J. 1983. "Baby Doe" regs thrown out by court. Science 220:479.

Federal Register. 1983. Nondiscrimination on the basis of handicap. Interim Final Rule. 48:9630.

President's Commission Report. 1983. The Study of Ethical Problems in Medicine and Biomedical and Behavioral Research. March 21, Washington, DC.

Appendix

Commentary 1

Anneliese F. Korner

The following are reflections on chapters in this volume by Gottfried, Gaiter, Avery, Linn et al., High and Gorski, Blackburn and Barnard, and Lawson and Turkewitz. There are many interesting and converging themes in these chapters. In their communality of findings, the studies described validate each other very nicely over a variety of settings. From these chapters it is clear that great progress has been made in our understanding of the physical and social environment of neonatal intensive care units (NICUs), and that all this happened in a very short time. Historically, it is interesting that, even though we became aware of the potential noise hazards in the NICU in the late 1960s and early 1970s (e.g., League et al., 1972; Seleny and Streczyn, 1969), the first systematic and broader exploration of the NICU environment was published as recently as 1977 by Lawson et al. (1977). Since then, investigations into the physical and social environment of preterm infants have flourished, coming to a peak in 1981, when many of the contributors to this volume presented their research at a Society for Research in Child Development Symposium.

One common theme in several of the chapters is the finding and concern over preterm infant exposure to continuous and high levels of illumination and noise. Although these are established facts by now, not much is known about how the preterm infant processes this massive stimulation. However, it is known from studies of adults that overstimu-

---

Preparation of Commentary 1 was supported by Grant MH 36884 of the Department of Health and Human Services, National Institute of Mental Health, Prevention Research Branch.

lation can have a disruptive and disorganizing effect on the physiologic and psychological functioning of the organism (e.g., Frankenhaeuser and Johansson, 1974). At the very least, then, the adults working in the NICU are affected by these conditions and, very likely, so are the small patients.

Engineers of intensive care nurseries (ICNs) certainly could do a great deal to modify the nursery environment. It should not be insurmountable to build incubators generating much lower noise levels than are currently available. Perhaps a clever engineer will someday build a one-way vision incubator for use with very small preterm infants. These infants would not have been exposed to light at all had they not been born prematurely. A one-way vision incubator would shield these infants from the bright lights and, at the same time, make them clearly visible to the attending personnel. Meanwhile, much can be done to at least attenuate the illumination levels. For example, in one of the nurseries housing growing preterm infants observed by Lawson and Turkewitz (this volume), lights were dimmed during the night. At the Stanford University Medical Center's nurseries, bright lights are routinely kept out of the infants' eyes by placing blankets over the top end of the isolette.

Another recurring theme reflected in these chapters is that the nursing care provided in the nurseries is not sufficiently contingent on the infants' state and behavioral signals, particularly of distress. In a prior paper, Gorski (1983) described how easily preterm infants become overwhelmed and show physiologic and behavioral signs of distress in response to multiple medical ministrations administered in rapid succession. He advised that medical ministrations be staggered to give the infant a chance to recover between procedures. Such changes will, of course, complicate the routine of the nurses and other medical personnel, but the results may well be worth the inconvenience. Along similar lines, it may be fruitful to determine whether some of the traditional routine nursing procedures given every 2 or 3 hours could be reduced in frequency without jeopardizing the infant's care. This certainly should be possible in the case of the older and healthier babies. Controlled studies are obviously needed in this area.

Except for the time prior to discharge from the hospital, feeding schedules in most nurseries are not contingent on the infants' state of hunger or satiation. Both Brazelton and Barnard observed that, when awakened from a deep sleep, preterm infants do not feed as well as when they are closer to wakefulness. Brazelton (1979, personal communication) suggested that older, stable preterm infants should be fed not so much by the clock but somewhat on demand, as indicated by an increase in the infant's activity. When the busy nurses objected that they could not watch the state of the baby that closely, Brazelton suggested that they attach a bell to one of the infant's limbs that would "ring for service" as the infants became more active. This suggestion is not as radical as it would seem at first. As far back as 1952, a study conducted by Horton et al. showed that most of the 20 vigorous, healthy preterm infants ranging in weights between 1.55 and 2.21 kilograms gained adequate weight on a self-demand feeding schedule.

Blackburn and Barnard, in Chapter 6, raise the question of whether caregiving in the ICN should incorporate the concept of state modulation. Gaiter, in Chapter 4, observes that there are few nursery activities that lower the infant's state of arousal. On the basis of our experience with intervention, it is our belief that the issue of state modulation of the infants is a very important one. In a sequence of three studies, we repeatedly found that waterbeds that gently oscillated in the temporal pattern of a maternal biologic rhythm are soothing to preterm infants and are conducive to modulating their motility (Edelman et al., 1982; Korner et al., 1982, 1983). In the two sleep studies, quiet sleep was maintained significantly longer and irritability was reduced in one and waking activity in the other study while the infants were on the waterbed. In the sleep study that involved infants receiving theophylline (a widely used stimulant drug that frequently causes sharp reductions in sleep and motor agitation), the duration of quiet sleep was significantly increased, as was active sleep to a lesser extent. State changes, restlessness during sleep, latencies to falling asleep, and jittery and unsmooth movements all were significantly reduced while the infants were on the waterbed. In a longitudinal pilot study of a small sample of very young, sick preterm infants who were raised from the fourth day of life on waterbeds, the infants in the experimental group performed significantly better in attending and pursuing animate and inanimate visual and auditory stimuli, demonstrated better modulated spontaneous activity, showed significantly fewer signs of irritability and/or hypertonicity, and were more than twice as often in the visually alert, inactive state as the control group. The infants were examined when they were between 34 and 35 weeks conceptional age by a neurologist who was unaware of the group status of the subjects. Although the results of this last study are preliminary, the combined results of the three studies dovetail so well that it is safe to say that waterbeds that oscillate gently in the temporal pattern of maternal biologic rhythms soothe preterm infants in that they increase quiet sleep and reduce irritability and unmodulated activity.

Another recurrent theme in several chapters of this text is that NICU preterm infants get neither enough nor the appropriate social and sensory stimulation from their caregivers. For example, High and Gorski describe in Chapter 7 how briefly the nurses interact with the infants in general and how sick infants receive more attention than healthy ones. The latter was also shown by Gottfried in Chapter 3. Gottfried also stressed that much of the social approach to preterm infants lacked sensory integration between tactile, visual, and auditory stimulation. Linn et al. (Chapter 5 in this volume) found that when the nursery census dropped, nurses did not spend more time in social interaction with the infants than when they were busier coping with a larger census. These observations could be explained in part by differences in the interest patterns of the nurses. In my experience, there are some nurses who derive most of their satisfaction from saving lives and enjoy the challenge of intensive care therapy, whereas others are more fulfilled by helping older, healthier infants and their families with social and psychological support. Frequently, nurses interested in intensive care are bored with discharge planning tasks and, conversely, nurses who feel committed to the psychological and social care of infants and families may be stressed in caring for the acutely sick. The obvious solution to this problem is to carefully select the nurses for each type of nursery task on the basis of their interests and commitments.

Social and sensory stimulation of preterm infants obviously should be age and stage related. Much is yet to be learned in this domain. Controversy still exists as to whether or not stimulation of preterm infants should be compensatory in nature, i.e., should make up for an experiential deficit of the types of patterned stimulation highly prevalent in utero. Investigators who adhere to this view have primarily used vestibular-proprioceptive stimulation in their interventions. Other investigators have used visual, auditory, and highly social forms of stimulation to which preterm infants *begin* to respond. Without solid research evidence as to which type of stimulation is most relevant at what age, it may make sense to provide compensatory types of stimulation to small preterm infants and to expose infants closer to term to more complex social stimulation. This does not imply, however, that older preterm infants should be treated like term infants. It is hoped that from the studies in this volume, which compared the level and kinds of stimulation received by preterm and term infants, the inference will not be drawn that preterm infants are deprived and should be treated more like term infants. In my view, such comparisons are purely of intrinsic interest. We know from a growing literature that most preterm infants do not respond like term infants, even at the expected date of their birth. Papers such as those by Brown and Bakeman (1980), DiVitto and Goldberg (1979), and Field (1979) make it clear that preterm infants tend to become overwhelmed, unresponsive, and/or disorganized when treated like term infants. The unfortunate result is that parents experience them as very unrewarding.

The issue at hand really is that stimulation requirements vary with the age, medical condition, and individual physiologic and behavioral make-up of the infant. This is why approaches to infant stimulation deemed invariably appropriate for different conceptional ages may be very much misguided. Although research studies are usually designed to find a main effect of a standard form of stimulation, the approach in clinical practice stimulation and readiness to respond. A very good example of such a sensitive approach is described in VandenBerg's (1982) recent chapter on "Humanizing the Intensive Care Nursery."

In conclusion, the research studies presented in this volume reflect an enormous advance in understanding the nursery environment. Many of the chapters point to a number of changes that could be made to improve this environment. To sell these changes on the basis that they may improve the long-range developmental outcome of preterm infants may not be the best strategy, and this should not be the main criterion for making them. Long-range effects of any intervention are difficult to measure, particularly when the effects of prematurity and differing familial circumstances in which the nursery graduates are raised confound the picture. More contingent caregiving, for example, may not be measurable in differences of later developmental quotients or school achievement, but may produce subtle changes, such that infants gradually learn that the environment is predictable and that their state and behavior have some effect on the environment. However, such considerations should not be the only reason for modifying the nursery environment. If these changes give greater comfort to infants, their parents, and the nursery personnel *while* the infants are in the nursery, they are well worth making.

References

Brown, J. V., and Bakeman, R. 1980. Relationships of human mothers with their infants during the first year of life; effects of prematurity. In: R. W. Bell and W. P. Smotherman (eds.), Maternal Influences and Early Behavior. SP Medical and Scientific Books, New York.

DiVitto, B., and Goldberg, S. 1979. The effects of newborn medical status on early parent-infant interaction. In: T. Field, A. Sostek, S. Goldberg, and H. H. Shuman (eds.), Infants Born at Risk. SP Medical and Scientific Books, New York.

Edelman, A. M., Kraemer, H. C., and Korner, A. F. 1982. Effects of compensatory movement stimulation on the sleep-wake behaviors of preterm infants. J. Am. Acad. Child Psychiatry 21(6):555–559.

Field, T. M. 1979. Interaction patterns of preterm and term infants. In: T. Field, A. Sostek, S. Goldberg, and H. H. Shuman (eds.), Infants Born at Risk. SP Medical and Scientific Books, New York.

Frankenhaeuser, M., and Johansson, G. 1974. On the psychophysiological consequences of understimulation and overstimulation. Reports from the Psychological Laboratories of the University of Stockholm, Supplement 25.

Gorski, P. A. 1983. Premature infant behavioral and physiological responses to caregiving interventions in the intensive care nursery. In: J. D. Call, E. Galenson, and R. L. Tyson (eds.), Frontiers of Infant Psychiatry. Basic Books, New York.

Horton, F. H., Lubchenco, L. O., and Gordon, H. H. 1952. Self-regulatory feeding in a premature nursery. Yale J. Biol. Med. 24:263–272.

Korner, A. F., Ruppel, E. M., and Rho, J. M. 1982. Effects of water beds on the sleep and motility of theophylline-treated preterm infants. Pediatrics 70:864–869.

Korner, A. F., Forrest, T., and Schneider, P. 1983. Effects of vestibular-proprioceptive stimulation on the neurobehavioral development of preterm infants: A pilot study. Neuropediatrics 14:170–175.

Lawson, K., Daum, C., and Turkewitz, G. 1977. Environmental characteristics of a neonatal intensive care unit. Child Dev. 48:1633–1639.

League, R., Parker, J., Robertson, M., Valentine, V., and Powell, J. 1972. Acoustical environments in incubators and infant oxygen tents. Prev. Med. 1:231–239.

Seleny, F. L., and Streczyn, M. 1969. Noise characteristics in the baby compartment of incubators. Am. J. Disabled Child. 117:445–450.

VandenBerg, K. A. 1982. Humanizing the intensive care nursery. In: A. Waldstein (ed.), Issues in Neonatal Care. Westar, Special Education Programs, United States Department of Education.

Appendix
Commentary 2
John H. Kennell and Marshall H. Klaus

The authors and editors of this book have taken on the difficult task of attempting to work out what to prescribe for the environment of the small, sick premature infant. What should be the light, sound, and movement as well as the human contact for such infants? In large part, this is now medically determined. Most important, what set of standards should we use as guideposts?

1. Should the end point be the largest weight gain in the infant?
2. Is the baby quiet or active?
3. What is the milk intake?
4. What is the number of stools?

Between 1933 and 1958, the incubators of most infants were set at a temperature that resulted in a decrease in the incidence of diarrhea and an increase in weight gain. Between 1926 and 1933 Blackfan and Yaglou (1933), working with a group of fully clothed infants weighing between 1300 and 2200 grams, observed that high relative humidity and an air temperature of 25°C were required to maintain an equilibrium of body temperature. When a comparable group of infants was placed in slightly warmer thermal environments with a lower relative humidity (both variables changed) wider fluctuations in temperature, an increase in the incidence of diarrhea, a decrease in weight gain, and an increase in mortality were noted. Because of this study, for 25 years, incubators in the United States were flooded with humid air without an understanding of the relationship of temperature and humidity.

It was the patient work of Silverman and colleagues (Silverman and Agate, 1964; Silverman and Blanc, 1957; Silverman et al., 1958, 1963) and the physiologic observations of Burnard and Cross (1958), Hill (1959; Hill and Rahimtulla, 1965) and others that finally unraveled the complex mystery of humidity and temperature control. The results of their careful studies elucidated the significance of neutral thermal environmental temperature and positively affected infant survival rates and probably the quality of survival. Several conclusions might be drawn from this work. Once physiologic processes were understood, the clinical applications became obvious. From an understanding of the physiology, the caretakers were no longer simply attentive to the temperature of the infant but realized the advantage of placing the infant in an environment in which he or she had minimal oxygen consumption and the least activity. Thus, as a biologic understanding of the process emerged, the clinical recommendations appropriately followed.

Problems of the physical environment of the preterm infant can be approached in somewhat the same fashion as temperature control. Environmental variables may be far more difficult to investigate in detail because many controlling set-points may not be so easily fathomed. The infant's brain is developing; thus, it will be necessary to follow patients for long periods of time to determine the positive and negative effects of an environmental alteration. The following suggestions should be noted:

1. The end points, in general, should not only be the immediate effects but should also include long-term observations and evaluations of the well-being of the growing infant.
2. Because the effects of interactions between two individuals, the mother and the infant, are in focus, it is very easy to forget the other partner in the dyad. It will be necessary to investigate the effects on the mother and her needs during this early experience because some interventions may interfere with her taking on the care of the infant. In the human species, the mother is typically the caretaker responsible for the baby's survival and the mediator for his or her development.
3. New methods and procedures for assessing the needs of the infant must be explored. Just as investigators have successfully asked newborns to choose their mother's face or voice from those of other mothers, the infant might be able to choose the most favorable auditory input by changing the pattern of sucking bursts on a nipple attached to a source of sounds with varying qualities and intensities. Is it possible that infants at a postconceptional age of 36 to 40 weeks could somehow indicate their preferred sound environment? One way to check this approach would be to see if the infant can choose the neutral thermal temperature of his or her isolette by sucking on a nipple, thereby raising or lowering the incubator temperature, which could be recorded precisely.
4. Instead of looking for "quick and dirty solutions," an attempt must be made to evaluate what might be going on overall, both positive and negative, and to consider the effect on other aspects of the infant's neurosensory system. In this regard, the work of Field (1977) and others should be kept in mind. They have shown that at 2 to 3 months

imitation of an infant rather than stimulation is much more effective at gaining the baby's attention. Should we try to get the infant's attention? How much stimulation and how much imitation should be used?

5. There is a tendency on the part of most researchers to adultomorphize the infant and thus be unable to perceive and appreciate his or her needs. This is in contrast to the ability of most mothers to identify and sense their infants' requirements. Thus, methodology should be open to experimental approaches in which the mother and infant try procedures to help themselves adapt to the situation in the nursery.
6. There should be constant alertness for the problem of overutilization of NICUs for a number of complex medical, social, and economic reasons (Whitby et al., 1982). Many infants never required this special type of hospital care, and these separated infants and mothers should have been kept together. Because most premature babies are greater than 4 pounds and only a small number (less than 1%) have a weight below 1000 grams (2.2 pounds), the focus should be on this large group of more mature premature infants who may inadvertently be separated and exposed to conditions that could, over a period of time, be detrimental to their developmental needs.

From past history in this century, the environmental care of preterm infants has been a treacherous matter. Clinicians and researchers should be cautious, requiring replication of every study before making definitive statements and clinical recommendations.

The environment not only contains oxygen, sound, light, and the infant, but also physicians, nurses, and parents. In the past, many changes in the environment were made without evaluating these multiple effects. Parents are so significant for the ongoing and future care of infants that it is necessary to study the effects of the nursery environment on parents. It has been less than 2 decades since discussions began about allowing parents into the premature nursery to touch and hold their infants, a move stimulated by studies at Stanford University (Barnett et al., 1970) and Case Western Reserve University in Cleveland (Klaus and Kennell, 1970).

Nurseries throughout the United States have made changes in their policies and have instituted a number of procedures especially for parents. These interventions may help parents become acquainted with and attached to their premature infants. Such care for parents may ultimately improve infant outcome, and provide promising new directions for research. The following are some improvements in parental care and support that may have benefits for infants:

1. *Maternal transport*—There has now been considerable experience

transporting the mother from the outlying hospital to be near the infant in the NICU. Does this make a difference? If so, can this be made available to all mothers?
2. *Maternal day care and rooming in*—Maternal day care for premature infants allows a mother to participate in caretaking, which may help her to develop an attachment to the infant as well as to directly benefit the baby. There needs to be more systematic investigation of the benefits and the problems of the mother rooming in and providing care for her premature infant. When Tafari (Tafari and Sterky, 1974) in Ethiopia required mothers to live in, care for, and breastfeed their premature infants, it was possible to care for 3 times as many infants, the number of surviving infants increased 500%, and the cost of care dropped significantly. There were similar results when poor mothers in Baraqwanath, South Africa were required to live in the premature nursery and breastfeed their premature infants (Kahn et al., 1954). Can there be similar advantages to involving parents more extensively in the care of their infants in industrialized nations? The nursery of Donald Garrow at High Wycombe in England provides a room for each mother to live in adjacent to her premature infant's cubicle. This offers one possible model for future research consideration.
3. *Nesting*—We have seen improved confidence and competence of mothers who lived in and provided total care for their premature infants for 3 days prior to discharge (Kennell et al., 1973, 1975). However, in a structured randomized study conducted 1 month after discharge, no differences between mothers who participated in the "nesting" intervention and control mothers were found.
4. *Transporting infant to mother*—The authors' experience transporting healthy premature infants from the NICU to spend an hour in the mother's bed in the maternity unit of the same hospital the first 3 days has been limited (Klaus and Kennell, 1982). This procedure for maintaining contact between mother and baby merits further careful study.
5. *Home-based intervention*—The disproportionate number of developmental problems and neurosensory disturbances in the infants who are discharged to low socioeconomic level homes provides a compelling challenge for future research. Based on the research of Larson (1980), would community programs that provide home-based interventions and support for parents of low socioeconomic status, when started as early as possible, lead to more favorable outcomes for infants?
6. *Postdischarge review with parents*—Discussions with parents to review their experiences in the hospital approximately 1 month after

their preterm infant was discharged seem to be helpful. Parents often have a distorted view of the condition of the baby and of what went on during the period of intensive care (Klaus and Kennell, 1982). Does this have any long-term effects on infant development?

7. *Value of support*—The studies by investigators such as Minde and his colleagues (Minde et al., 1978, 1980a, 1980b) have demonstrated that when mothers of prematures met in discussion-support groups their interest and interaction with their infant improved. This intervention appears to be promising.

8. *Grandparents and other family support*—In the next 10 years, should there be a much stronger effort to bring grandparents and other supportive family members into the NICUs to help anxious, depleted, and bewildered parents through the long trying period of hospitalization? Study of the benefits and hazards should be undertaken.

The last 20 years have been a prelude to exciting opportunities in the challenge to improve the environment for premature infants and their families through the types of research reported in this book.

During the last decade, while behavioral studies of premature infants and their parents were being conducted, there was a major shift in the population in the premature nursery and dramatic changes in the NICU environment attributable to progress in medical management. In the last 10 years, there has been a striking increase in the amount of caretaker time and effort devoted to very low birth weight infants, particularly those weighing less than 1000 grams. Two decades ago, it was rare for any of these infants to survive, but in the 1980s, 50% or more are surviving in NICUs (Hack et al., 1979, 1982). These infants not only require a disproportionate amount of time and effort from the nurses, physicians, and other caretakers, but also require the extensive use of increasingly complex technologic devices that may be frightening to parents. In addition, these infants do not look like babies the parents expected, and most develop some life-threatening problems. In view of these recent changes, it is necessary to take a fresh look at what parents of very sick and very low birth weight babies can tolerate and to reappraise what can be done to lessen the stress and support them through the difficult period of NICU care. With the extensive use of mechanical ventilation, intravenous hyperalimentation, repeated concerns about patent ductus arteriosis, heart failure, septicemia, and necrotizing enterocolitis, one must be concerned about how much parents can tolerate, and how much should be expected of them.

The changes in the patient population and the characteristics of the ICN require a new generation of studies that will be more difficult and require more interdisciplinary teamwork between neonatologists and behavioral scientists. As a result of the heavy pressure for admission of sick preterm infants to the Level III ICN, babies have been discharged earlier and at lower and lower weights. Some infants seem quite fragile at the time of discharge. Is there a correlation between vigor, responsiveness, and physiologic maturity of the infant at discharge and the type of neurosensory abnormalities and school adjustment problems reported by Klein et al. (1983)? It is clear from recent studies that, although the graduates of the ICN seem to score well on some developmental tests, these same infants may have neurosensory difficulties, i.e., problems of visual motor integration, spatial relations, and speech and language, and passive, withdrawn behavior that may have adverse effects on school performance (Klein et al., 1983). Thus, using one measure, the results would be acclaimed; using another measure, the verdict would be different. How many of these problems are attributable in part to the effects of the NICU environment on the parents rather than on the infant? How long do these effects persist? Can they be modified? How?

References

Barnett, C. R., Leiderman, P. H., Grobstein, R., and Klaus, M. H. 1970. Neonatal separation: The maternal side of interactional deprivation. Pediatrics 45:197–205.

Blackfan, K., and Yaglou, C. 1933. The premature infant: A study of the effects of atmospheric conditions on growth and development. Am. J. Dis. Child 46:1175.

Burnard, E., and Cross, K. 1958. Rectal temperature in the newborn after birth asphyxia. Br. Med. J. 2:1197.

Field, T. M. 1977. Effects of early separation, interactive deficits and experimental manipulations on infant-mother face-to-face interaction. Child Dev. 48:763–771.

Hack, M., Fanaroff, A. A., and Merkatz, I. R. 1979. The low-birth-weight infant—evolution of a changing outlook. N. Engl. J. Med. 301:1162–1166.

Hack, M., Merkatz, I. R., Gordon, D., Jones, P. K., and Fanaroff, A. A. 1982. The prognostic significance of postnatal growth in very low-birth-weight infants. Am. J. Obstet. Gynecol. 143:693–699.

Hill, J. 1959. The oxygen consumption of newborn and adult mammals: Its dependence on the oxygen tension in the inspired air and on environmental temperature. J. Physiol. 149:346.

Hill, J., and Rahimtulla, K. 1965. Heat balance and the metabolic rate of newborn babies in relation to environmental temperature; and the effect of age and of weight on basal metabolic rate. J. Physiol. 180:239.

Kahn, E., Wayburne, S., and Fouche, M. 1954. The Baragwanath premature baby unit—an analysis of the case records of 1000 consecutive admissions. S. Afr. Med. J. 28:453–456.

Kennell, J. H., Chesler, D., Wolfe, H., and Klaus, M. H. 1973. Nesting in the human mother after mother-infant separation. Pediatr. Res. 7:269.

Kennell, J. H., Klaus, M. H., and Wolfe, H. 1975. Nesting behavior in the human mother after prolonged mother-infant separation. In: P. Swyer and J. Statson, (eds.), Current Concepts of Neonatal Intensive Care. Warren H. Green, St. Louis.

Klaus, M. H., and Kennell, J. H. 1970. Mothers separated from their newborn infants. Pediatr. Clin. North Am. 17:1015–1037.

Klaus, M. H., and Kennell, J. H. 1982. Parent-Infant Bonding. Mosby, St. Louis.

Klein, N., Hack, M., Gallagher, J., and Fanaroff, A. 1983. School performance of normal intelligence very low birthweight children. Pediatr. Res. 17:98A.

Larson, C. 1980. Efficacy of prenatal and postpartum home visits on child health and development. Pediatrics 66:191–197.

Minde, K., Trehub, S., Corter, C., Boukydis, C., Celhoffer, L., and Marton, P. 1978. Mother-child relationships in the premature nursery: An observational study. Pediatrics 61:373–379.

Minde, K., Marton, P., Manning, D., and Hines, B. 1980a. Some determinants of mother-infant interaction in the premature nursery (abstract). J. Am. Acad. Child Psychiatry 19:1–21.

Minde, K., Shosenberg, B., Marton, P., Thompson, J., Ripley, J., and Burns, S. 1980b. Self-help groups in a premature nursery—a controlled evaluation. J. Pediatr. 96:933–940.

Silverman, W., and Agate, F. 1964. Variation in cold resistance among small newborn animals. Biol. Neonate 6:113.

Silverman, W., and Blanc, W. 1957. The effect of humidity on survival of newly born premature infants. Pediatrics 20:477.

Silverman, W., Fertig, J., and Berger, A. 1958. The influence of the thermal environment upon the survival of newly born premature infants. Pediatrics 22:876.

Silverman, W., Agate, F., and Fertig, J. 1963. A sequential trial of the nonthermal effect of atmospheric humidity on survival of newborn infants of low birth weight. Pediatrics 31:719.

Tafari, N., and Sterky, G. 1974. Early discharge of low birth-weight infants in a developing country. Environ. Child Health 20:73–76.

Whitby, C., DeCates, C. R. and Roberton, N. R. C. 1982. Infants weighing 1.8–2.5 kg.: Should they be cared for in neonatal units of postnatal wards? Lancet 1:322–325.

Appendix
Commentary 3
T. Berry Brazelton

This volume is timely and even overdue. It is time to look closely at the environments provided for high-risk infants in light of current knowledge and major advances in neonatal intensive care therapy (see Chapter 1). By improving neonatal technology, not only can survival of infants with increasingly shorter gestations be expected, but many will have intact central nervous systems, eyes, and lungs. No longer are the great majority of such children crippled as a result of specialized care. Retrolental fibroplasia and bronchopulmonary dysplasia are becoming increasingly rare sequelae. The incidence of cerebral palsy and generalized retardation are decreasing as survival rates of extremely immature babies increase, despite complicated and tortuous hospital courses. It is time to look carefully at newborn experiences in nursery environments so that treatment for them will further their future organization toward successful cognitive and affective outcomes.

The neuropsychologic literature has begun to document the phenomenal plasticity of the nervous system to recovery of adequate functioning even after central nervous system (CNS) damage. St. James Roberts (1979) defined five pathways by which an immature nervous system can achieve functional reorganization after cerebral insult:

1. *Vicarious functioning*—A separate or functionally dormant brain area takes over the function of the damaged area, thereby permitting the resumption of normal behavior. This model, described by Munk in 1881, does not require environmental intervention but does demand an immature brain.
2. *Equipotentiality*—Proposed by Lashly in 1983, this model assumes considerable redundancy in the CNS and mass action of the many units rather than specified centers. It allows for takeover by substitution of equipotential centers. The extent of recovery by this process depends on the site and extent of lesions. Luria et al. (1969)

described a similar process of inhibited pathways that are redundant with damaged functions. The redundancy of pathways, coupled with their relative lack of differentiation in an immature central nervous system, makes it more likely that substitution of an intact set of pathways can replace those impaired or damaged. This redundancy becomes an asset in that the undifferentiated pathways have time to define themselves in favor of the new demands of replacement. However, opportunities for an immature nervous system to reorganize or improve its functioning depend on appropriate stimuli from nurturant environments.

3. *Substitution*—Behavioral substitution can achieve the same goals as the function that has been lost. Meyer (1974) reviewed ways that lesioned areas can be compensated for by the substitution of functions from intact areas. An environment that permits regression and allows time for recovery would increase the likelihood of effective substitution.

4. *Regrowth and Supersensitivity of neurons after injury*—Regenerative sprouting of damaged axons involving the original neuron may help compensate for an injury. The idea of supersensitive neurotransmitters that "leak" into the damaged area and activate post-lesion pathways with restoration of normal action is intriguing but still controversial. If the leakage is too great, overcompensation and hypersensitivity with resultant ineffectual functioning can occur. Perhaps such overcompensation occurs in an overwhelming environment. This possibility fits well with the notion that "inappropriate stimulation" is an overload that interferes with recovery.

5. *Diaschisis*—This model rests on the idea that trauma interferes with neural systems by causing general disruption of the CNS (surrounding irritation or hematoma, changes in cerebrospinal fluid and composition, edema, vascular supply changes, and so on). As the disruptive reactions subside, the neural systems of an immature CNS may have a better chance of recuperation and even of invasion and takeover by surrounding plastic systems. In this model, the environment's capacity to provide stimuli that will help the infant organize his or her behavior is critical.

Sameroff and Chandler (1975) suggested a sixth model: a succession of stages in which spurts of progress are followed by a period of regression and reorganization. This "jagged progress" model includes successive spurts and reorganizations not only of the baby's internal function but also of the environment's efforts to achieve "normalcy" or "optimality." It rejects a critical period hypothesis as too rigid and proposes a dynamic theory of reorganization, regression, and re-energizing before each spurt of improvement.

Because the brain of a preterm infant is subjected to the physiologic stress of immaturity and CNS insult, several important questions arise: How long can the organism maintain availability for reorganization? Does a critical period for redundancy exist? After an insult, does the opportunity diminish for functional differentiation? Indeed, does function follow use or experimental opportunities (as suggested by Huebel et al., 1977)? The possibility for failure in the system by providing negative or less-than-optimal experience for immature and disordered organisms may be increasing. Nurseries for high-risk infants are certainly overwhelming in their demands on the newborn's ability to shut out relentless light, noncontingent noises, and many negative interactional experiences (see Chapters 2–5 in this volume).

In studies of the neonate's capacity for regulation after reacting to stimuli from the environment, evidence shows both a capacity for using habitation and a sleep state to shut out overwhelming or repeatedly disturbing stimuli (Brazelton, 1961). The shutting out of stimulation is effective as a form of protection, but is probably an expensive and demanding mechanism for the infant. If it is assumed that a disordered or immature nervous system is vulnerable and needs a shutdown mechanism, the need for sleep and withdrawal by the infant as a refuge from disturbing environmental stimulation can be understood. For example, a preterm infant in an incubator will seem highly reactive when aroused. As the infant is picked up, not only will he or she overreact by throwing his or her shoulders and head back as if to avoid interaction with the examiner, but if the examiner tries to cuddle the infant, the infant will either stiffen or sag. If the examiner tries to engage the infant in eye-to-eye contact, the infant's eyes may avert and move away. If the examiner continues, the infant may try to sleep, shut out the examiner, have a bowel movement, experience rapid respirations, or have acrocyanotic color changes. After a period of reduced stimuli, the baby may recover and begin to take in stimuli from the examiner. There is a physiologic cost in this initial period of shutting out stimulation because the infant uses an inexperienced system.

If it is postulated that disorganized nervous systems can process stimulation at their own pace, it is time to rethink the structure and function of nursery environments. In working with infants who are small for their gestational age, Als et al. (1976) saw that their behavior during the neonatal period was dominated by hypersensitivity to stimuli from the environment. Not only were they likely to shut out stimulation by crying or sleeping, but they were overwhelmed by cues that soothe and stimulate a normal or term infant to respond in an organized, positive manner.

If the threshold for an infant's receptivity is respected, infants who might otherwise be in constantly habituated states of receptivity can be reached. "Sleeping" infants therefore might be seen as defended infants (Brazelton, 1961). Accordingly, if the "need" of a high-risk infant to shut out overwhelming environments is respected, the search for appropriate levels of stimulation should be pursued in order that those infants might have a chance to receive and organize information.

Recent work with Down's syndrome infants has demonstrated that impaired infants can be brought to alert states and then taught amazing accomplishments (Peuschel et al., 1978). In other words, their capacity to organize and their alert states of consciousness become the basis for learning experiences because the nervous system can respond with increasing organization and complexity. If this concept is applied to high-risk preterm infants or to otherwise stressed infants, an attempt could be made to provide organizing environments with sensitive experiences. The goal for any organizing, developing infant might be represented by the forces in Figure A.1.

The recovering central nervous system is the primary force for recovery and future development. Two sources provide the required energy: 1) an internal feedback system; and 2) positive reinforcement from the external environment. Piaget (1953) referred to feedback systems programmed in the small infant as "circular processes." For example, a 5-month-old infant who brings a thumb to his or her mouth or an object into visual space to explore glows with achievement and a sense of having accomplished an act by himself or herself. White (1959) proposed an "inner sense of competence" resulting from a purposeful effort. This sense of competence becomes a source for fueling its repetition, and as the infant becomes more proficient, the awareness of having achieved and learned builds on itself. As a consequence, motivation for learning is facilitated.

To provide for this type of learning experience, environments that nurture the infant's recovery systems must be provided. Thus, noise levels in the ICN need to be closely monitored. Buffers that divert the circularization and magnification of sound might be instituted. Changing levels of illumination so that they reflect a diurnal cycle of day and night would be a major innovation in preterm nurseries. Gorski et al. (1980) recommended a simple maneuver of covering the incubator with a cloth at night. As the crib is covered, the infant's eyes open, his or her face alerts and he or she seems to begin to look around for stimuli. That he or she is less defended and more alert in reduced light seems obvious. For an infant being intensely observed for cyanosis, even milder reduction of illumination in some sort of rhythmic but systematic way might also be effective. Nurseries sensitive to the individual recovery of the infant are using waterbeds (Korner et al., 1975) and mild kinesthetic stimulation programmed to be contingent to the infant's own movement (Barnard, 1973).

Primary nursing (each nurse consistently in charge of his or her own set of infants) provides an opportunity for caregivers to gain an

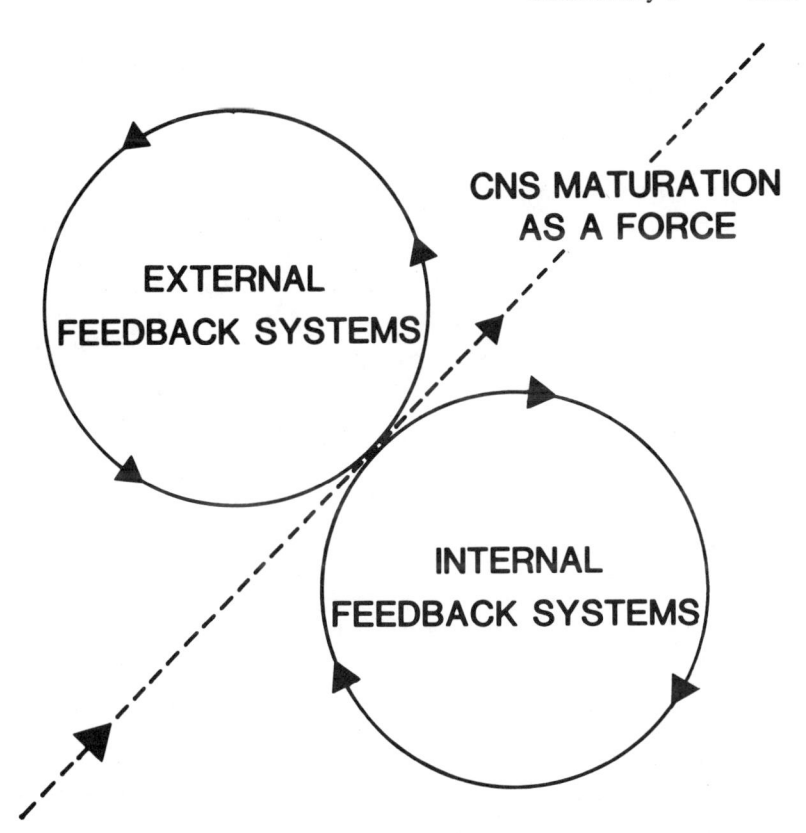

Figure A.1. The goal for any organizing, developing infant.

understanding of each infant's individualized level of responsiveness. Keeping Cardex records of the level of recovery of responsiveness in the motor, autonomic, state, and responsive systems is helpful information to pass on to each nursing shift. This cooperation encourages increased involvement of the nursing and pediatric staff and alerts them to the individuality of each baby. Moreover, nursing supervisors suggest that this involvement reduces "burnout" (see Chapter 10 in this volume) and rapid turnover in staff.

A firm research base will support the conviction that recovery and improved organization (autonomic, state, and behavioral) can be fostered in preterm infants if their environments are changed to be adaptive to their level of organization and functioning. The more alert and responsive infants are more likely to experience sensitive and effective parenting in the home environment.

References

Als, H., Tronick, E., Adamson, L., and Brazelton, T. B. 1976. Behavior of the full-term but underweight newborn infant. Dev. Med. Child Neurol. 18:590–602.

Barnard, K. E. 1973. The effect of stimulation on the sleep behavior of the premature infant. Commun. Nurs. Res. 6:12.

Brazelton, T. B. 1961. Observations of the neonate. J. Acad. Child Psychiatry 1:38.

Gorski, P. A., Davidson, M. F., and Brazelton, T. B. 1980. Stages of behavioral organization in the high risk neonate: Theoretical and clinical considerations. In: P. M. Taylor (ed.), Parent Infant Relationship. Grune and Stratton, New York.

Hubel, D. H., Wiesel, T. N., and Levay, S. 1977. Plasticity of ocular dominance columns in monkey striate cortex. In: H. B. Barlow and R. N. Gaze (eds.), A Discussion on Structure and Functional Aspects of Plasticity in the Nervous System. Philosophical Transactions of the Royal Society, London.

Korner, A., et al. 1975. Effects of waterbed flotation on premature infants. Pediatrics 56:361.

Lashley, K. S. 1983. Factors limiting recovery after central nervous system lesions. J. Nerv. Ment. Dis. 88:733.

Luria, A. R., et al. 1969. Restoration of cortical function following local brain damage. In: P. J. Vinken and C. V. Euyer (eds.), Handbook of Clinical Neurology, Vol. 3. North Holland Press, Amsterdam.

Meyer, P. M. 1974. Recovery of function following lesions of the subcortex and neocortex. In: D. G. Stein, J. J. Rosen, and N. Bulters (eds.), Plasticity and Recovery of Function in the Central Nervous System. Academic Press, New York.

Peuschel, S. M., Canning, C. D., Murphy, A., and Zausmer, E. 1978. Down Syndrome: Growing and Learning. Andrews and McMeel, Fairway, KS.

Piaget, J. 1953, The Origins of Intelligence in the Child. Rutledge, London.

St. James Roberts, I. 1979. Neurological plasticity, recovery from brain insult, and child development. In: H. Reese and L. Lipsitt (eds.), Advances in Child Development, p. 254. Academic Press, New York.

Sameroff, A., and Chandler, M. 1975. Reproductive risk and the continuum of caretaking casualty. In: F. Horowitz, M. Hetherington, S. Scarr-Salapatek, and G. Siegel (eds.), Review of Child Development Research, Vol. 4. University of Chicago Press, Chicago.

White, R. W. 1959. Motivation reconsidered: The concept of competence. Psychol. Rev. 66:297.

Index

Acidosis, 172
Activity, 24-hour pattern, 121–123
Activity level, 58, 132, 133
   caregiver-infant activity relationship, 119–121, 124–125
Administation
   relationship with neonatologists, 244
   support of nursing, 233, 234
Age
   chronological
      vs. postmenstrual age, 138
   estimated gestational, 103–105, 108
      circadian rhythmicity, 158
   at observation, 103–105, 108
   postmenstrual, 134, 138
   specificity, 127
Air flow, 184
Alertness, 58, 148–149
   bright, 136
   lidded, 136
Aminoglycoside antibiotics, 24, 25, 204, 205
Animate background sound, term vs. preterm infant, 100
Apnea, 86
Arm movement, with oral orientation, 125
Arousal, 77, 123, 267
   continued, 126
Autonomic organization, 283–284
Awake state, 148–149
   active, 136
   nonfussing state, 134, 148–149
   relation to age, 139–140

Baby Doe rule, 260
Bacteria, resistant strains, 216–217
Bassinet, 176
Behavioral organization, 56–57, 78, 114, 283–284
   infant-caregiver interaction, 123
   term vs. preterm infant, 99–103
Behavioral responsivity, 132
Bifactor environmental model, 127
Birth weight, 103–105, 108
Body movement, gross, 125
Body temperature, 2–3, 173, 176
   at birth, 175
Brainstem, 137
Brazelton 6-state system, 134
Breastfeeding, 218
Bright alert state, 149
Bronchopulmonary dysplasia, 211, 241, 279
Bunting, 190–191
Burn, 206, 210
Burnout, 108, 109, 232, 233, 234, 283

Caloric intake, 3–4
Cap, 190–191
Caregiver
   burnout, 108, 109, 232, 233, 234, 283
   contingent responsivity to infant, 105–108, 109
   education to research, 88
   effects on infants, 74–75
   emotional stress, 8
   environment of, 25
   infant observation, 152

285

286 Index

Caregiver *(continued)*
  looking, 106–108
  time present, 151
    medical condition effect, 152
  touching, 106–108
  transport nurse specialist, 12
Catecholamine, 173
Categorization, by degree of illness, 103–105, 108
Catheter
  central venous, complications, 211–212
  umbilical vessel, complications, 211–212
Central nervous system, 279–281
  circadian periodicity, 158
  diaschisis, 280
  equipotentiality, 279–280
  hypothermia, 173
  "jagged progress" model, 280
  of preterm infant, 131–132
  regrowth and supersensitivity, 280
  substitution, 280
  vicarious functioning, 279
Cerebral cortex, 137
Cerebral palsy, 279
Child abuse, 5
Chronic lung disorder, 241
Circadian periodicity, 8
  central nervous system, 158
  endocrine system, 158
  establishment of, 158
  gestational age, 158
  neonatal intensive care unit, 157–169
    lighting, 16, 253–254
  rhythmicity of state, 158
Clinical nurse, 232
Clinical nurse specialist, 243
Computer tomography procedure, heat loss in, 193
Computerized continuous observational system, 132–133
Conduction, 173
Conduction heat loss
  dry mattress, 177–178
  water mattress, 178
  wet mattress, 178
Contingency perception, 115
Convection, 173
Convection heat transfer, 180–181
Cooling rate, 175
Cross-modal stimulation, 86
Crying, 58, 73, 115, 137
  caregiver response to, 39, 40, 49
  term vs. preterm infant, 100–102
Custodial intervention, 132, 133

Death, 245–246
  team approach, 245–246
Delivery room, 191–192
  bowel bag, 191–192
  heat loss in, 191
  radiant warmer, 191
Developmental delay, 5
Developmental research, 84
Diapering, 117, 119, 133
  activity prior to, 119–125
Disinfectants, complications of, 217
Diurnal variation, 25–26, 143, 157–159
  handling, 161, 167
  light level, 161, 167, 168
  regularity, 36
  rhythmic, 115
  sound level, 161, 167, 168
Down's syndrome, 282
Drowsy state, 134
Drug therapy, complications, 218–219

Education program, 12–13
Electrical hazards, 210–211
  microshock, 211
Endocrine system, circadian periodicity, 158
Environment
  animate, 114
    defined, 114
  inanimate, 114
    defined, 114

neonatal intensive care unit vs.
    home, 99–103, 108
  study method, 84–85
Environmental intervention, 85, 133,
    251–256, 266
  defined, 251–252
  studies of, 24
Environmental model, bifactor, 127
Environmental periodicity, infant state
    periodicity, 163–166, 167–168
Environmental specificity, 127
Environmental temperature, 176, 184
Esophageal temperature, 174–175
Ethical decisions, 237–238, 242,
    259–263
  team approach, 244, 246–247
Ethicist, medical, 20–21
External stimulus barrier, 126
Eye movement, 134
  rapid, 136, 145

Family
  emotional support of, 19–20
  exclusion of, 1, 2
  home care of term infant, 152–153
  increased social stimulation,
    255–256
  support, 275
Feedback system, internal, 282
Feeding, 60, 117, 119, 133, 134
  activity prior to, 119–125
  critically ill preterm, 68
  distress, 115
  early, 4
  energy loss due to, 183
    control, 184
  healthy preterm, 68
  historical aspects, 3–4
  noncontingent, 266–267
  preterm infant, 60
  term infant, 68
Fluid administration, intravenous,
    complications, 218
Fluid balance, 3–4
Foster grandparent program, 256
Fussiness, 73

active, with cry, 137
mild, 136

Gas regulation, 215
  complications, 215–216
Gaseous pollutants, 216
Grandparent support, 275
Grieving, 245–246

Habituated state, 281–282
Handling, 30, 37, 38, 48, 58, 74–75,
    76, 127, 151, 160, 205–208
  benefits, 86
  constant, 4
  diurnal variation, 161, 167
  historical aspects, 3, 4
  hypoxemia, 8
  intermediate vs. intensive care, 167
  preterm infant,
    critically ill, 65, 67
    healthy, 65, 67–68
  quality, 208
  term newborn, 63–65, 67–68
Healthdyne Transport Incubator,
    189–190
  battery systems, 189
  incubator, 189
  life-support module, 189–190
  monitoring module, 189–190
Hearing impairment, 24–25
  aminoglycoside antibiotics, 204,
    205
  due to incubator noise, 205
  prematurity, 47, 85
Heart rate, 132, 133
Heartbeat, 115
  recorded, 86
Heat loss, clothing for control,
    190–191
Heat release, metabolic, 172, 173
Hexachlorophene, 217
Home environment, lower class,
    descriptive study, 99–103
Home-based intervention, 274
Humidity, 176, 183, 184, 186

288 Index

Humidity *(continued)*
  radiant warmer, 186, 190, 191
  thermal environment, 271–272
Hyaline membrane disease, 241
Hyperalertness, 136
Hyperbilirubinemia, 60, 201, 203–204
Hyperoxemia, 75
Hypersensitivity, 281
Hypothermia, 172–173
  central nervous system, 173
  mortality rate, 172
  sympathetic nervous system, 173
Hypovolemia, 172
Hypoxemia, 8, 75, 172
  associated with handling, 8, 206–208

Iatrogenic complications, 23, 56
  of neonatal intensive care unit procedures, 199–219
Inanimate background sound, term vs. preterm infant, 100
Inanimate stimulation, 58
Incubator, 176, 184–185, 209–210, 271
  access vs. thermal control, 185
  auditory level, 28–29
  high relative humidity, 271
  historical aspects, 1, 2, 3
  humidity control, 184–185
  light level, 28–29
  noise level in, 204–205
  one-way vision, 266
  open-type radiant heat, 186, 187
  transport
    access, 187
    closed isolette, 187
    forced-air "closed" type, 187
    in-hospital use, 192
    requirements, 187–188
Infant
  activity, 70–71, 76–77
  behavior, 70–74
  body movement, 74
  checking, 68

contingent responsivity to caregiver, 105–108, 109
directed environment, 272
dying, 263
effects on caregivers, 75–76
looking behavior, 71–72
morbidity rate, 199–200
normal term, 57
preterm, 57
  individual differences, 125–126
smiling, 72
time in various positions, 151, 152
very low birth weight, 56, 241
  mortality rate, 199, 275
  parents, 275
Infant state classification, 134–137
Infant state modulation, 125
Infant state periodicity, environmental periodicity, 163–166, 167–168
Infant-caregiver interaction, 33–46, 56–57, 57–58, 63–70, 93
  acute medical status, 45
  behavioral organization, 123
  diurnal rhythmicity, 36, 42
  duration, 35–36
  frequency, 35–36
  gender differences, 40
  handling, 37, 38, 48, 58, 74–75, 76, 127, 151, 160, 205–208
  looking, 106–108
  medical-nursing contact, 37, 38, 42
  neonatal intensive care unit vs. home, 152–153
  noncontingent, 266
  reduction of, 266
  response to crying, 39, 40, 49
  sensory coordinated experiences, 41–43, 49–50
  social interaction, 37, 38–40, 42
  synchronization of, 158
Infant-caregiver ratio, 13, 98
Infant-family interaction, 35, 50, 78, 261–262, 272, 273
Infant-mother interaction, 272, 273
Infection, 216–217
  control, historical aspects, 1, 4
  cytomegalovirus, 217

Ingestion of mass, 173
Institutional review board, 260, 261
Integrated sensory experience, 115
Intellectual deficits, 85
Intensive care, 59–61
 incidence, 23
 transport incubator, 187
  requirements, 187–188
Intermediate care, 59–61, 77–78, 88, 150, 159
Intubation, 77–78
 complications, 211
Irritability, 58, 134
Isolation, 23–24
Isolette, 185
 sound level in, 100
Isopropyl alcohol, 217

Laboratory service, 17
Level I facility, 10, 60–61
 defined, 11
Level II facility, defined, 11
Level III facility, 60–61, 88, 116
 defined, 11–12
 educational programs, 12–13
 neonatology staffing patterns, 13
 nursing staffing patterns, 13–14
 personnel, 18–21
  role overlap, 19–20
 radiology, 17
 structural elements, 14–17
 transport, 12
Lighting
 circadian rhythm, 158
 fluorescent, 200–201
 level, 265–266
 needed modifications, 253–254
  circadian rhythm, 253–254
  full spectrum, 253
 for visual monitoring, 7–8
Limb movement, 73–74, 125
Looking, term vs. preterm infant, 100–102
Lung, in hypothermia, 172

Maternal transport, 273–274

Mattress
 dry, 177
 water, 178
 wet, 178
Medical status, effects of, 45
Medical/legal considerations, 247
Medical-nursing interaction, 37, 38, 58, 69–70, 85, 115, 132, 133, 151
Medication, energy loss due to, 183
 control, 184
Metabolic rate, 176
Monitoring alarm, 16
 activation, 74
Mortality, neonatal intensive care unit vs. small hospital, 9
Mother, 272, 273
 day care, 274
 discussion-support group, 275
 emotional support of, 19–20
 high risk, 9–10, 12
 in neonatal intensive care unit, 85
 rooming in with, 114–115, 274
Mother's milk, 218
Mouthing, 72–73

Neck stretching, 125
Neonatal care
 cost benefit analysis, 259–260
 historical aspects, 1–5
Neonatal intensive care unit
 average length of stay, 23
 circadian periodicity, 157–169
 effect on parents, 273–275
 environment mapping, 87–92
  continuous-interval recording technique, 87
  continuous real time recording technique, 87–92, 99–103, 105, 108
  duration, 87, 92–93
  frequency of interval, 87
  sequence, 87
 goals, 7, 9, 262–263
 harmful effects, 261–262
 vs. home environment, 99–103, 108

290 Index

Neonatal intensive care unit *(cont.)*
  iatrogenic complications, 23
  infant population characteristics, 96
  overutilization, 273
  physical layout, 14–17, 96, 159, 168, 251
    cabinet, 16
    effects of change, 97–98
    lighting, 16
    location within hospital, 16
    room temperature, 16–17
    single vs. multiple rooms, 16
    sink, 17
    sound level, 15
    spacing, 15, 16
    window, 16
  research goals, 272–273
  staff characteristics, 96
  see also Level III care
Neonatologist, 13, 18
  academic, 240–247
  clinical care, 240
  ethical decisions, 242
  frustration, 241
  house staff relationship, 241–242
  relationship with administration, 244
  relationship with neonatology group, 242
  relationship with nursing staff, 243–244
  relationships with other hospital personnel, 242–243
    research material, 243
    space requirements, 242–243
  relationship with social workers, 243
  research, 240–241
    funding, 240–241
  as role model, 242
  priorities, 240
  teaching, 240, 242
Neonatology, 4
  environmental, defined, xi
Neurologic problems, 85
Neurosensory problems, 276
Newborn convalescent care unit, 25

Newborn nursery, 114–115
Noise level, *see* Noise pollution; Sensory stimulation, auditory
Noise pollution, 24–25, 47, 204–205, 254–255, 265–266
Nurse clinician, 232
Nurse specialist, 232
Nurse-patient ratio, 13, 98
Nursery routine, historical aspects, 1–2, 4
Nursing, 18–20
  administrative support, 233, 234
  burnout, 108, 109, 232, 233, 234, 283
  charge nurse, 231, 232
  ethical decisions, 227, 228
  first year, 231–232
  frustration, 232
  historical aspects, 1–2, 4, 19
  interest pattern, 268
  job satisfaction, 232, 233
  more than three years, 233–234
  neonatal intensive care unit desirability, 228–229
  novice, 230–231
  as patient advocate, 233
  primary, 283
  professional growth, 229–233
  relationship with neonatologists, 243–244
  research projects, 228
  role expansion, 232–233
  second and third years, 232–233
  staffing pattern, 233–234
    re-entry, 234
  stress, 228, 230–231
    control of, 231
  technological demands, 228, 229
  transport team, 232
  turnover, 233–234

Objective risk scoring system, 105
Observation code, 89
Organismic specificity, 127–128
Oxygen consumption, 172, 208–209, 272

Index **291**

due to cold, 208–209
Oxygen level, 132, 133
Oxygenation abnormality, 48, 75

Parent
   emotional support of, 19–20
   home care of term infant, 152–153
   neonatal intensive care unit effects on, 273–275
   postdischarge review, 274–275
   very low birth weight infant, 275
Parenteral alimentation, 217–218
   complications, 218
Pediatric house officer, 235–239
   coping behaviors, 238
      inappropriate, 238–239
   vs. internship year, 235
   neonatal intensive care unit rotation modifications, 239
   stress, 235–236
      consoling parents, 236–237
      education, 235–236
      ethical decisions, 237
      expectations, 236
      fatigue, 235
      medical complexity, 236
      pressure, 236
   support systems, 237–238
      attending physicians, 238
      interpersonal skills training, 237
      other house officers, 237
      nurses, 237
      personal resources, 238
      social workers, 237–238
Phase synchrony, 114, 124, 125
Phenolic compounds, 217
Phototherapy, 201
   adverse effects, 201–204
   DNA damage, 202
   effect on physical growth, 203
   hematologic effects, 202
   hypocalcemia, 203
   retina damage, 202–203
   water loss in, 193–194, 201–202
Physical therapist, 20
Play, 126

Position deformity, 206
Predischarge care, 59–61
Premature Infant Refocus Project, 115–128
Prenatal care, 10
President's Commission for the Study of Ethical Problems in Medicine and Biomedical and Behavioral Research, 260–261
Primary care, *see* Level I care

Radiant warmer, 179, 185–186, 209–210
   in delivery room, 191
   high water loss, 186
   plastic bubble wrap, 186, 190, 191
   in surgical theater, 192–193
   water loss, 177
Radiation, 173
Radiation exposure, 210
   ultrasound, 210
Radiation heat transfer, 178–180
   control of, 180
Radiology service, 17
Recording method
   computerized continuous observational system, 132–133
   24-hour continuous, 33
   continuous-interval, 87
   continuous real time, 87–92, 99–103, 105, 108
   time-lapse video, 116
Recovery system, 282
Rectal temperature, 174–175
   vs. skin temperature, 177
Regional center, *see* Level III facility
Regionalization, 4, 9–13
Research, 240–241
   funding, 240–241
Respiratory distress syndrome, 185
Respiratory evaporation, 173
Respiratory problems, 85
Respiratory rate, 132, 133
Respiratory therapist, 20
Retardation, 279

Index

Retina, damage due to phototherapy, 202–203
Retrolental fibroplasia, 279
Review board, institutional, 260, 261
Rocking, 30, 43, 48, 49, 69, 86, 115
Rooming in, 274
   with consistent nurse caregiver, 114–115
   with mother, 114–115
Rooting, 125

School adjustment problems, 276
Sensory coordinated experience, 30–33, 41–43, 49–50, 256, 268
Sensory deficit hypothesis, 252
Sensory stimulation, 99, 115, 126, 167–168, 267–269
   animate social, 126, 127
   auditory, 9, 24–25, 25–29, 46, 47, 93, 108, 114, 125, 204–205, 265–266
     animate, 100
     for caregivers, 7–8
     diurnal variation, 161, 167, 168
     inanimate, 100
     in incubator, 28–29
     needed modifications, 254–255
     reduction of, 254–255
     sleep, 205
     in utero, 113
   aversive tactile, 93
   cyclic, in utero, 114
   deprivation, 23–24, 85–86, 108, 252
   description of, 56
   disjunctive, 24
   individual differences, 268–269
   kinesthetic
     needed modifications, 255
     in utero, 113
   light, 25–29, 46–47, 200–201
     diurnal variation, 158, 161, 167, 168, 200–201
     in incubator, 28–29
     measurement, 160
     needed modifications, 253–254
   newborn intensive care unit vs. newborn convalescent care unit, 25–46, 47–49
   overstimulation, 24, 86, 108
   painful, 93
   rhythmic, in utero, 114
   social, 108
   tactile, 8, 9, 48, 108, 127, 205–208
     hypoxemic episode, 8
     increased, 256
     quality, 208
     term vs. preterm infant, 100
     in utero, 113
   temperature, 9, 208–210
   term vs. preterm infants, 268
   vestibular, 93, 108
     needed modifications, 255
     in utero, 113
   visual, 9, 108, 114, 265–266
     circadian periodicity, 158
     diurnal variation, 158, 161, 167, 168, 200–201
     light level measurement, 160
     needed modifications, 253–254
Separation effect, 5
Skin, of infant, 172
   transepidermal water loss, 182–183
   water permeability, 176
Skin infection, 206
Skin temperature, 174–175, 176
   vs. rectal temperature, 177
Skin trauma, 206
Sleep
   active, 134, 136
     term vs. preterm infants, 145–148
   to avoid stimuli, 281
   disturbance, 158
   interruptions in neonatal intensive care unit, 206–208
     harmful effects, 206–208
   noise during, 205
   quality, 145–148
   quantity, 141–145

Index

quiet, 134, 136
   diurnal variation, 145
   term vs. preterm infant, 145–148
   relation to age, 137, 138–139
   transitional, 145
   undisturbed, 263
Sleep state, 134, 141–148
Sleep/wake state organization, 132, 134, 137–150
   medical condition effects, 149
   postmenstrual age influence, 149
   term vs. preterm infants, 137
Social interaction, 25–26, 29–33, 37, 38–40, 46, 48–49, 58, 115, 132, 133, 134, 151
   family, 35, 50, 78, 261–262, 272, 273
   staffing pattern effects, 98–99
Social stimulation, 105–108, 109, 267–269
   individual differences, 268–269
   needed modifications, 255–256
   term vs. preterm infants, 268
Social stroking, 117, 119, 127
   activity level and, 121–125
Social worker, 18, 19, 20
   perinatal, 11
   relationship with other hospital personnel, 237–238, 243
Sound, *see* Noise; Sensory stimulation, auditory
Staffing pattern
   nurse, 233–234
   social interaction and, 98–99
State modulation, 267
State organization, 283–284
Steady state, thermal, 177
Stimulation
   disjunctive, 168
   fixed interval, 115–116
   quasi-self-activating, 115–116
   soothing, 126
   temporally organized, 115–116
Stress
   caregiver, 228, 230–231
      control of, 231
Sucking, 125, 133

Surgical gown, transparent polyethylene, to control heat loss, 192–193
Surgical theater, heat loss in, 192–193
   air-fluidized bed, 193
   plastic drape, 192–193
   radiant warmer, 192
Sympathetic nervous system, hypothermia, 173

Temperature regulation, 171–194
Theophylline, 267
Thermal environment, humidity, 271–272
Thermal modeling, 171, 173–175
Thermodynamics, 173–174
Thermogenesis, 172
   oxygen consumption, 172
   peripheral vasoconstriction, 172
Time-sampling analysis, 25
Touching, 108
Toy, 93
Transactional model, 56
Transepidermal evaporation, 173
Transport, 12
   air transport, 12
   maternal transport, 12
   vehicle, 12

Ultradian periodicity, 157

Vaporization, 174
Vasoconstriction, peripheral, 172
Ventilation, complications, 211
Video recording, 116
Vital signs, 69–70
Vocalization
   caregiver, 106–108
      to infant, 68–69, 93
   increased, 256
   infant, 58, 73, 115, 137
      distress, 106–108
      positive, 106–108

Vocalization *(continued)*
  term vs. preterm, 100–102
  noncontingent adult speech, 108

Wakefulness
  quality, 148–149
    term vs. preterm infants, 148–149
  quantity, 148
Waking, transitional, 136
Water loss
  evaporate, 174, 181–183, 209
  respiratory, 181–182
  high, 186
  plastic bubble wrap, 186, 190, 191
  during phototherapy, 201–202
  topical agents for control, 190
  transepidermal, 175, 181, 182
Waterbed, 86, 267, 282
  increased quiet sleep, 267
Workweek, 5-day vs. 4-day, 233–234

X-Ray procedure, heat loss in, 193